MANAGEMENT GUIDELINES FOR NURSE PRACTITIONERS WORKING WITH CHILDREN AND ADOLESCENTS

MANAGEMENT GUIDELINES FOR NURSE PRACTITIONERS WORKING WITH CHILDREN AND ADOLESCENTS

Second Edition

Nancy L. Herban Hill, *RN, DSN, PNPC, APN*
Professor Emeritus, formerly Director
Graduate Program in Nursing
Mississippi University for Women
Columbus, Mississippi
Former consultant to Delta State University
School of Nursing and Arkansas State University School of Nursing
Pediatric Nurse Practitioner
Mountain View, Arkansas

Linda M. Sullivan, *RN, CS, DSN, FNPC, PNPC*
Nurse Practitioner
Children's Health Center, Inc.
Columbus, Mississippi
Professor
Mississippi University for Women
Columbus, Mississippi

F. A. DAVIS COMPANY | Philadelphia

F. A. Davis Company
1915 Arch Street
Philadelphia, PA 19103

Printed in Canada

Last digit indicates print number: 10 9 8 7 6 5 4 3 2 1

Acquisitions Editor: Joanne Patzek DaCunha, RN, MSN
Developmental Editor: Diane Blodgett
Cover Designer: Louis J. Forgione

As new scientific information becomes available through basic and clinical research, recommended treatments and drug therapies undergo changes. The authors and publisher have done everything possible to make this book accurate, up to date, and in accord with accepted standards at the time of publication. The authors, editors, and publisher are not responsible for errors or omissions or for consequences from application of the book, and make no warranty, expressed or implied, with regard to the contents of the book. Any practice described in this book should be applied by the reader in accordance with professional standards of care used with regard to the unique circumstances that may apply in each situation. The reader is advised always to check product information (package inserts) for changes and new information regarding dose and contraindications before administering any drug. Caution is especially urged when using new or infrequently ordered drugs.

Library of Congress Cataloging-in-Publication Data

Hill, Nancy Herban, 1934–
    Management guidelines for nurse practitioners working with children and adolescents/ Nancy Herban Hill, Linda M. Sullivan.—Rev. ed.
    p. ; cm.
    Rev. ed. of: Management guidelines for pediatric nurse practitioners, c1999.
    Includes bibliographical references and index.
    ISBN 0-8036-1102-1
    I. Pediatric nursing. 2. Nurse practitioners. I. Sullivan, Linda, 1947– II. Hill, Nancy Herban, 1934–. Management guidelines for pediatric nurse practitioners. III. Title.
    [DNLM: 1. Pediatric Nursing—methods. WY 159 H6475m 2003]
    RJ245.H55 2003
    610.73′62—dc21

2003053075

To pathfinders and visionaries who
"saw the Vision of the world,
and all the wonder that would be."
Alfred, Lord Tennyson
Locksley Hall

PREFACE

Pediatric clients are not small adults, but persons with unique needs—developmentally, physically, and emotionally. The practice of the nurse practitioner deals not only with the identified client, but also with the parent or guardian as the practitioner seeks to elicit a history of the illness as well as the meaning of the illness for that client and family. The degree of difficulty, because of the lack of verbal ability in most pediatric clients, presents nurse practitioners with a unique opportunity as they listen to presenting complaints, elicit signs and symptoms, evaluate information in light of current knowledge, and arrive at diagnoses and treatment plans. The process is often much like swimming in deep, murky water, with only glimpses of daylight.

Therefore, pediatric nurse practitioners and students have a need for a concise manual to assist in their assessment, evaluation of signs and symptoms, and initiation of treatment. The purpose of this book is to meet that need. The material presented has been drawn from a variety of sources—medical and nursing—which is appropriate because the nurse practitioner is both a nurse and a primary provider of health care.

N. L. H. H. and L. M. S.

ACKNOWLEDGMENTS

Our heartfelt gratitude goes to those who "aided and abetted" this endeavor: with special regard to our editor, Joanne DaCunha, who has patiently seen us through all the "misadventure" of the past 4 years; to our husbands and families, who have waited, watched, wondered, and encouraged; to Drs. Jacob Skiwski, James Zini, and David Burnette, who welcomed us to their practices and have encouraged us in our professional endeavors; to other mentors, students, and colleagues, including Dr. Barry McCraw, who have added comments and given support.

N. L. H. H. and L. M. S.

BIOGRAPHICAL SKETCHES

Nancy H. Hill, RN, DSN, PNCP, APN, is professor emeritus, Mississippi University for Women in Columbus, Mississippi, where she initiated the family nurse practitioner program in 1975. She is a graduate of Missouri Valley College in Marshall, Missouri, with a joint BSN (1956) and a diploma in nursing from St. Luke's Hospital School of Nursing (1955), St. Luke's Hospital, Kansas City, Missouri. She holds graduate degrees from Tulane University in New Orleans, Louisiana (1967), and the University of Alabama at Birmingham (1982, 1986), as well as a postmaster's certificate as a pediatric nurse practitioner from Mississippi University for Women (1994). She has been a consultant in nursing education and, since her retirement in 1994, has taught part-time at Delta State University and been in practice as a pediatric nurse practitioner in Mountain View, Arkansas. She holds national certification as a pediatric nurse practitioner and a license in Arkansas as an advanced practice nurse. Among her publications is *Community Health: A Systems Approach* (1976, with Carrie Braden). She is a widow, has one son, and since retirement occupies her time with writing and painting.

Linda M. Sullivan, RN, CS, DSN, FNCP, is a professor at Mississippi University for Women in Columbus, Mississippi, where she teaches part-time in the family and pediatric nurse practitioner program. She also maintains a full-time collaborative pediatric practice in Columbus with Dr. Jacob Skiwski. Dr. Sullivan graduated from Hunter College in New York City in 1969, where she received her BSN. In 1986, she received her master's degree from Mississippi University for Women. She holds national certification as a family nurse practitioner and as a pediatric nurse practitioner, along with certification from the state of Mississippi. She received her DSN from the University of Alabama at Birmingham in 1993. Among her publications is her latest book, titled *The Impact of Homelessness on Children*. She serves on multiple statewide and community committees and is an advisor and primary caregiver for several shelters in the area. She also works closely with local law enforcement agencies on the care of abused and neglected children. Dr. Sullivan is married and has three children and two granddaughters.

CONSULTANTS

Terry A. Hall Buford, RN, MN
Clinical Instructor
University of Missouri
Kansas City, Missouri

Gail M. Kiechhefer, RN, PhD
Assistant Professor and Coordinator, FNP Program
University of Washington
Seattle, Washington

Mary Ann Krammin, RN, PhD, PNP
Professor of Nursing
Oakland Community College
Waterford, Michigan

Mary Ann Ludwig, RN, PhD, PNP
Clinical Associate Professor
University of Buffalo School of Nursing
Buffalo, New York

CONTENTS

HOW TO USE THIS BOOK

This book focuses on ambulatory care pediatrics and the conditions most often encountered in such a pediatric practice. The format assists the nurse practitioner in the diagnosis and treatment of these conditions.

The book is organized by systems. The flow charts and diagrams included will assist the nurse practitioner in the diagnostic and treatment process. The resource section in the Appendix is an aid to locating resources for the nurse as well as the family.

F. A. DAVIS COMPANY • Philadelphia

THE HEALTHY CHILD AND ADOLESCENT

Chapter 1

HEALTH PROMOTION

Health promotion of children can be broadly defined as providing services and direction, supervision and suggestions, and surveillance and evaluation that promote the health of a child. These services can assist in detecting and treating problems that are symptomatic and asymptomatic in a child.

New Patient	ICD-9 CM: 99381
Periodic Comprehensive Preventive Visit	ICD-9 CM: 99391

NEONATES: BIRTH TO 1 MONTH

History

Obtain prenatal and birth history from caregiver. Asking the following questions can facilitate this history.

Prenatal and Birth History

Were there any problems during your pregnancy?

Were there any problems at the birth of your infant?

Was the pregnancy full term?

Did the infant require any special interventions or procedures at birth?

Was the newborn discharged at the same time that you were?

Since being home, have there been any special problems or concerns?

Is the infant using any special monitoring, assistive device, or medication at this time?

Social History

Who is currently living in your household?

Are there any smokers in the home?

Who is currently providing care for your infant?

Is the infant in day care?

Family History

Are there any illnesses or inheritable diseases in your family, and if so what are they, and who has them?

 Clinical Pearl: The construction of a genogram may be valuable in assessing family history and explaining its importance to caregivers.

Review of Systems

The review of systems provides an opportunity to assess the current health status of the infant and pinpoint any current problems. For a sick visit, determine the chief complaint or reason for the visit.

Sleep History

Identify sleep patterns of the neonate. Include length of time and sleep position. Infants should be sleeping on their backs and normally sleep 16 to 18 hours per day. Problems associated with sleep can be discussed here and are helpful in discerning disorders related to sleep (Fig. 1–1).

Nutritional History

Ask how much and how often the infant is being fed. Current nutritional requirements are as follows:

Adequate growth requires   100–120 kcal/kg per day for the full-term infant

115–130 kcal/kg per day for the preterm infant

150–180 kcal/kg per day for the very-low-birth-weight infant

 Clinical Pearl: Formula and breast milk contain 20 calories/ounce. Feeding the infant 2–4 ounces per feeding is normal.

Supplement Vitamin D 200 IU/day for:

1. All breastfed infants unless they were weaned to at least 500mL/day of vitamin D–fortified formula or milk;
2. All non-breastfed infants who are ingesting less than 500 mL/day of vitamin D–fortified formula or milk;
3. Children and adolescents who do not get regular sunlight exposure, do not ingest at least 500 mL/day of vitamin D–fortified milk, or do not take a daily multivitamin supplement containing at least 200 IU of vitamin D.

The following questions help the practitioner in obtaining an accurate and comprehensive nutritional history.

Does your infant feed well?

How much does the infant take per feeding?

Are there any identifiable problems associated with feeding (i.e., spitting up, falling asleep, poor sucking)?

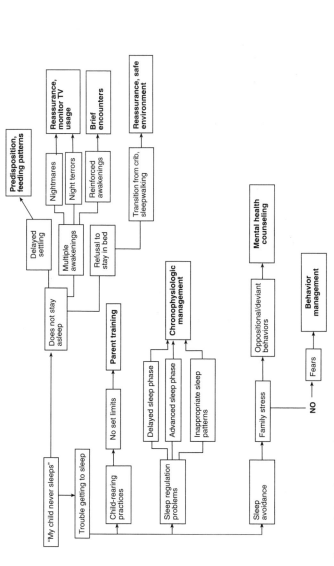

Figure 1–1. Evaluation of sleep disorders. (Adapted from Berman, S: Pediatric Decision Making, ed 2. BC Decker, Philadelphia, 1991, with permission.)

Clinical Pearl: Feeding problems can suggest a possible neurodevelopmental disorder, cardiac problems, and reflux or formula intolerance.

Note: Detailed feeding advice for the preterm infant can be obtained at: www.ellysatter.com.

Measurements

When a complete history has been obtained, the practitioner should begin a thorough assessment of the infant. The first part of the examination includes obtaining the infant's measurements. Measurements include height, weight, and head circumference and should be assessed at each visit and recorded on the medical record. These measurements should be plotted on an appropriate growth chart and compared at each visit to assess if the infant is growing at an acceptable and appropriate rate. Growth charts can be obtained at: http//:www.cdc.gov/nchs/about/major/nhanes/growthcharts/clinical_charts.html.

 Clinical Pearl: Average weight gain for an infant is 1 ounce per day for the first 3 months. Average birth weight is currently 7.5 pounds (range 5.5–10 pounds). Weight should double by the first 6 months of life and triple by 10 to 12 months of age. Average newborn length is 20 inches (range 18–22 inches). Length increases about 1 inch per month with an expected gain in the first year of 10 to 12 inches. Average head circumference is 14 inches (34 cm); the head is disproportionately large compared with the body. By about 6 months, the head circumference is about 44 cm, and by 1 year, 47 cm.

Sensory Screening

The newborn:

- Should respond to sound (hearing)
- Lifts head when prone (neurodevelopment)
- Fixates on human faces and can track 45 to 90 degrees

Developmental/Behavioral Assessment

Assessing behavioral/developmental health is essential (Tables 1–1 through 1–3 and Fig. 1–2). The following areas should be addressed.

Normal pattern of development, developmental milestones, and normal reflexes should be assessed each visit.

The infant should respond to sound, light, and noxious odors by either a physical or a physiologic response (i.e., increase in heart rate).

The infant's ability to maintain flexion should be assessed.

Denver II should be performed at each visit, and all delays should be referred for further evaluation.

Table 1-1   Normal Pattern of Development

Gross Motor Skills

Birth	Reflex head turn; moves head side to side
1 mo	Lifts head when prone
3 mo	Lifts shoulders up when prone
4 mo	Lifts up on elbows; head steady when upright
5 mo	Lifts up on hands; rolls from front to back; no head lag when pulled to sitting supine position
6 mo	Rolls back to front
7 mo	Sits alone 30 seconds or more
8 mo	Crawls/sits well
9 mo	Pulls to stand
10 mo	Cruises
13 mo	Walks
30 mo	Walks backwards
2 yr	Runs; kicks a ball
2.5 yr	Walks up and down stairs (taking one step at a time and holding on; stands on one foot)
3 yr	Walks up stairs alternating steps; rides a tricycle
4 yr	Walks down stairs alternating steps/hops on one foot
3 yr	Skips

Fine Motor/Adaptive Skills

1 mo	Tracks horizontally to mid line
2 mo	Tracks past midline/tracks vertically
3 mo	Unfisted for >50% of the time; tracks 180 degrees; visual threat; discovers midline
3 mo	Reaches for bright object; brings object to mouth
4 mo	"Rakes" at bright object
5 mo	Transfers object from one hand to the other
8 mo	Three-finger pincer grasp
9 mo	Neat pincer grasp; bangs cubes in midline
15 mo	Tower of two cubes; scrib bles spontaneously
18 mo	Tower of four cubes
2 yr	Copies vertical and horizon tal line; tower of six cubes
3 yr	Copies circle
4 yr	Copies "+" (3.5 yr)
4.5 yr	Copies square; draws per son with three parts
5 yr	Copies triangle; draws per son with six parts

Personal/Social Skills

Newborn	Regards face
6 wk	Spontaneous social smile
6 mo	Discriminates social smile
7 mo	Displays stranger anxiety; plays peek-a-boo (7-9 mo)
12 mo	Drinks from a cup
15-18 mo	Uses a spoon, spilling a little
2 yr	Washes and dries hands
3 yr	Uses a spoon well; uses but tons
4 yr	Washes and dries face; engages in cooperative play
5 yr	Dresses without assistance

Language Skills

Newborn	Alerts to bell
2 mo	Cooing; searches with eyes for sound
4 mo	Turns head to sound of voice or bell; laughs (3 mo)
6 mo	Babbles
8 mo	Mama/dada nonspecific
9 mo	Understands the word "no"
12 mo	Mama/dada specific; follows one-step command with gesture/3-5 word vocabulary
14 mo	Follows one-step command without gesture
16 mo	Can point to several body parts
2 yr	50-word vocabulary; 2-word sentences; uses pronouns indiscriminately
2.5 yr	Gives first and last names; uses plurals
3 yr	250-word vocabulary; 3-word sentences; speech intelligible to strangers 75% of time; uses pro- nouns discriminately

Cognitive Skills

Newborn–2 yr	Sensorimotor
2-6 yr	Preoperational
6-11 yr	Concrete operational
>11 yr	Formal operations

Miscellaneous Cognitive Milestones

24 mo	Concept of today
30 mo	Concept of tomorrow
36 mo	Concept of yesterday
7 yr	Concept of right and left

Source: Berkowitz, C: Pediatrics: A Primary Care Approach. WB Saunders, Philadelphia, 1996, with permission.

Table 1–2   Milestones of Development—A Summary*

Newborn	When prone, pelvis is high, knees are under abdomen
2–4 wk	Watches mother intently as she speaks to him
1 mo	Ventral suspension (held prone, hand under abdomen)—head up momentarily, elbows flexed, hips partly extended, knees flexed
4–6 wk	*Smiles at mother in response to overtures*
6 wk	*Ventral suspension—head held up momentarily in same plane as rest of body; some extension of hips and flexion of knees and elbows* *When prone, pelvis is largely flat, hips mostly extended* (but when sleeping, the infant lies with pelvis high, and knees are under abdomen, like a newborn) Pulls to sit from supine position—much head lag, but not complete; hands often open When supine, follows object 90 cm away over angle of 90 degrees
2 mo	Ventral suspension—maintains head in same plane as rest of body Hands are largely open When prone, chin is off couch; plane of face is 45 degrees to flat surface (e.g., bed or floor) Smiles and vocalizes when talked to Eyes follow a moving person
3 mo	Ventral suspension—holds head up long time beyond plane of rest of body When prone, plane of face is 45–90 degrees from flat surface When pulled to sit, there is only a slight head lag Hands loosely open *Holds rattle placed in hand* Vocalizes a great deal when talked to Follows object for 180 degrees (lying supine) *Turns head to sound (3–4 mo) on a level with the ear*
4 mo	When prone, plane of face is 90 degrees to flat surface Hands come together Pulls dress or shirt over face Laughs aloud
5 mo	When prone, weight is on forearms When pulled to sit, there is no head lag When supine, feet come to mouth; plays with toes *Able to go for object and get it*
6 mo	When prone, weight is on hands; extended arms When pulled to sit, there is no head lag *When supine, lifts head spontaneously* Sits on floor, hand forward for support When held in standing position, full weight is on legs Rolls, prone to supine Begins to imitate (e.g., a cough) *Chews* Transfers cube from one hand to another
7 mo	*Sits on floor seconds, no support* Roll, supine to prone When held standing, bounces Feeds self with biscuit Attracts attention by cough or other methods Turns head to sound below level of ear
8 mo	Sits unsupported; leans forward to reach objects Turns head to sound above level of ear
9 mo	Stands, holding on; pulls to stand or sitting position Crawls on abdomen

Table 1–2 **Milestones of Development—A Summary***

9–10 mo	*Uses index finger approach* *Uses finger-thumb apposition—picks up pellet between tip of thumb and tip of forefinger*
10 mo	Creeps on hands and knees; abdomen off flat surface Can change from sitting to prone and back Pulls self to sitting position *Waves goodbye* *Plays pat-a-cake* Helps to dress—holding arms out for coat, foot for shoe, or transferring object from one hand to another for sleeve
11 mo	Offers object to mother, but will not release it Utters one word with meaning When sitting, pivots around without overbalancing Walks, holding on to furniture; walks with two hands held
12 mo	Utters two to three words with meaning When prone, walks on hands and feet like a bear Walks, one hand held Casting objects, one after another, begins *Gives object to mother*
13 mo	*Walks, no support* Mouthing of objects stopped Slobbering largely stopped
15 mo	Creep up stairs; kneels Makes tower of two cubes Takes off shoes *Feeds self, picking up an ordinary cup, drinking, putting it down* Imitates parent in domestic work ("domestic mimicry") Jargon
18 mo	*No more coasting* Gets up and down stairs, holding rail Jumps, both feet Seats self in chair Makes tower of three to four cubes Throws ball without falling Takes off gloves and socks; unzips Manages spoon well Points to three parts of body on request Turns pages of books, two or three at a time Points to some objects on request Toilet control—tells parent that he wants to go potty; largely dry by day
21–24 mo	*Spontaneously joins two or three words together to make sentence*
24 mo	Picks up object from floor without falling Runs Kicks ball Turns doorknob Makes tower of six or seven cubes Puts on shoes, socks, pants; takes off shoes and socks Points to four parts of body on request Imitates vertical and circular strokes with a pencil Turns pages of a book singly Is mainly dry at night Climbs stairs, two feet per step

(*Continued on the following page*)

Table 1-2   Milestones of Development—A Summary* *(Cont'd.)*

	Motor
	Gross: Runs well, no falling
	Walks up and down stairs alone
	Kicks large ball on request
	Fine: Turns pages of book singly
	Adaptive
	Builds tower of six to seven cubes
	Aligns cubes for train
	Imitates vertical and circular strokes with pencil
	Language
	Uses pronouns
	Uses three-word sentences; jargon discarded
	Carries out four directions with ball ("on the table," "to mother," "to me," "on the chair")
	Personal-Social
	Verbalizes toilet needs consistently
	Pulls on simple garments
	Inhibits turning of spoon in feeding
	Exhibits domestic mimicry
30 mo	**Motor**
	Gross: Jumps up and down
	Walks backward
	Fine: Holds crayons in fist
	Adaptive
	Copies crude circle, closed figure
	Names some drawings: house, shoe, ball, dog
	Language
	Refers to self as "I"
	Knows full name
	Personal-social
	Helps put things away
	Unbuttons large buttons
3 yr	**Motor**
	Gross: Alternates feet going upstairs
	Jumps from bottom step
	Rides tricycle, using pedals
	Fine: Holds crayon with fingers
	Pincer grasp
	Adaptive
	Builds tower of 9–10 cubes
	Imitates three-cube building
	Names own drawing
	Copies circle and imitates cross
	Language
	Uses plurals
	Names action in picture book
	Gives sex and full name
	Obeys two prepositional commands (e.g., "on" and "under")
	Personal-Social
	Feeds self well
	Puts on shoes
4 yr	**Motor**
	Walks downstairs alternating feet
	Does broad jump
	Throws ball overhand
	Hops on one foot

Table 1–2   Milestones of Development—A Summary*

	Adaptive

Adaptive
Draws person with two parts
Copies cross
Counts three objects with correct pointing
Imitates five-cube gate
Pick longer of two lines
Language
Names one or more colors correctly
Obeys five prepositional commands (e.g., "on," "under," "in back,"
   "in front," "beside")

Personal-Social
Washes and dries face and hands; brushes teeth
Distinguishes front from back of clothes
Laces shoes
Goes on errands outside of home

5 yr
Motor
Skips, alternating feet
Stands on one foot more than 8 sec
Catches, bounces ball
Adaptive
Builds two steps with cubes
Draws unmistakable person with body and head
Copies triangle
Counts 10 objects correctly
Language
Knows four colors
Names penny, nickel, dime
Gives descriptive comment on pictures
Carries out three commands (e.g., "go under the table, get the
   penny, and give it to me.")
Personal-Social
Dresses and undresses without assistance
Asks meaning of words
Prints a few letters

6 yr
Motor
Has advanced throwing
Stands on each foot alternately, eyes closed
Walks line backward, heel-toe
Adaptive
Builds three steps with blocks
Draws person with neck, hands, and clothes
Adds and subtracts within 5
Copies drawing of diamond
Language
Uses Stanford-Binet items (vocabulary)
Defines words by function or composition (e.g., "house is to live in")
Personal-Social
Tie shoelaces
Differentiates AM from PM
Knows right from left
Counts to 30

* Most important milestones in italics.
Souce: Adapted from Palmer, FB: Streams of development. In Oski, FA, et al (eds): Principles and Practice of Pediatrics. JB Lippincott, Philadelphia, 1990, pp. 606–615.

Table 1–3 Normal Reflexes in Infants and Children

Response	Age at Time of Appearance	Age at Time of Disappearance
Reflexes of Position and Movement		
Moro reflex	Birth	1–3 mo
Tonic neck reflex (unsustained)	Birth	5–6 mo (partial up to 2–4 yr)
Neck righting reflex	4–6 mo	1–2 yr
Landau response	3 mo	1–2 yr
Palmar grasp reflex	Birth	4 mo
Adductor spread of knee jerk	Birth	7 mo
Plantar grasp reflex	Birth	8–15 mo
Babinski response	Birth	Variable
Parachute reaction	8–9 mo	Variable
Reflexes to Sound		
Blinking response	Birth	
Turning response	Birth	
Reflexes to Vision		
Blinking to threat	6–7 mo	
Horizontal following	4–6 wk	
Vertical following	2–3 mo	
Optokinetic nystagmus	Birth	
Postrotational nystagmus	Birth	
Lid closure to light	Birth	
Macular light reflex	4–8 mo	
Food Reflexes		
Rooting response—awake	Birth	3–4 mo
Rooting response—asleep	Birth	7–8 mo
Sucking response	Birth	12 mo
Handedness	2– 3yr	
Spontaneous Stepping	Birth	
Straight Line Walking	5–6 yr	

Physical Examination

All examinations should be performed with the infant fully undressed. The practitioner should evaluate the following.

Skin

- Skin color, hydration, any signs of trauma, and rash or other skin abnormalities

Head, Neck, and Face

- Head for symmetry
- Eyes for position and alignment, red reflex, and pupillary response
- Position of ears, visualize eardrum, ability to hear, and patency of nasal canal and mouth (check palate, gums, and other abnormalities)

Chest

- Symmetry of chest and respiratory rate (normal for newborn is 30–60/minute) (Tables 1–4 and 1–5 and Fig. 1–3)
- Heart rate, rhythm (normal heart rate 140 beats/minute), and respiratory sounds by auscultation with diaphragm and bell of stethoscope

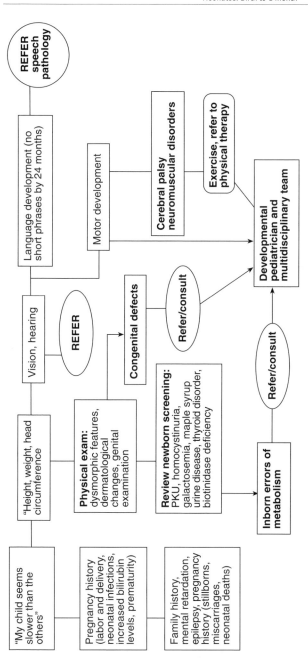

Figure 1–2. Evaluation of developmental delays. (PKU, phenylketonuria.)

Table 1–4   Range of Normal Vital Signs

Age	Pulse (beats/min)	Respirations (breaths/min)	Systolic Blood Pressure (mm Hg)
Newborn	125	64–70	
1 yr	120	35–40	
2 yr	110	31–35	96
4 yr	100	26–31	96
6 yr	100	23–36	96–98
8 yr	90	21–23	104
10 yr	90	21	110
12 yr	85–90	21	115
14 yr	80–85	21–22	118–120
16 yr	75–80	20	120–124

Abdomen

- Check umbilicus and stump for healing or cord (should fall off by 14 days of life), hepatosplenomegaly (liver can be 2 cm below costal margin *but* spleen should not be palpable)
- Auscultation of bowel sounds

Genitourinary

- Check position and patency of anus
- In males, check penis for hypospadias or epispadias. If circumcised, check for healing of circumcision. If not circumcised, do *not* retract foreskin, but observe for ability to urinate
- In males, examine testicles to see that they are both descended into scrotal sac and examine inguinal area for hernias
- Ask caregiver about urinary or bowel problems or concerns

 Clinical Pearl: An infant who has had an undescended testicle has an increased risk for testicular cancer in later life.

Musculoskeletal

- Check for hip dysplasia using either Barlow's or Ortolani maneuver
- Check clavicles for fractures (palpate along the clavicle, and if a bump or misalignment is found, order a radiograph)
- Check for evidence of pain on palpation or movement of any part of the body
- Observe for asymmetry and misalignment of extremities

Table 1–5   Variations in Vital Signs by Age

Age	Temperature (°F)	Pulse (beats/min)	Respiration (breaths/min)
3 mo	99.4	130	30–80
1 yr	99.7	115	20–40
3 yr	99.0	105	20–30
5 yr	98.6	95	20–25
9 yr	98.1	95	17–22
13 yr	97.8	85	17–22

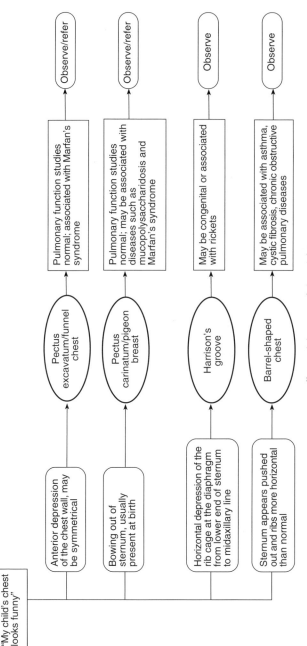

Figure 1–3. Differential diagnosis of chest deformities.

Neurologic

- Evaluate muscle tone, head control, and head lag
- Elicit Moro response (make a loud noise, infant should extend then flex arms, clench hands, and flex hips and knees)
- Note cry (pitch)
- Check for grasp, rooting, stepping, and sucking response (see Table 1–3)

Overall Appearance

- Check hygiene
- Appropriateness of clothing (overbundling, underdressing)
- Relationship between caregiver and infant (bonding and eye contact, demeanor of caregiver and infant)
- Check for any signs of abuse

Diagnostic Tests

Appropriate tests should be ordered and evaluated by examination, history, or state law. Some tests that may be indicated are as follows.

Test	Results Indicating Disorder	CPT Code
Hereditary or metabolic screen	Inborn errors of metabolism	80048
Thyroid panel	Low TSH = hyperthyroid	84443
	High TSH = hypothyroid	
PKU	Abnormal results indicate disease	84030

TSH, thyroid-stimulating hormone; PKU, phenylketonuria.

Procedures

Immunizations

Immunizations that may be started at birth include hepatitis B (recommended to be started between newborn and 2 months of age) and palivizumab (Synagis) for respiratory syncytial virus (seasonal, October to March) in high-risk infants only. See Tables 1–6 through 1–8.

Anticipatory Guidance

Parents of newborns need certain guidelines to know how to prevent injuries and illness. The practitioner should address the following items at the newborn visit and at each subsequent visit.

- The use of car seats (rear facing and center back seat position is safest)
- Sleep positions ("Back to Sleep")—should be on the back or on the side with no comforters or pillows
- Smoke-free environments
- Appropriate temperature maintenance of the home
- Stress never leaving infant alone—this safety precaution provides safety from pets and other children and accidental injuries

- Identifying signs and symptoms of illness
- Parental adjustment to the new child
- Age-appropriate toys

INFANTS: 1 TO 12 MONTHS

History

The 1- to 12-month-old infant presents a unique challenge for the nurse practitioner because this is a time of tremendous growth and change. The history can often provide much-needed clues in the overall diagnosis of the infant. The following is an outline for the nurse practitioner to follow.

If this is an initial visit, review all *prenatal, birth, and family history* of both birth parents. Ask appropriate questions to elicit a thorough history (see History under Neonates).

Review social history at each visit because situations may change often. Check on who lives in the home, where the infant is cared for and by whom, where the infant sleeps, and if there are any smokers in the home.

Review of Systems

What is the chief reason for the visit? Is child ill or is this a well checkup?

Have any changes occurred in the home or are any new stressors currently being experienced in the home?

Nutritional History

Evaluate weight gain and discuss eating habits of the infant. Infants should gain about 1 ounce per day. Calorie requirements are approximately 110 kCal per day for a full-term, normal infant. Feeding should be about every 2 to 4 hours with no more than 5 hours between feedings. Breastfeeding infants should feed about 10 minutes per breast at each feeding, and the mother should be encouraged to alternate breasts at each feeding. Formula choices are varied, and parents should be aware that there are many appropriate choices available (Table 1–9).

Measurements

Weight should be plotted at each visit. Birth weight is regained by 2 weeks of age, doubles by 6 months, and triples by 12 months. For the premature infant, subtract weeks of prematurity from postnatal age when plotting measurement to avoid misdiagnosing a failure to thrive.

 Clinical Pearl: If weight is below the third percentile or varies more than 2 standard deviations from previous visit, further investigation should be done.

Table 1-6 Recommended Childhood Immunization Schedule, United States, 2003

Vaccine ▼ / Age ▶	Birth	1 mo	2 mo	4 mo	6 mo	12 mo	15 mo	18 mo	24 mo	4-6 yr	11-12 yr	13-18 yr
Hepatitis B[1]	Hep B #1	only if mother HBsAg (−)	Hep B #2		Hep B #3						Hep B series	
Diphtheria, tetanus, pertussis[2]			DTaP	DTaP	DTaP		DTaP	DTaP		DTaP	Td	
Haemophilus influenzae type b[3]			Hib	Hib	Hib	Hib	Hib					
Inactivated polio[4]			IPV	IPV		IPV	IPV	IPV		IPV		
Measles, mumps, rubella[5]						MMR #1				MMR #2	MMR #2	MMR #2
Varicella[6]						Varicella	Varicella				Varicella	
Pneumococcal[7]			PCV	PCV	PCV	PCV	PCV			PCV	PPV	
Hepatitis A[8]										Hepatitis A series		
Influenza[9]										Influenza (yearly)		

Legend: Range of Recommended Ages | Catch-Up-Vaccination | Preadolescent Assessment

Vaccines below this line are for selected populations

18

This schedule indicates the recommended ages for routine administration of currently licensed childhood vaccines, as of December 1, 2001, for children through age 18 years. Any dose not given at the recommended age should be given at any subsequent visit when indicated and feasible. ▉ Indicates age groups that warrant special effort to administer those vaccines not previously given. Additional vaccines may be licensed and recommended during the year. Licensed combination vaccines may be used whenever any components of the combination are indicated and the vaccine's other components are not contraindicated. Providers should consult the manufacturers' package inserts for detailed recommendations.

Approved by the Advisory Committee on immunization Practices (www.cdc.gov/nip/acip) the American Academy of Pediatrics (www.aap.org), and the American Academy of Family Physicians (www.aafp.org).

Recommended Childhood and Adolescent Immunization Schedule- United State, 2003. Pediatrics (2003) Vol. III

[1] **Hepatitis B vaccine (Hep B).** All infants should receive the first dose of hepatitis B vaccine soon after birth and before hospital discharge; the first dose may also be given by age 2 months if the infant's mother is HBsAg-negative. Only monovalent hepatitis B vaccine can be used for the birth dose. Monovalent or combination vaccine containing Hep B may be used to complete the series; four doses of vaccine may be administered if combination vaccine is used. The second dose should be given at least 4 weeks after the first dose, except for Hib-containing vaccine which cannot be administered before age 6 weeks. The third dose should be given at least 16 weeks after the first dose and at least 8 weeks after the second dose. The last dose in the vaccination series (third or fourth dose) should not be administered before age 6 months.

Infants born to HBsAg-positive mothers should receive hepatitis B vaccine and 0.5 mL hepatitis B immune globulin (HBIG) within 12 hours of birth at separate sites. The second dose is recommended at age 1–2 months, and the vaccination series should be completed (third or fourth dose) at age 6 months.

Infants born to mothers whose HBsAg status is unknown should receive the first dose of the hepatitis B vaccine series within 12 hours of birth. Maternal blood should be drawn at the time of delivery to determine the mother's HBsAg status; if the HBsAg test is positive, the infant should receive HBIG as soon as possible (no later than age 1 week).

[2] **Diphtheria and tetanus toxoids and acellular pertussis vaccine (DTaP).** The fourth dose of DTaP may be administered as early as age 12 months, provided that 6 months have elapsed since the third dose and the child is unlikely to return at age 15–18 months. **Tetanus and diphtheria toxoids (Td)** is recommended at age 11–12 years if at least 5 years have elapsed since the last dose of tetanus and diphtheria toxoid-containing vaccine. Subsequent routine Td boosters are recommended every 10 years.

[3] **Haemophilus influenzae type b (Hib) conjugate vaccine.** Three Hib conjugate vaccines are licensed for infant use. If PRP-OMP (PedvaxHIB → [Merck]) is administered at ages 2 and 4 months, a dose at age 6 months is not required. DTaP/Hib combination products should not be used for primary immunization in infants at age 2, 4, or 6 months, but can be used as boosters following any Hib vaccine.

(Continued on the following page)

Infants: 1 to 12 Months **19**

[4] **Inactivated poliovirus vaccine (IPV).** An all-IPV schedule is recommended for routine childhood poliovirus vaccination in the United States. All children should receive four doses of IPV at age 2 months, 4 months, 6–18 months, and 4–6 years.

[5] **Measles, mumps, and rubella vaccine (MMR).** The second dose of MMR is recommended routinely at age 4–6 years but may be administered during any visit, provided that at least 4 weeks have elapsed since the first dose and that both doses are administered beginning at or after age 12 months. Those who have not previously received the second dose should complete the schedule by the visit at age 11–12 years.

[6] **Varicella vaccine.** Varicella vaccine is recommended at any visit at or after age 12 months for susceptible children (i.e., those who lack a reliable history of chickenpox). Susceptible persons aged ≥ 13 years should receive two doses, given at least 4 weeks apart.

[7] **Pneumococcal vaccine.** The heptavalent **pneumococcal conjugate vaccine (PCV)** is recommended for all children aged 2–23 months and for certain children aged 24–59 months. See *MMWR* 2000;49(RR-9):1–37.

Pneumococcal polysaccharide vaccine (PPV) is recommended in addition to PCV for certain high-risk groups.

[8] **Hepatitis A vaccine.** Hepatitis A vaccine is recommended for use in selected states and regions and for certain high-risk groups; consult your local public health authority. See *MMWR* 1999;48(RR-12):1–37.

[9] **Influenza vaccine.** Influenza vaccine is recommended annually for children age ≥ 6 months with certain risk factors (including but not limited to asthma, cardiac disease, sickle cell disease, HIV and diabetes; see *MMWR* 2001;50(RR-4):1–44) and can be administered to all others wishing to obtain immunity. Children aged ≤12 years should receive vaccine in a dosage appropriate for their age (0.25 mL if age 6–35 months or 0.5 mL if aged ≥ 3 years). Children aged ≤ 8 years who are receiving influenza vaccine for the first time should receive two doses separated by at least 4 weeks.

Additional information about vaccines, vaccine supply, and contraindications for immunization, is available at www.cdc.gov/nip or at the National Immunization Hotline, 800-232-2522 (English) or 800-232-0233 (Spanish).

**Table 1–7   Schedule of Immunizations for Children *not*
Immunized Within the First Year of Life**

Children Under 7	Immunization
First visit to provider	Hep B, DTaP, OPV, MMR, Hib (if child is 15 mo or <6 yr), Varicella (if >12 mo)
1 mo after first visit	Hep B, DTaP
2 mo after first visit	DTaP, IPV, Hib
>8 mo after first visit	DTaP, HB, IPV
4–6 yr	DTaP, IPV, MMR
11–12 yr	MMR (if not received at 4–6 yr)
14–16 yr	Td (repeat every 10 yr)

Children Over 7	Immunization
First visit	HB, Td, IPV, MMR, Varicella
4 weeks after first visit	HB
16 weeks after first dose	HB
1 mo after first visit	HB, Td, IPV
6–14 mo after first visit	HB, Td, IPV
10 yr	Td (repeat every 10 yr)
11–12 yr	MMR
if > 13 yr	2-dose series of varicella 4 wk apart

Table 1–8   CPT Codes for Immunizations

Immunization	CPT Code
DtaP	90723
Hepatitis B	90704–747
Comvax	90748
MMR	90710
Varicella	90716
DT	90719
HIB	90645–648
IPV	90713
Rotavirus	90680
Hepatitis A & B	90636
Influenza	90657–660
Measles	90705
Rubella	90706
Mumps	990704
Tetanus toxoid	90703

Height and head circumference should be plotted each visit. Head
circumference increases 2 cm per month (0–3 months), 1 cm per
month (3–6 months), and 1 inch per month (6–18 months).

Sensory Screening

Verbalization and responsiveness skill should be evaluated at each
visit (see Tables 1–2 and 1–3).

Assess response to light and sound at each visit.

Table 1-9 Approximate Composition of Infant Formulas*

	Kilocalories/ Ounce	Protein Source	Protein g/dL	Fat Source	Fat g/dL	Carbohydrate Source	Carbohydrate g/dL	Sodium (mEq/ dL)	Potassium (mEq/dL)	Phosphorus (mg/dL)	Calcium (mg/dL)	Osmolality (mOsm/ kg water)
Human Milk												
Mature human milk	20	Human Milk	1.0	Human milk	4.4	Lactose	6.9	0.7	1.3	14	32	300
Premature Formulas (Hospital and Transitional)												
Enfamil Human Milk Fortifier (3.8 g) added to 100 mL preterm milk (Mead Johnson)	24	Preterm human milk plus fortifier, whey and caseinate	2.3	Preterm human milk fat	3.5	Preterm human milk, lactose, fortifier, corn syrup solids	10.1	1.5	1.7	60	117	410–440
Enfamil Premature (Mead Johnson)	24	Nonfat milk, whey	2.4	Soy, MCT (40%), coconut oils	4.1	Corn syrup solids, lactose	9.0	1.4	2.1	67	134	310
Similac NeoCare (Ross)	22	Nonfat milk, whey	1.9	Soy, coconut, MCT (25%) oils	4.1	Corn syrup solids, lactose	7.7	1.0	2.7	46	78	290
Similac Natural Care Human Milk Fortifier (Ross)	24	Nonfat milk, whey	2.2	MCT (50%), soy, coconut oils	4.4	Lactose, polycose	8.6	1.5	2.7	85	171	280
Similac Special Care (Ross)	24	Nonfat milk, whey	2.2	MCT (50%), soy, coconut oils	4.4	Lactose, polycose	8.6	1.5	2.7	73	146	280
SMA-Preemie (Wyeth Ayerst)	24	Whey, nonfat milk	2.0	Coconut, oleic, oleo, soy, MCT (10%) oils	4.4	Lactose, glucose polymers	8.6	1.4	1.9	40	75	280

Table 1–9 Approximate Composition of Infant Formulas*

	Kilocalories/ Ounce	Protein Source	g/dL	Fat Source	g/dL	Carbohydrate Source	g/dL	Sodium (mEq/dL)	Potassium (mEq/dL)	Phosphorus (mg/dL)	Calcium (mg/dL)	Osmolality (mOsm/ kg water)
Cow's Milk–Based Formulas												
Bonamil (Wyeth Ayerst)	20	Nonfat milk	1.5	Soy, coconut, soy lecithin oils	3.6	Lactose	7.1	0.8	1.6	36	46	290
Enfamil (Mead Johnson)	20	Whey, nonfat milk	1.4	Palm olein, soy, coconut, high-oleic sunflower oils	3.8	Lactose	7.0	0.8	1.9	36	53	300
Gerber (Gerber)	20	Nonfat milk	1.5	Palm olein, soy, coconut, high-oleic sunflower oils	3.7	Lactose	7.2	0.9	1.9	39	51	320
For Special Feeding Problems												
Portagen (Mead Johnson)	20	Sodium caseinate	2.4	MCT (86%), corn oil	3.3	Corn syrup solids, sucrose	7.8	1.6	2.2	48	64	230
Monodisaccharide-free diet powder Product 3232A (Mead Johnson)	13 Using 81.0 g powder and water to make 1 quart	Casein hydrolysate with added amino acids	1.9	MCT (85%), corn oil	2.9	Modified tapioca starch, may add 59 g CHO/quart, corn syrup solids, sucrose, glucose, fructose	2.8 6.3	1.2	1.9	43	64	Dependent on additional CHO source: 250 without CHO source

(Continued on the following page)

Table 1-9 Approximate Composition of Infant Formulas* *(Cont'd.)*

	Kilocalories/ Ounce	Protein Source	Protein g/dL	Fat Source	Fat g/dL	Carbohydrate Source	Carbohydrate g/dL	Sodium (mEq/dL)	Potassium (mEq/dL)	Phosphorus (mg/dL)	Calcium (mg/dL)	Osmolality (mOsm/ kg water)
Protein Vitamin Mineral Formula Component (Ross)	Add 30 g powder, CHO, and fat to 900 mL water	Casein	2.2	Coconut oils: may add corn, soy, safflower, MCT oils	Tr	May add sucrose, polycose, dextrose, fructose	Tr	1.6	2.5	51	72	Dependent on source and amount of CHO
RCF CHO-Free Formula Base	12 Dilute 1 : 1 without added CHO	Soy protein isolate with L-methioninc	2.0	Soy, coconut oils	3.6	May add sucrose, polycose, dextrose, fructose	—	1.3	1.9	50	70	Dependent on source and amount of CHO
For Feeding Beyond 4–Months of Age with Solids Added to Diet												
Follow-Up (Carnation)	20	Nonfat milk	1.8	Palm olein, soy, coconut, high-oleic safflower oils	2.8	Corn syrup, lactose	8.9	1.2	2.3	61	91	326
Follow-Up Soy (Carnation)	20	Soy protein isolate with L-methioninc	2.1	Soy oil	3.7	Sucrose, tapioca dextrin	6.8	1.2	2.0	61	91	270
For Feeding Beyond 1 Year of Age												
Whole cow's milk	20	Cow's milk	3.3	Cow's milk	3.7	Lactose	4.7	2.1	3.9	93	119	288
Next Step (Mead Johnson)	20	Nonfat milk	1.8	Palm olein, soy, coconut, sunflower oils	3.4	Corn syrup solids, lactose	7.5	1.2	2.2	57	81	270

Table 1–9 Approximate Composition of Infant Formulas*

	Kilocalories/ Ounce	Protein g/dL	Protein Source	Fat g/dL	Fat Source	Carbohydrate g/dL	Carbohydrate Source	Sodium (mEq/dL)	Potassium (mEq/dL)	Phosphorus (mg/dL)	Calcium (mg/dL)	Osmolality (mOsm/ kg water)
Next Step Soy (Mead Johnson)	20	2.2	Soy protein isolate with L-methioninc	3.0	Palm olein, soy, coconut, high-oleic sunflower oils	8.0	Corn syrup solids, sucrose	1.3	2.6	61	78	260
Similac Toddler's Best (Ross)	20	2.4	Nonfat milk	3.2	High-oleic safflower, coconut, soy coils	7.4	Sucrose, lactose	1.2	2.6	64	105	360
Nutrient Dense												
Kindercal (Mead Johnson)	30	3.4	Calcium caseinate, sodium caseinate, milk protein concentrate	4.4	Canola, high-oleic sunflower, corn, MCT (20%) oils	13.5	Maltodextrin, sucrose, soy fiber	1.6	3.4	85	85	310
PediaSure (Ross)	30	3.0	Caseinate, whey proteins	5.0	High-oleic safflower, soy, MCT (20%) oils	11.0	Corn syrup solids, sucrose	1.7	3.4	80	97	310
PediaSure with Fiber (Ross)	30	3.0	Caseinate, whey proteins	5.0	High-oleic safflower, soy, MCT (20%) oils	11.0	Corn syrup solids, sucrose, soy fiber	1.7	3.4	80	97	345

25

Developmental Assessment

Normal patterns of growth and development, accomplishment of developmental milestones, and normal reflexes should be assessed at each visit (see Tables 1–2 and 1–3).

The Denver II should be done on all children, and referrals should be made for all abnormal findings.

Physical Examination

The practitioner should first observe the general appearance of the infant and the interaction between the caregiver and infant. The examination should be performed in an organized fashion, but the practitioner should take advantage of the infant's periods of quiet for parts of the examination that require auscultation. The entire examination should be done in good light with the infant fully unclothed and should consist of the following.

- Assess the muscle tone, hearing, and visual tracking of the infant
- Assess the position of the eyes, elicit the red reflex and check for strabismus
- Assess the cardiac and respiratory status of the infant preferably when the infant is quiet or asleep
- Check hips and evaluate extremities and joints for abnormalities, unequal size, pain, or decreased range of motion
- Assess skin and evaluate hygiene
- Evaluate the abdomen, genitalia, and anus; observe particularly for any signs of hernias or injuries that might be suspicious of abuse
- Inspect and examine the ears, nose, and throat
- Assess the neurologic system (see Table 1–4)
- Presence of teeth should be noted (Table 1–10)

Table 1–10   Eruption of Teeth

Primary Teeth	Age of Eruption in Months
Central incisor	6–7.5
Lateral incisor	7–9
Cuspid	16–18
First molar	12–14
Second molar	20–24

Permanent Teeth	Age of Eruption in Years
Central incisor	6–8
Lateral incisor	7–9
Cuspid	9–12
First bicuspid	10–12
Second bicuspid	10–12
First molar	6–7
Second molar	11–13

Diagnostic Tests

Test	Results Indicating Disorder	CPT code
Hematocrit or hemoglobin (done between 6 and 9 months)*	<11 indicates anemia	83036
Urinalysis (done at 9 months)	Blood, bacteria, white blood cells	81000
For children at risk		
Lead screening (12 months)	>10	83665
Tuberculin test: PPD	Positive	86580–85
Cholesterol	LDL high; HDL low	82465

* Hemoglobin electrophoresis may be repeated at 6 months if suspicious results obtained at birth.
PPD, purified protein derivative; HDL, high-density lipoprotein; LDL, low-density lipoprotein.

Procedures

Immunizations
Immunizations should be administered according to the recommended guidelines (see Tables 1–6 and Table 1–7).

Anticipatory Guidance

Injury
Infants are vulnerable to injury. Caregivers must remain vigilant in their protection of the infant, and this includes watching toys selected for age appropriateness. Poisons, household cleansers, and medications should all be stored away from children. Water safety includes setting the bath water heater at less than 120°F; never leaving the child unattended in bath or pool, and emptying all pools and buckets to prevent accidental drowning. Baby walkers should not be used.

Violence
Children need to be protected from obvious dangers such as firearms. All firearms should be stored unloaded and out of children's reach.

Sleep Positioning
"Back to Sleep" is the American Academy of Pediatrics statement that children should be put to sleep on their backs to decrease the possibility of an apparent life-threatening event. Children should not be put to bed with pillows or thick comforters because these also increase the possibility of suffocation.

Nutrition
Caution parents that solids should not be introduced until about 6 months of age.
Infants should be encouraged to drink from a cup by 6 months and be weaned from the bottle by 12 months.

Table foods, chopped, can be introduced at 8 months, and transition from baby food to table foods is usually accomplished by 12 months.

Juice should be limited. The American Academy of Pediatrics has come out strongly against the overuse of juices because they have too high a carbohydrate and calorie content. Juices should be limited to 4 to 6 ounces per day.

Foods that might lead to aspiration, such as peanuts, popcorn, hot dogs, and pieces of raw fruit and vegetables, should not be given to infants younger than 12 months.

EARLY CHILDHOOD:1 TO 4 YEARS

History

If this is the initial visit, all *prenatal, birth, and family history* should be reviewed.

A history of illnesses, hospitalizations, surgeries, and medications, now and in the past, should be elicited.

Review *social history*. Discuss any changes or new stressors in the home or family.

Ascertain reason for visit. Is child ill or is this a well checkup?

Review immunizations.

Are they up to date? If not, explain the catch-up schedule (see Table 1–7).

Have any new immunizations been added to the schedule that would be of benefit or are now required for the child?

Because of all the media controversy about immunizations, the nurse practitioner should be prepared to answer any questions or concerns the caregiver may have regarding immunizations.

Social History

Assess any changes in living arrangements in the home.

Check if there are any smokers in the home.

Ask if the child is now attending day care.

Check if there are any other changes or stressors in the home or family.

Family History

Review family history of illnesses or other inheritable diseases if this is a new patient.

Check if there are any changes now in the family history.

Sleep History

Identify patterns of sleep, where the child sleeps, and if there are any problems associated with sleep (see Fig. 1–1).

Review of Systems

It is helpful to assess current health status.

Ask if there have been any visits to another health care provider, any accidents or other traumas, or visits to emergency departments since the last visit.

Ask if there are any medicines being taken at this time and if previously prescribed medicines that were supposed to be continued are being taken.

Ask if there are any new allergies or other problems.

Nutritional History

Discuss usual eating habits of the child.

Discuss weaning form the bottle because this should be accomplished by 1 year of age.

Ask if the child is doing some self-feeding and drinking from a cup.

When formula has been discontinued (9–12 months), the child ideally should be started on 2% milk.

Review food choices, stressing the avoidance of foods that may cause choking.

Encourage a balanced diet and nutritional snacks and drinks, limiting sugar and keeping juice to a maximum of 4 to 6 ounces per day (Fig. 1–4).

Measurements

Measurements for every child should be obtained at each visit and plotted on a growth chart. The following are acceptable measurement parameters for the nurse practitioner to look for.

During early childhood years, the average yearly weight gain is 4.4 to 6.6 pounds.

Height increases about 4.8 inches between 1 and 2 years and 2.4 to 3.2 inches between 2 and 3 years.

 Clinical Pearl: At 2 years of age, height of the child is approximately half the adult height they will be expected to obtain.

Sensory Screening

Beginning at the 3-year-old visit, objective measurement of hearing and vision should be done.

Developmental Assessment

Developmental assessment should be done at each visit, and a Denver II should be performed.

Note: Simply observing the child from the moment he or she enters the clinic can be an important part of developmental screening.

Ask the parents or observe the following major areas for each of the following age groups.

DAILY FOOD GUIDE PYRAMID

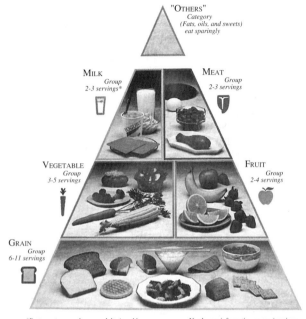

"OTHERS"
*Category
(Fats, oils, and sweets)
eat sparingly*

MILK
*Group
2-3 servings**

MEAT
*Group
2-3 servings*

VEGETABLE
*Group
3-5 servings*

FRUIT
*Group
2-4 servings*

GRAIN
*Group
6-11 servings*

*Preteens, teens, and young adults (age 11 to 24) and pregnant and lactating women need 4 servings from the Milk Group to meet their increased calcium needs.

Need more information on serving sizes or the variety of foods in each group? Ask for a copy of Dairy Council's GUIDE to GOOD EATING.

Figure 1–4. Daily food guide pyramid.

At 2 years of age, the child should:

- Be able to climb steps one at a time
- Make a stack of five blocks
- Have at least a 20-word vocabulary and be able to make 2-word phrases
- Imitate circular strokes with a crayon or pencil
- Follow a two-part command

At 3 years of age, the child should:

- Be able to ride a bicycle
- Tell you their first name, age, and sex
- Feed and dress self
- Balance on one foot and jump in place

At 4 years of age, the child should:

- Be able to sing a song
- Draw a person with three parts

- Build a 10-block tower
- Hop on one foot
- Throw a ball overhand
- Tell you their first and last name

Physical Examination

At each visit, a thorough head-to-toe physical examination should be performed with the child undressed. Beginning at age 3 years, blood pressure should be measured at least annually and ideally at each visit. Other vital signs should be taken as well, including pulse, respirations, temperature, and heart rate (see Tables 1–4 and 1–5). The child should be examined for signs of child abuse. If abuse is suspected, the child should be asked if anyone has ever hurt them, if anyone has asked them to keep secrets, if anyone has ever touched them when they did not want to be touched, and finally if they are afraid of anyone. Any positive answers should be followed up with more probing questions, and all suspected abuse should be reported to the police and the local Department of Human Services office.

The presence and position of teeth should be noted (see Table 1–10). A referral to a dentist is recommended at age 3 years.

Diagnostic Tests

Test	Results Indicating Disorder	CPT code
Urinalysis (ideally at age 5) can be performed at age 4	Presence of bacteria, glucose, ketones, or other abnormal findings	81000–009
For children at risk PPD Lead screening	Positive >10	86580–85 83655

Procedures

Immunizations

Between ages 4 and 6 years, children need to receive all their required preschool immunizations (see Tables 1–6 and 1–7).

Anticipatory Guidance

The nurse practitioner should address the following areas to assist parents in understanding what they can do to help protect their child.

- Injury prevention
- Use a car seat (back seat only)
- Supervised play inside and outside the home
- Recheck the hot water heater and maintain the temperature less than 120°F
- Have at least one smoke detector in the home
- Provide coverage for all electrical outlets to avoid injuries

- Put all medicines and chemicals out of children's reach
- Strategies to prevent drowning (age 4 is an appropriate time to offer swimming lessons)
- Gun safety, including storage in locked closet, unloaded weapons with ammunition in places other than where the gun is stored

MIDDLE CHILDHOOD: 5 TO 10 YEARS

History

As the child continues to grow and mature and become more independent, the history continues to be an important part of every examination. Often a history can provide significant clues to the overall health of the child and family. The following are guidelines for obtaining the history of the 5- to 10-year-old child.

For all new patients, a review of prenatal, birth, and family history should be obtained.

A review of any illnesses, either for the child or within the family, should be obtained.

Review past or present injuries, surgeries, and medical diagnosis.

Review social history.

Ascertain reason for visit. Is child ill or is this a well checkup?

Review immunizations. Are they up to date?

Discuss sexuality education issues with parents and child. Inquire if there is age-appropriate sexual education literature available in the home. At age 10, discuss puberty and related sexuality issues with parents and children.

Social History

Assess any changes in living arrangements in the home.

Check if there are any smokers in the home.

Ask what grade the child is in and how they are progressing in school.

Check if there are any other changes or stressors in the home or family.

Family History

Review family history of illnesses or other inheritable diseases if this is a new patient.

Check if there are any new changes or stressors in the family.

Sleep History

Identify patterns of sleep, where the child sleeps, and if there are any problems associated with sleep (see Fig. 1–1).

Review of Systems

At each visit, it is essential that a review of systems be performed. This should also include the following.

Ask if there have been any visits to another health care provider, any accidents or other traumas, hospitalizations, or visits to emergency departments since the last visit.

Ask if there are any medications being taken at this time or if previously prescribed medications were completed or continued as scheduled.

Nutritional History

Ask about the child's eating habits and appetite.

Encourage nutritional snacks, including fruits and vegetables, and drinks; stress limiting juice to a maximum of 4 to 6 ounces per day.

Ask if the family eats their meals together.

Determine the percentage of fat in the child's diet. Less than 30% of a child's diet should be fat because it contributes to obesity (see Fig. 1–4).

 Clinical Pearl: Obesity is the number one problem related to nutrition that is reported in children today.

Dental History

Check fluoridation of the drinking water and supplement as needed (for ages 3–6 years, if the fluoride is <0.3 ppm, give 5 mg/day; 0.3–0.6 ppm, give 0.25 mg/day; for ages 6–16 years, if the fluoride is <0.3 ppm, give 1 mg/day; 0.3–0.6 ppm, give 0.5 mg/day).

Encourage brushing teeth at least twice a day and flossing once a day by the age of 8.

Measurements

Measurements for every child should be obtained at each visit and plotted on a growth chart. A change of more than 2 standard deviations may indicate a problem and should be examined further. Height generally increases during the school-age years at a rate of about 2.5 inches per year. During this time, weight increases by approximately 5 to 7 pounds per year. The head circumference increases in size slowly, reaching its adult size by 12 years of age.

Sensory Screening

A vision and hearing screening test should be performed at yearly intervals when none are provided at school. Parents should be encouraged to obtain a yearly vision test either at the clinic or at a private physician because poor school performance is often linked to either vision or hearing problems.

Developmental/Behavioral Assessment

The child and the parent should be included in the obtaining and providing of the history. By age 6, children are able to respond and be reliable historians. The nurse practitioner may choose to divide developmental screening into two sections—one in which the child is the respondent and one in which the parent is the respondent.

The nurse practitioner should ask the child questions in the following areas:

- Questions related to family, such as how is the relationship among family members; what, if any, activities does the family do for enjoyment; and how the child gets along within the family
- Questions related to friends, including if their parents know or have met most of their friends and families, what they do for fun with their friends, and if they have a best friend
- Questions related to school, such as what grade they are in, how their grades are, what they do and do not like about school, and who their teacher is
- Questions related to their own activities outside of school and degree of independence from their parents

The nurse practitioner should ask the parent questions in the following areas:

- Any major changes within the family that may be causing stress for the parent or child
- The relationship between them, other siblings, and the child
- How they view the child's friendships
- If there are any problems at school and whether the parents maintain contact with the child's teacher
- How their child spends time outside of school

Physical Examination

A head-to-toe physical should be performed each visit. Along with this, the following should be included:

- Measure and plot weight and height for age
- Vision, hearing, and blood pressure assessments
- Scoliosis screening starting at age 8 years
- Tanner staging should be done each visit (Table 1–11)
- Observe for any evidence of abuse; all positive findings should be followed up
- Presence and position of permanent teeth should be noted (see Table 1–10)

Table 1-11   Stages of Puberty—Tanner Stages

| | Female | Female and Male | Male | |
Stage	Breasts	Pubic Hair	Penis	Testes
1	Diameter of areolae increases	None	Prepubertal	Prepubertal
2	Breast buds develop	Light, straight, sparse	Enlarges	Testes enlarge, scrotum becomes red and coarse
3	Areolae and breasts enlarge	Darker, curling, slight increase in amount	Lengthens	Continuation of stage 2
4	Contour differentiates between areola and breast	Coarse, curly, moderate amount	Increases in diameter	Scrotum darkens
5	Breasts fully developed	Adult distribution and amount, spread to medial thighs; thickening will continue	Fully developed	Testes and scrotum fully developed

Source: Adapted from Tanner, JM: Growth at Adolescence, ed 2. Blackwell Scientific, Oxford, 1962.

Diagnostic Tests

Test	Results Indicating Disorder	CPT Code
Urinalysis (at 5 years)	Presence of bacteria, blood, nitrites, protein, glucose	81000-009
For children at risk Tuberculin test: PPD Cholesterol screening	Positive HDL low LDH high	86580-85 82465

Procedures

Immunizations
Assess that immunizations appropriate for age have been given.

Anticipatory Guidance
Parents and children can be assisted in learning how to keep their child and themselves safe if they attend to the following areas and incorporate the following measures in their health maintenance routines.

Keep the child's environment smoke-free.

Use smoke detectors in the home and have a family escape plan in the event of a fire.

Keep all medications and noxious substances out of the child's reach, and reinforce with the child the importance of not ingesting any dangerous substance.

Always supervise the child in or around water to prevent drowning.

Use sunscreen if the child is in the sun, but stress the importance of avoiding the sun and the dangers of sunbathing to parents and children.

Ensure that all dangerous objects such as knives and guns are out of the child's reach and that the child is taught the dangers of weapons.

Use seat belts on all car trips, and stress that children should not be riding in the front seat of the car.

ADOLESCENCE: 11 TO 21 YEARS

History

Whenever possible, the adolescent should have all or part of the examination done in privacy without a parent or sibling present. Because the need for confidentiality and privacy becomes greater during this period, the adolescent needs reassurance that he or she can confide in the nurse practitioner to insure a successful relationship with the health care practitioner. If this is an initial visit, obtain appropriate history from parents, such as prenatal, birth, infancy, and early childhood history and family history. Other areas to include in the history are as follows.

Obtain information related to nutrition, appetite, and diet.

Ask about sleep patterns and related problems.

Ask about immunization status.

Ask about the adolescent's relationships with family members.

Evaluate the adolescent's understanding of puberty and the changes that occur during this time.

Screen for any history of abuse.

Ascertain the reason for this visit.

Inquire about any past or current illnesses, medications, or other therapies.

Ask about herbal or other alternative medications that may be currently used.

Measurements

Physical, psychological, and social states of well-being are all intimately linked during adolescence. Continued surveillance of growth is an important part of each visit, so measure height, weight, Tanner staging (see Table 1–11), blood pressure (see Tables 1–4 and 1–5), and pulses. As the child enters puberty, girls generally have a predictable growth spurt at age 12 and boys have one at age 14. The following are guidelines for the nurse practitioner:

Weight generally increases about 5 pounds per year and height increases 2.5 to 3 inches per year until maturity.

Increased weight in girls is usually accounted for by an increase in body fat; increased weight in boys is usually due to an increase in muscular tissue.

Dentition should be evaluated because the third set of molars erupts between age 18 and 22.

Sensory Screening

All adolescents should have an annual vision screening.

Hearing screening should be performed when available at a clinic or when there are reported signs and symptoms that suggest a hearing problem.

Developmental/Behavioral Assessment

A good developmental history can be obtained from the adolescent. The following areas should be explored with the adolescent:

- Birth order in the family
- Relationship with other family members
- What type of discipline is used in the home
- What responsibilities in the family do they have (i.e., chores)
- What is their relationship with peers? Do they have friends, do they have a best friend, and what do they like to do with their friends
- Have they begun dating and if so have they become sexually active
- Have they experimented with any drug or alcohol and if so how often and how much
- Ask the adolescent how school is going for them and if there are any problems currently with grades, teachers, or other students
- Ask about the adolescent's level of activity such as exercise, participation in sports, or other recreational activities
- Ask if the adolescent has any concerns about self, family, or friends

It is important to ask parents questions related to development. These questions may include the following areas:

- Changes or stressors in the home, family, or school
- Parental concerns about friends
- Parental concerns about drug or alcohol use
- Parental concerns about school
- Parental observations about recreational or physical activity of the adolesecent

 Clinical Pearl: The HEADSS interview is an efficient way to address areas of concern with adolescents. The HEADSS interview addresses areas related to *Home, Education, Activities, Drugs, Sex,* and *Suicide.*

Physical Examination

The physical examination of the adolescent should include the following:

A head-to-toe examination should be performed in privacy.

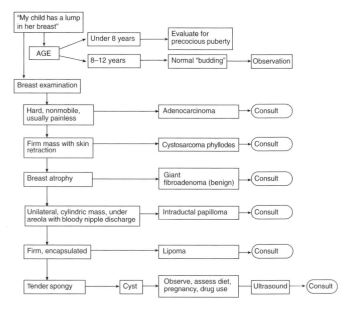

Figure 1–5. Evaluation of breast lumps in female patients.

Girls who are sexually active should receive a Pap smear and screening for chlamydia, rapid plasmin regain (RPR), and human immunodeficiency virus (HIV) test.

Scoliosis screening should be done at each visit.

Examine the skin and assess for acne; offer treatment when appropriate.

Tanner staging should be done at each visit. Girls should be evaluated for breast lumps (Fig. 1–5). Boys should be evaluated for gynecomastia and hernias. Testicular self-examination should be taught, and testes should be checked for masses.

Diagnostic Tests

Test	Results Indicating Disorder	CPT code
Hemoglobin or hematocrit (13 years)	<11 indicates anemia	83036
Urinalysis	Positive for bacteria, blood, glucose, nitrites, protein	81000–009
Children at risk Tuberculin test: PPD	Positive	86580–085
Cholesterol screening	HDL low LDL high	82465

Test	Results Indicating Disorder	CPT code
STD screening		
Chlamydia	Positive	87710
Yeast	Positive for *Candida*	87106
Bacterial	Positive for bacteria	87073–076
Herpes	Positive for herpes	87207
HIV	Positive	86701–703
RPR	Positive	86592–593
Pelvic examination	Abnormal cells	57410
Pap smear	Abnormal cells	88141-155 88164-167

STD, sexually transmitted disease.

Procedures

Immunizations

Immunizations should be given as schedule requires (see Tables 1–6 and 1–7).

Anticipatory Guidance:

There are many areas of concern, especially related to safety, with adolescents. Some areas that merit attention include:

- Use of seat belts when driving or being driven in a car
- The use and misuse of alcohol
- Drug use
- Avoidance of all tobacco products
- Wearing appropriate safety apparatus at work and at play
- The importance of learning to swim to avoid drowning

Because homicide is the second leading cause of death in this age group, stress avoidance of carrying or using weapons and associating with gangs or peers involved in unlawful activities.

Other areas in anticipatory guidance include:

- The importance of seeing the dentist two times a year
- Brushing teeth two times a day
- Eating properly and avoiding stringent diets that may injure health
- The need for regular exercise
- Listening to their own feelings and getting help when they feel that their emotions are out of control
- Learning to deal with stress

INTERNATIONAL ADOPTION: GUIDELINES FOR HEALTH CARE PROVIDERS

International adoption is becoming more common, and the health care provider needs to know which tests and evaluations are appropriate.

Also, guidelines for immunizations are important to help parents feel reassured that their child will have the optimal health potential possible. The following are some guidelines for the nurse practitioner to follow.

Appropriate Tests

- Complete blood count with differential
- Hemoglobin electrophoresis (Asian and Latino)
- Glucose-6-phosphate dehydrogenase (Asian and Latino)
- Urinalysis with microscopic examination
- Three stool specimens for ova and parasites, *Giardia* antigen, *Cryptosporidium* direct fluorescent antibody (probably not necessary for Korean children)
- One stool specimen for bacterial culture (not necessary for Korean children)
- Hepatitis B surface antigen and antibody and core antibody (IgG total)
- Hepatitis C antibody
- Repeat hepatitis B and C 6 months after arrival
- RPR, fluorescent treponemal antibody absorption
- HIV-1, HIV-2 enzyme-linked immunosorbent assay now and repeat in 6 months
- Total thyroxine, free thyroxine, and TSH
- Rickets screen (not imperative because this can usually be diagnosed clinically)
- All state-mandated tests if less than 6 months of age (routine newborn screening)
- Lead (venous)
- PPD (use 10 mm of induration as cutoff for chest radiograph and preventive therapy); repeat in 6 months
- Hearing and vision evaluation
- Dental visit if child is older than 18 months
- Developmental evaluation (Denver II)
- Subspecialty consultations as indicated by examination or test results

Immunizations

History is usually unreliable and it is suggested that immunizations be repeated. The *Haemophilus influenzae* type B, pneumococcus, and varicella vaccines are not regularly given outside the United States.

REFERENCES

American Academy of Pediatrics Clinical Report: Prevention of Rickets and Vitamin D Deficiency: New guidelines for vitamin D intake. Pediatrics 111(4):908, 2003.

American Academy of Pediatrics: Selecting and using the most appropriate car safety seats for growing children. Pediatrics 109:550, 2002.

American Academy of Pediatrics, Committee on Children with Disabilities: Developmental surveillance and screening of infants and young children (RE0062). Pediatrics 108:192, 2001.

American Academy of Pediatrics, Committee on Injury and Poison Prevention: Injuries associated with infant walkers. Pediatrics 108:790, 2001.

American Academy of Pediatrics, Committee on Injury and Poison Prevention: Falls from heights: Windows, roofs, and balconies (RE9951). Pediatrics 107:1188, 2001.

American Academy of Pediatrics, Committee on Injury and Poison Prevention: Reducing the number of deaths and injuries from residential fires (RE9952). Pediatrics 105:1355, 2000.

American Academy of Pediatrics, Committee on Injury and Poison Prevention: Firearm-related injuries affecting the pediatric population (RE9926). Pediatrics 105:888, 2000.

American Academy of Pediatrics, Committee on Injury and Poison Prevention: Bicycle helmets. Pediatrics 108:1030, 2001.

American Academy of Pediatrics, Committee on Nutrition: The use and misuse of fruit juice in pediatrics (RE0047). Pediatrics 107:1210, 2001.

American Academy of Pediatrics, Committee on Practice and Ambulatory Medicine: Recommendations for preventive pediatric health care (RE9939). Pediatrics 105:645, 2000.

American Academy of Pediatrics, Committee on Sports Medicine and Fitness and Committee on Injury and Poison Prevention: Swimming programs for infants and toddlers (RE9940). Pediatrics 105:868, 2000.

American Academy of Pediatrics: Recommended childhood and adolescent immunization schedule—United States, 2003. Pediatrics 111:212, 2003.

American Academy of Pediatrics: 2001 Family shopping guide to care seats: Safety and product information. Pediatrics 106:986, 2001.

Aronson, J: Medical evaluation and infectious considerations on arrival. Pediatr Ann 29:218, 2000.

Betchel, B: First year in the U.S. critical for international adoptees. Infect Dis Child 15:47, 2002.

Dickey, R: Managing Contraception Pill Patients. Enis Medical Publications, Durant, Okla., 1998.

Johnson, D: Long-term issues in international adoptees. Pediatr Ann 29:284, 2000.

Miller, L: Initial assessment of growth, development, and the effects of institutionalization in internationally-adopted children. Pediatr Ann 29:224, 2000.

Ogden, C, et al: Centers for Disease Control and Prevention 2000 Growth Charts for the United States: Improvements to the 1977 National Center for Health Statistics Version. Pediatrics 109:45, 2002.

Stroop, J: The family history as a screening tool. Pediatr Ann 29:279, 2000.

Tanner, J: Growth at Adolescence. Blackwell Scientific Publication, Oxford, 1962.

Vincent, M, and Adeyeles, E: Are you comfortable taking the sexual history? Fam Pract 20:87, 1998.

Chapter 2
SPORTS

INCIDENCE

It is estimated that more than 35 million children and adolescents participate in an organized sport. The American Academy of Pediatrics does not recommend that young athletes limit themselves to one sport before adolescence. The American Academy of Pediatrics has categorized sports by degree of contact and by intensity.

BENEFITS

Participation in a sport has been found to contribute to self-esteem, to establishing friendships, and to learning the importance of practice with regard to performance. Participating in sports is an opportunity for the child to interact with authority figures other than parents and to learn self-discipline. If the emphasis is on "win at all costs," however, the child can become depressed and be exposed to inappropriate adult behavior.

PREPARTICIPATION TRAINING

Preparticipation strength and endurance training has been recommended for all age groups. A preseason conditioning program would include aerobic, flexibility, and strength-building exercises. Conditioning programs contribute to overall health and fitness and may lower the athlete's potential for injury.

PREPARTICIPATION PHYSICAL EXAMINATION

The purpose of the preparticipation physical examination is to ensure the safe participation in the athletic activity, to identify health problems that may interfere with or become worsened by the athletic activity or would increase the risk of injury. Ideally the preparticipation examination should be scheduled 6 weeks before the start of the season. Many students forget, however, and either the clinic is deluged with last-minute requests for examinations or the coach schedules a mass screening in the gymnasium at the school. Neither of these options is the best for the nurse practitioner or the student. Suggested guidelines for optimizing the preparticipation examination follow.

Contact the school system to determine the "age" of the physical examination required. Does the examination have to be done just a few days before participation, or can it be done during the summer before the start of the season?

Find out whether cheerleaders are included as part of the athletic program.

Find out who reviews the completed forms or whether they are merely filed for future reference.

Preparticipation Physical Examination, a guide for sports examinations, can be obtained from the American Academy of Family Physicians, PO Box 8723, Kansas City, MO 64114 (800-274-2237).

EXAMINATION

History

Family History

Is there a family history of cardiac problems, particularly sudden death?

Student History

Is there a history of chest pains, syncope, or exercise-induced asthma?

What is the past history of injuries?

What is the anticipated level of sports involvement, and what is the sport?

Are there any chronic health problems?

What is the nutritional history?

Is there a history of substance abuse?

What is the status of immunizations?

Physical Examination

The physical examination should be conducted with the child in his or her underwear and should contain the following elements.

- Head to toe, observing particularly height and weight (comparison to monitor growth spurts)
- Vision screening

Table 2–1 Two-Minute Orthopedic Examination

Instructions	*Observations*
Stand facing observer	Acromioclavicular joints, general habitus
Look at ceiling, floor, over both shoulders; touch ears to shoulders	Cervical spine motion
Shrug shoulders (examiner resists)	Trapezius strength
Abduct shoulders 90 degrees (examiner resists at 90 degrees	Deltoid strength
Full external rotation of arms	Shoulder motion
Flex and extend elbows	Elbow motion
Arms at sides, elbows 90 degrees flexed, pronate and supinate wrists	Elbow and wrist motion
Spread fingers; make fist	Hand or finger motion and deformities
Tighten (contract) quadriceps; relax quadriceps	Symmetry and knee effusion; ankle effusion
"Duck walk" (4 steps away from examiner with buttocks on heels)	Hip, knee, and ankle motion
Back to examiner	Shoulder symmetry, scoliosis
Knees straight, touch toes	Scoliosis, hip motion, hamstring tightness
Raise up on toes; raise heels	Calf symmetry, leg strength

Source: Sports Medicine: Health Care for Young Athletes, American Academy of Pediatrics, Elk Grove Village, Ill, 1991, with permission.

- Heart (resting and exercise [15% have mitral valve prolapse]) and lungs
- Blood pressure (1–3% of teenagers have hypertension)
- Orthopedic examination (Table 2–1)
- Tanner staging (female athletes have onset of menarche 2.3 years later than average with no change in secondary characteristics)
- Presence or absence of hernias
- Presence of skin lesions

Laboratory Evaluation

Routine urinalysis and blood counts are usually not necessary. If these tests are performed, the nurse practitioner should be aware of the physiologic changes found in athletes. Urinalysis may reveal stress-induced hematuria and albuminuria (particularly if the athlete just came from a practice session), and blood counts may show exercise-induced anemia.

Counseling

Assessment of self-worth includes two questions: How does the student feel about participating in the sport? How does the student feel about himself or herself? This assessment is particularly important for female athletes, who are particularly susceptible to eating disorders.

Nutrition

Meeting normal guidelines for adolescents, as suggested by the food pyramid, should be stressed. The student should be asked about use of nutritional supplements.

Table 2–2   Stretching Basics

1. Warm up entire body (short, light jog) before *any* stretching
2. Breathe normally throughout stretching session
3. Devote 10–15 minutes solely to stretching
4. Concentrate
5. Stretch with a partner if possible
6. Hold each stretch for 20–30 seconds; avoid bouncing
7. Stretch all muscle groups first; then work specifically on those used most for the chosen sport
8. Stretch at least 5 minutes after cool down
9. Lessen stretch if pain occurs
10. Avoid comparisons to other people

Source: Adapted from Stretching Principles, Institute for Athletic Medicine, Minneapolis, Minn, 1992, with permission.

Body Function and Health Maintenance

Female athletes are vulnerable to menstrual disorders.

Injury Risk and Prevention

Which sports are played, and what activities do these sports demand (e.g., running, jumping)? Before practice and competition, a good warm-up routine helps to prevent injury. The nurse practitioner can provide information about basic stretching and condition exercises (Table 2–2). The practitioner should review the safety measures taken, such as types of protective equipment, and what health care facilities are available.

MEDICAL CONDITIONS

Some medical conditions warrant exclusion from sports participation. For other conditions, the child may need further evaluation before participating.

Exclusions include carditis; eye problems, such as one-eyed vision, only one eye, or previous history of eye injury or surgery; spleen if enlarged; liver if enlarged; and hypertension in weightlifting.

The following are problems that require further evaluation.

- Instability of cervical vertebrae 1 and 2 (risk of spinal injury)
- Bleeding disorders
- Hypertension (secondary or essential)
- Congenital heart disease (moderate or severe forms or children who have had surgery)
- Arrhythmia (children with chest pain, syncope, dizziness, shortness of breath, mitral valve regurgitation)
- Heart murmur (mitral valve prolapse, congenital heart disease)
- Cerebral palsy
- Kidney, loss of one (evaluate for contact, collision, and limited contact sports)

- Liver, if chronically enlarged (evaluate for contact, collision, and limited contact sports)
- Cancer
- Musculoskeletal or neurologic condition if history of spinal or head injury or concussion
- Organ transplant
- Sickle cell disease (may participate in all but high exertion, collision, and contact sports)

Children with diabetes, asthma, and seizures should be evaluated to ensure they are taking their medicine properly. Diabetic athletes should monitor their blood glucose every 30 minutes during continuous exercise and 15 minutes after completion of the activity.

If a child is excluded for a health reason, and the parent wishes the child to participate, it is wise to get a written release from the parents and the child that signifies they are aware of the risks they take.

RISK FOR INJURY

Sports injuries have been separated into two main categories: macrotrauma, or a sudden acute trauma from a major collision with an unreliable playing surface, and microtrauma, which primarily comprise overuse injuries. Results of microtrauma are stress fractures, "shin splints," tendinitis, shoulder impingement, and epicondylitis. Sports most responsible for microtrauma include sports requiring endurance or a high level of limb repetition (e.g., distance running), sports with quick stop-start and jumping action (e.g., basketball), sports using a hard surface area, and sports involving repetitive single limb action (e.g., tennis/racket sports, skiing, swimming, baseball).

Contributing factors identified in sports-related injuries include:

- Inadequate preparticipation physical examination
- Hazardous surfaces in performance or practice areas
- Training and practice errors
- Lack of or improper safety equipment
- Inadequately trained coaches
- Performing while overly tired or injured
- Improper nutrition
- Limited awareness of possible risk or risk factors (Gottlieb, 1994)

CONTAGIOUS DISEASES

Athletes can contract a contagious disease in the locker room, during the sports event, and traveling to events as well as during their leisure time. The most common modes of transmission are person-to-person contact,

common source, and airborne or droplet. The following recommendations have been made for an athlete with a contagious disease.

Fever: The American Academy of Pediatrics has recommended that
athletes with fever not participate in sports.

Infectious mononucleosis: No participation in sports is
recommended until spleen returns to normal size. The athlete can
return to full participation gradually.

Human immunodeficiency virus (HIV): HIV-infected athletes may
play all sports. Routine testing of teammates is not suggested.

Impetigo/boils/furuncles: Infected athletes should not participate in
contact or water sports until lesions are healed. They should not
share equipment or towels.

Warts: The lesions should be treated. For wrestling, lesions must be
covered before participation, and the athlete must have been on
treatment for at least 3 days.

Tinea: Wrestlers are excluded from participation. The National
Collegiate Athletic Association guidelines for participation are 3
days of treatment for skin lesions and 2 weeks of treatment for
scalp lesions.

Prevention of the spread of contagious diseases among athletes is
imperative. The locker room, showers, and equipment such as mats
should be cleaned and disinfected regularly.

NUTRITION

Nutritional Needs

Athletes need increased protein, calcium, iron, and carbohydrates.
Athletes should be encouraged to eat a balanced diet with an increase in
protein-, iron-, and calcium-rich foods.

Protein: The recommended daily requirement for protein is 0.8
g/kg. The increase in daily requirements for endurance athletes is
1.2 to 1.4 g/kg and for resistance-trained athletes is 1.4 to 1.8
g/kg. Increasing dietary intake of protein should suffice.

Calcium: The recommended daily requirement for calcium is 1200
to 1500 mg for females age 11 to 24 years. Factors that are related
to calcium depletion include cigarette smoking, alcohol
consumption, increased intake of caffeine, and a high-phosphorus
diet. Daily ingestion of calcium carbonate antacid tablets is an
inexpensive means of calcium supplementation. Drugs for treating
osteoporosis, such as raloxifene, are not recommended because
they can cause harm to the fetus.

Iron: The recommended daily requirement for iron is 15 to 18 mg
in females age 11 to 24, 12 mg in males ages 11 to 18, and 10 mg

for males age 19 to 24. Supplementation should be used only in cases of "true" anemia. Increase in daily consumption of iron-rich foods is recommended.

Carbohydrates: Foods are more economical than the sports drinks and bars that are popular. Suggested foods are pastas, cereals, breads, fruits, vegetables, yogurt, and cookies.

Nutritional Supplements

Substances labeled as a nutritional supplement are not regulated by the Food and Drug Administration. The quality, quantity, and purity of the active substance are unknown. Although not recommended for the young athlete, nutritional supplements are taken to build body mass, to increase alertness, to reduce fatigue, and to lose weight.

Creatinine: Creatinine, a nitrogenous compound, is found naturally in meat and fish. This is a popular supplement, and users are found even in the sixth and seventh grades. The total recommended daily allowance is 2 g, but athletes often take three to four times the daily requirement. Usual dosages are 20 to 30 g per day divided into four doses for 5 days, then a maintenance dose of 2 to 3 g per day (0.3 g/kg). The supposed benefit of supplementation is in sports that require repetitive efforts. Caffeine inhibits uptake, whereas exercise and carbohydrates enhance the activity. Creatinine use is not recommended for anyone younger than age 18 years.

Anabolic steroids: Dehydroepiandrosterone (DHEA) and androstenedione ("andro") are the performance enhancers most requested by youth and may have some effect on muscle mass. The dose is 300 mg per day for 7 days. As hormones, they can produce gynecomastia in males, hirsutism in females, acne, labile moods (testosterone rage), and premature epiphyseal closure in physically immature athletes. Anabolic steroids put the athlete at risk for liver cancer and heart disease. An athlete tests positive at a drug screen. Athletes should not use this supplement.

Amino acids: Although athletes require greater intake of protein, there is little evidence that ingestion of protein or amino acid supplements results in improved performance.

Minerals: The only minerals that might need supplementation are calcium and iron. Athletes lose iron through sweat, feces, and urine. There is a "pseudoanemia" that is the result of a physiologic increase in plasma volume secondary to increased exercise. Endurance athletes seem to have an increased need for iron. Calcium deficiency can lead to osteoporosis and to an increase in stress fractures. This is especially true for girls who participate in gymnastics, figure skating, and equestrian events.

Carbohydrates: In many sports, athletes eat large amounts of carbohydrates before the athletic event ("carbo loading") and within 1 to 2 hours after the event. This is done to increase glycogen storage in the muscle and to replace what is lost during the exercise.

REFERENCES

American Academy of Pediatrics, Committee on Sports Medicine and Fitness: Intensive training and sports specialization in young athletes (RE 9906). Pediatrics 106:154, 2000.

American Academy of Pediatrics, Committee on Sports Medicine and Fitness: Medical conditions affecting sports participation (RE0046). Pediatrics 107:1205, 200l.

American Academy of Pediatrics, Committee on Sports Medicine and Fitness: Mitral valve prolapse and athletic participation in children and adolescents (RE9523). Pediatrics 95:789, 1995.

American Academy of Pediatrics, Committee on Sports Medicine and Fitness: Athletic participation by children and adolescents who have systemic hypertension (RE9715). Pediatrics 99:637, 1997.

American Academy of Pediatrics, Committee on Sports Medicine and Fitness: Risk of injury from baseball and softball in children (RE0032). Pediatrics 107:782, 2001.

American Academy of Pediatrics, Committee on Sports Medicine and Fitness: Injuries in youth soccer: A subject review (RE9934). Pediatrics 105:659, 2000.

American Academy of Pediatrics, Committee on Sports Medicine and Fitness: Strength training by children and adolescents (RE0048). Pediatrics 107:1470, 2001.

American Academy of Pediatrics, Committee on Sports Medicine and Fitness: Safety in youth ice hockey: The effects of body checking (RE9835). Pediatrics 105:657, 2000.

American Academy of Pediatrics, Committee on Sports Medicine and Fitness: Human immunodeficiency virus and other blood-borne viral pathogens in the athletic setting (RE9832). Pediatrics 104:1400, 1999.

American Academy of Pediatrics, Committee on Sports Medicine and Fitness and American Academy of Ophthalmology Committee on Eye Safety and Sports Ophthalmology: Protective eyewear for young athletes (RE9630). Pediatrics 98:311, 1996.

American Academy of Pediatrics, Committee on Sports Medicine and Fitness and Committee on School Health: Organized sports for children and preadolescents (RE0052). Pediatrics 107:1459, 2001.

American Academy of Pediatrics, Committee on Sports Medicine and Fitness and Committee on School Health: Physical fitness and activity in schools (RE9907). Pediatrics 105:1156, 2000.

Andrews, J: Making the most of the sports physical. Contemp Pediatr 3, 1997.

Berul, C: Cardiac evaluation of the young athlete. Pediatr Ann 29:162, 2000.

Faigenbaum, A, and Micheli, L: Preseason conditioning for the preadolescent athlete. Pediatr Ann 29:156, 2000.

Feinstein, R, and McCambridge, T: The preparticipation physical examination: A pediatrician's responsibility. Pediatr Ann 31:18, 2002.

Gomex, J: Sideline medical emergencies in the young athlete. Pediatr Ann 31:50, 2002.

Gottlieb, A: Cheerleaders are athletes too. Pediatr Nurs 20:630, 1994.

Halstead, M, and Bernhardt, D: Common infections in the young athlete. Pediatr Ann 31:42, 2002.

Johnson, W: Nutritional supplements and the young athlete: What you need to know. Contemp Pediatr 18:63, 2001.

Kurowski, K: The preparticipation athletic evaluation. Am Fam Physician 61:2683, 2000.

Marx, R, and Delaney, S: Sideline orthopedic emergencies in the young athlete. Pediatr Ann 31:60, 2002.

Metzel, J: Performance-enhancing drug use in the young athlete. Pediatr Ann 31:27, 2002.

Metzel, J: Caring for the young dancer (gymnast, figure skater). Contemp Pediatr 6:134, 1999.

O'Connor, F, et al: Exercise-related syncope in the young athlete: Reassurance, restriction, or referral? Am Fam Physician 60:2001, 1999.

Patel, D, and Gordon, R: Contagious diseases in athletes. Contemp Pediatr 9:138, 1999.

Patel, D, et al: Youth sports: More than sprains and strains. Contemp Pediatr 3:45, 2001.

Unit **2**
MANAGING
ILLNESS

Chapter 3

COMMON PRESENTING SYMPTOMS AND PROBLEMS

CONSTIPATION

SIGNAL SYMPTOMS ▶ frequency of stools less than normal for the individual chronic, hard, dry stools

Constipation	ICD-9 CM: 564

Description: Constipation, the delay or difficulty in defecation for 2 or more weeks, can be categorized into four types: organic (structural and disease-oriented), nonorganic (functional or retentive), dietary, and related to drug or cathartic abuse. Normal stool frequency per week for infants up to 1 year is 5 to 28; for toddlers, 4 to 21; and for children older than age 3 years, 3 to 14.

Etiology: See Table 3–1.

Occurrence: Common.

Age: Occurs in all age groups.

Ethnicity: Ethnicity is not significant.

Gender: More common in males than females.

Contributing factors: Psychological factors, such as holding in anger; toilet training techniques; diet; and diseases that complicate defecation, such as hypothyroidism and cerebral palsy.

Signs and symptoms: The child presents to the clinic with the complaint of no stools for a variable number of days, straining at stool, fecal soiling, and possibly blood-tinged stool. Investigate the child's usual bowel pattern and the changes noted that caused the office visit. Obtain a history of diet and medicines taken. Findings reveal a normal abdomen or one with mild distention. Abdominal palpation reveals a firm colonic

Table 3–1 Causes of Constipation

Organic	Nonorganic	Drug-Induced	Metabolic	Neuro-muscular
Anal stenosis	Lack of privacy at school	Narcotics	Dehydration	Absent abdominal muscle
Anal stricture	Anxiety caused by social events	Antidepressants	Celiac disease	Mytonic dystrophy
Hirschsprung's disease	Ability to ignore sensation of rectal fullness	Psychotropics	Hypothyroidism	Spinal cord lesion
Pseudo-obstruction	Dietary: lack of bulk, excessive milk intake, underfeeding, malnutrition	Iron supplements	Renal tubular acidosis	
Rectal abscess fissure	Sexual abuse	Theophylline	Cystic fibrosis	
Collagen vascular disease				

mass. Rectal examination reveals firm-to-hard stool in the rectum. Rectal and perineal examinations may reveal anal fissures, perianal abscesses, and diaper dermatitis, all of which may make it painful to pass stools (Fig. 3–1).

Diagnostic tests: None. If history and physical examination warrant further follow-up:

Test	Results Indicating Disorder	CPT Code
Radiographic studies: anteroposterior and lateral abdomen, KUB	May reveal retained stool or signs of obstruction	74000–74022 74400
Colonic manometry for intractable constipation (refer)	May reveal myotonic dystrophy	91020

KUB, kidney, ureter, and bladder.

Differential diagnosis:

A ganglionic megacolon (Hirschsprung's disease) causes small, ribbon-like stools; rectal examination reveals no stool in the rectum.

Intestinal obstruction is suggested when a child is experiencing bile-colored vomitus and severe abdominal pain.

Treatment: The goal of treatment is to empty the large intestine, establish regular bowel habits, and eliminate pain of passing hard stools (Table 3–2).

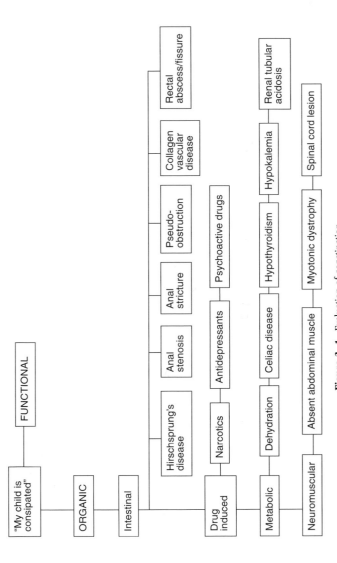

Figure 3–1. Evaluation of constipation.

Table 3–2   Treatment of Constipation

Nonpharmacologic	Pharmacologic
Dietary changes: increase fluids; increase bulk by adding fruits and vegetables (e.g., prune juice, tomatoes, olive oil, green vegetables) Manual removal of the impacted stool	Suppositories: Glycerin rectal suppositories Bisacodyl (Dulcolax) suppository, use 1 time, to facilitate the passage of stool Pediatric Fleet enema, use one time to help pass a hard stool and empty large intestine After through cleansing begin: stool softener (soft stool reduces or eliminates pain associated with bowel movements): Mineral oil, 15–30 mL by mouth. Not for children under 1 year of age. The best guide to adequacy is the appearance of oil seepage in underwear Polyethylene glycol 3350 (MiraLax) powder: 1/2 cap every other day for 2 weeks, then 1 or 2 times per week as needed

Clinical Pearl: Give mineral oil between meals to reduce interference in the absorption of fat-soluble vitamins.

Follow-up: If no bowel movement in 2 to 3 days, the child should return to the clinic for further evaluation.

Sequelae: Chronic stool retention with increasing reliance on laxatives; anal fissures and fistulas and urinary tract infections.

Prevention/prophylaxis: Changes in usual diet, increased fluid intake, and increased exercise are usually effective.

Referral: In cases of chronic constipation or fecal impaction, refer patient to the primary physician or psychiatrist.

Education: Have child, with proper foot support, sit on the commode for 5 minutes after the evening meal to assist in reestablishing regular bowel habits. Have parent keep a stooling diary and reward the child with "stars" on successful defecation. Teach parents what constitutes normal bowel habits. Teach parents how to make dietary changes and when to become concerned about changes in their child's bowel habits.

DIARRHEA

SIGNAL SYMPTOMS▶   passage of watery, loose stools

Diarrhea	ICD-9 CM: 787.91

Description: Diarrhea is an increase in the frequency, water content, and volume of feces that involves secretory, osmotic, and inflammatory processes. Usually more than eight stools occur in 24 hours, temperature is greater than 38°C, and abdominal pain is present. Causative agents may be viral, bacterial, chemical, or the condition may be concomitant with other conditions. Diarrhea may be accompanied by vomiting.

Etiology: See Table 3–3.

Table 3–3   Causes of Diarrhea

Hand-to-Mouth Contact	Common Drugs	Illnesses	Other
Rotavirus, echovirus, cocksackievirus, parvovirus; entertoxin strains of E. coli, cholera, Clostridium perfringens, Staphylococcus, Yersinia, nonenterotoxin Shigella, other strains of E. coli	Antibiotics	Otitis media	Neoplasms
Parasitic infections	Laxatives	Urinary tract infections	Aganglionic megacolon
	Stimulants		
		Pneumonia	

Occurrence: Common; by the age of 3 years, a child will have had one to three episodes.

Age: All age groups.

Ethnicity: Ethnicity is not significant.

Gender: Occurs equally in males and females.

Contributing factors: Environmental factors, such as exposure to others with the illness, especially in day care setting; poor hygienic measures, such as inadequate hand washing by caregivers.

Signs and symptoms: The child presents with a complaint of diarrhea. History includes a description of illness, including onset, amount, number, color, and frequency of stools; presence of blood or mucus in the stool; and presence of fever or vomiting. Fluid intake and urinary output are assessed. History of rash and other symptoms is investigated, as is history of exposure to similar illnesses (Fig. 3–2).

Findings may reveal generalized abdominal tenderness and hyperactive bowel sounds. Rebound tenderness indicates the possibility of appendicitis or peritonitis. If dehydrated, the child may be listless and lethargic, with dry mucous membranes, poor skin turgor, and weight loss (Table 3–4)

Diagnostic tests: None for diarrhea. Tests are ordered, if warranted, to determine the etiology of the diarrhea.

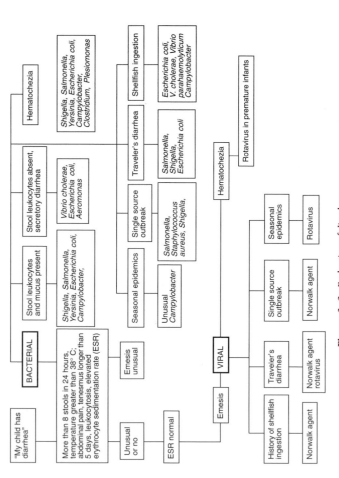

Figure 3–2. Evaluation of diarrhea.

Test	Results Indicating Disorder	CPT Code
Stool for occult blood	Blood in the stool	82270
Urinalysis with specific gravity	Dehydration	8100
White blood cells	Viral or bacterial infection	85048
Stools checked with Wright's stain	Presence of WBCs: *Shigella, Salmonella, Yersinia, Escherichia coli, Campylobacter*	87999
Stool for ova, cysts, and parasites	Indicative of parasitic infections	87177

Differential diagnosis:

Intussusception: There is a characteristic acute onset, right upper quadrant pain, and currant jelly–colored stools.

Appendicitis: In children, localized or point tenderness is diagnostically significant. Children with appendicitis often walk with a limp and lie with the right leg flexed; hyperextension of the right leg is painful (psoas sign).

Treatment: The goal is to restore and maintain fluid and electrolyte status.

Nonpharmacologic

First 12 hours: If an infant is breastfeeding, the mother should maintain infant at the breast and increase time at breast, but discontinue any supplemental feedings.

For older infants, parents should modify diet and formula and give small amounts of an oral rehydration solution (e.g., Pedialyte, Naturalyte, Rehydrolyte) in additiona to smaller amounts of formula. Parents should offer 4 to 8 ounces of oral rehydration solution for every loose or watery stool if child is not vomiting; otherwise, small amounts are given more frequently. Offer with teaspoon until child adapts to the slightly salty taste.

Table 3–4   Classification of Dehydration

Parameter	Mild	Moderate	Severe
Body weight	3–5%	8–10%	15–20%
Skin turgor	Normal to poor	Poor	Poor
Skin color	Normal	Pale	Pale
Mucus membrane	Normal	Dry	Parched
Pulse	Normal	Normal	Tachycardia
Blood pressure	Normal	Normal	Low
Perfusion	Normal	Normal	Circulatory collapse
Fontanel	Normal	Depressed	Severely depressed

Clinical Pearl: Do not give tea, juices, soft drinks, Kool-Aid, milk, or chicken broth, or plain water.

Some still introduce foods slowly with the BRAT diet (bananas, rice cereal, applesauce [not juice], and toast), then increase the number of foods in diet as tolerated. The BRAT diet is no longer considered appropriate because of the high sugar content, and the rice is not well tolerated by the intestine. Tea has no nutritional benefits. It is recommended, if no vomiting, to allow child his or her normal diet with the following restrictions: no ice cream or food high in fat or sodium content. Other suggested foods are starchy foods such as potatoes, breads, pastas, and noodles and cooked meats such as chicken. White grape juice may be given because it contains equal amounts of fructose and glucose and is well tolerated. Pear juice is also well tolerated.

Pharmacologic

Parents should increase child's fluid intake to rehydrate; if dehydration is severe, admit to the hospital for intravenous fluid replacement.

 Clinical Pearl: Antidiarrheal agents are usually unnecessary and can be dangerous in cases of inflammatory enteritis (shigellosis).

If diarrhea has a bacterial etiology, antibiotics specific for the organism may be given.

 Clinical Pearl: Do not treat *Salmonella* with antibiotics because they prolong the carrier state.

Treating shigellosis with antibiotics is usually indicated.

Follow-up: The child should return to the clinic if not improved in 48 hours, particularly if the child is younger than 3 years of age. Keep in contact with the caregiver by telephone.

Sequelae: Dehydration is a consideration. Milk intolerance may occur after recovery, probably as a result of secondary lactose intolerance.

Prevention/prophylaxis: Avoid overfeeding of infants. Maintain good hygienic measures, such as hand washing. Prepare and store foods properly.

Education: Instruct parents in recording fluid intake, the number and characteristics of the stools, and the frequency of urination. Instruct parent and child in good hand-washing techniques, and emphasize the importance of hand washing after diaper changing and defecation. Instruct parents to keep toileting and diaper changing areas separate from areas for food preparation. Clean floors and surfaces with a solution of quarter cup of household bleach in 1 gallon of water prepared daily and discarded after use to protect small children.

FEBRILE SEIZURES

SIGNAL SYMPTOMS abnormal muscle movements associated with a rapid onset of fever

Febrile Seizures	ICD-9 CM: 780.31

Description: Febrile seizures are generalized tonic-clonic episodes associated with high fevers; patients have little postictal confusion or weakness. Seizures usually last less than 15 minutes and occur once in a 24-hour period.

Etiology: Unknown, but the rapidity of onset of fever, 101°F or higher, appears to be related.

Occurrence: Febrile seizures occur in 3% to 4% of all children; 25% to 30% have a second occurrence, and less than 9% have more than three occurrences. Seizure recurrences occur within 6 to 12 months of the initial seizure.

Age: Onset typically occurs before age 3 years but may continue in children as old as 6 years.

Ethnicity: May be higher in African-Americans.

Gender: More common in males.

Contributing factors: Any underlying illness that increases body temperature.

Signs and symptoms: The child is brought to the clinic, and the parent reports that a seizure occurred when the child's temperature became elevated. The child has a history of a sudden increase in body temperature to greater than 101°F, onset of generalized tonic-clonic seizure activity, and loss of consciousness. The child had little or no postictal confusion (Fig. 3–3).

Diagnostic tests: None for the initial episode or repeated episodes when preceded by a fever and when the source of the fever is identified.

Test	Results Indicating Disorder	CPT codes
Spinal tap	Rule out meningitis	62270
Electroencephalography performed 2 weeks after seizure	Rule out seizure disorder	95816

Related episodes unrelated to fever require additional work-up for seizure disorder.

Differential diagnosis: Seizures due to epilepsy or a primary injury or disease of the central nervous system, such as head trauma or aneurysm. A description of the seizure may assist in the diagnosis: Complex seizures are focal, last longer than 15 minutes, and occur more than once in a 24-hour period.

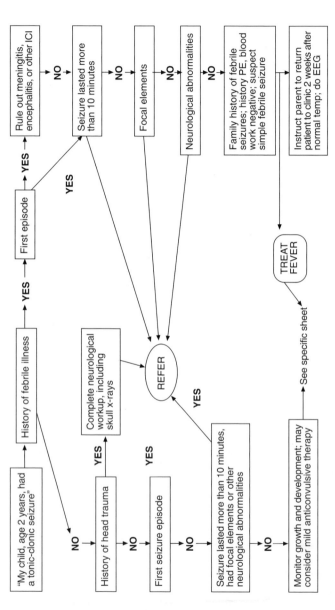

Figure 3–3. Febrile convulsions in young children. (EEG, electroencephalogram; ICI, intracranial infection; PE, physical examination.)

Table 3–5   Ibuprofen Suspension Dosages (100 mg/5 mL)

| Age | Weight | | Fever <102.5°F | Fever >102.5°F |
	lb	kg		
6–11 mo	13–17	6–7.9	1/4 tsp (25 mg)	1/2 tsp (50 mg)
12–23 mo	18–23	8–10.9	1/2 tsp (50 mg)	1 tsp (100 mg)
2–3 yr	24–35	11–15.9	3/4 tsp (75 mg)	$1^1/_2$ tsp (150 mg)
4–5 yr	36–47	16–21.9	1 tsp (100 mg)	2 tsp (200 mg)
6–8 yr	48–59	22–26.9	$1^1/_4$ tsp (125 mg)	$2^1/_2$ tsp (250 mg)
9–10 yr	60–71	27–31.9	$1^1/_2$ tsp (150 mg)	3 tsp (300 mg)
11–12 yr	72–95	32–43.9	2 tsp (200 mg)	4 tsp (400 mg)
Adult	96–154	44–70	2 tsp (200 mg)	4 tsp (400 mg)

Treatment: Acetaminophen or ibuprofen can reduce the fever. Further treatment depends on the underlying cause. See Tables 3–5 and 3–6 for dosing.

Clinical Pearl: It is not recommended to alternate antipyretics.

Follow-up: Have caregiver report any further seizures. Consider initiating anticonvulsant therapy if patient has more than three episodes, if the seizures last longer than 15 minutes, if there is a family history of nonfebrile seizures, or if neurologic abnormalities are present or persist.

Sequelae: A seizure episode that lasts for a long time may result in Todd's paralysis. The paralysis is transient (1 hour to 1 month) and affects one side and the extremities.

Prevention/prophylaxis: Children with a history of febrile seizures may be given diazepam rectal gel (Diastat), 0.5 mg/kg in children age 2 to 5 years and 0.3 mg/kg in children age 6 to 11 years, at the onset of a fever (one dose). Children should be treated with ibuprofen (Advil) or acetaminophen (Tylenol) appropriate for age.

Referral: For repeated episodes, consult with or refer patient to a primary care physician or neurologist for definitive diagnosis and treatment.

Education: Explain to caregivers that, although frightening, febrile seizures are usually self-limiting with little or no significant sequelae. Most children have only one episode.

FEVER

SIGNAL SYMPTOMS▶   increased body temperature

Fever	ICD-9 CM: 780.6.

Description: Fever is a rectal temperature greater than 38°C (100.4°F), oral temperature greater than 37.5°C (99.5°F), and axillary temperature greater than 37°C (98.6°F). The three categories of fever are as follows:

Table 3-6 Recommended Acetaminophen Dosages

Age	Weight (lb)	Weight (kg)	Suspension Drops and Original Drops (80 mg/0.8 mL) Dropperful [dpprl]	Chewable Tabs (80-mg tabs)	Suspension Liquid and Original Elixir (160 mg/5 mL)	Junior Strength (160-mg caps/chewables)	Regular Strength (325 mg) Caps/Tabs	Extra Strength Caps/Gelcaps (500 mg) 0–3 mo
0–3 mo	6–11	2.5–5.4	½ dppr (0.4 mL)					
4–11 mo	12–17	5.5–7.9	1 dppr (0.8 mL)					
12–23 mo	18–23	8.0–10.9	1½ dppr (1.2 mL)					
2–3 yr	24–35	11.0–15.9	2 dppr (1.6 mL)	2 tab	½ tsp			
4–5 yr	36–47	16.0–21.9		3 tab	¾ tsp			
6–8 yr	48–59	22.0–26.9		4 tab	1 tsp	2 cap/tab		
9–10 yr	60–71	27.0–31.9		5 tab	1½ tsp	2½ cap/tab		
11 yr	72–95	32.0–43.9		6 tab	2½ tsp	3 cap/tab		
Adults and Children ≥ 12 yr	96+	44.0+			3 tsp	4 cap/tab	1 or 2 caps/tabs	2 caps/gel

- Fever of short duration with localizing signs
- Fever without localizing signs and with a duration of less than 1 week
- Fever of unknown origin (FUO), with a duration of more than 14 days, that remains undiagnosed; in adolescents, FUO is a sustained fever lasting more than 21 days with 7 days' hospitalization that remains undiagnosed

Fever should be distinguished from hyperthermia, which is an abnormal rise in body temperature that is not due to a disease process (Figs. 3–4 and 3–5).

Etiology: The body's natural response to infection or certain disease processes.

Occurrence: Common.

Age: Any age group.

Ethnicity: Ethnicity is not significant.

Gender: Occurs equally in males and females.

Contributing factors: Contributing factors include the child's immune status (e.g., nonimmunized, immunosuppressed, diagnosed with sickle cell anemia) and environmental factors, such as enrollment in a day care center, history of family illness, presence of pets, and recent travel.

Signs and symptoms: The child presents with a history of fever, or the parent complains that the child feels hot. The history should include queries related to the immune system, immunization status, recent hospitalizations, environmental factors, and the presence of rashes.

Specific physical findings may or may not be present; they are not present in cases of nonspecific fever. The presence of rashes, organomegaly, painful joints, and murmurs may provide clues to diagnosis. Assess the level of illness. The Yale Observation Scale (Table 3–7) and the Rochester Criteria (Table 3–8) are useful for determining who can be treated as an outpatient.

Diagnostic tests:

Test	Results Indicating Disorder	CPT Code
Complete blood count with differential, peripheral smear	<15,000 cells/mm^3 and 10% bands	850014
Erythrocyte sedimentation rate	Elevated	85651
Urinalysis with culture (particularly for boys <6 mo and girls <2 yr)	Presence of pathogens	87088
Blood culture (takes 24–48 hr for results)	Presence of pathogens	87040
Spinal tap	Rule out meningitis	62270
Stool for blood and culture	White cells, enteric pathogens	82270/ 87045

(continued on the following page)

Test	Results Indicating Disorder	CPT Code
Radiograph of chest	Pneumonia	71020
Serum transaminase	Monitor liver function	84450/84460
Alkaline phosphatase		84075
Serologic tests: Venereal Disease Research Laboratory (VDRL)	Rule out syphilis	86592
Antinuclear antibodies, rheumatoid factor, and complement	Rule out collagen diseases	86038/86039, 86430, 86162

Differential diagnosis:

- Bacterial infections, leukemia, lymphoma, juvenile rheumatoid arthritis, and enteric fever
- "Fevers" reported by unreliable caretakers
- Elevations in body temperature owing to normal deviations, such as physical activity, ovulation, environmental heat, and excess clothing
- Temperature elevations resulting from diseases that increase heat production or cause defective heat loss or central nervous system diseases that affect the hypothalamus
- "Fevers" reported as a result of an incorrectly taken temperature or a thermometer that is unreliable

Treatment: Take immediate measures to reduce fever in the following cases:

- Child less than 2 to 3 months old
- Child is having an active seizure
- Temperature greater than 106°F to 107°F
- Child has altered mental status
- Child is immunocompromised
- Alteration in vital signs: hypotension or extremely fast pulse and respiratory rate
- Suspicion of non–interleukin-1 fever as a result of underlying central nervous system disease
- Fever is a result of burns or exposure

Tepid sponges reduce the temperature by 0.5°F to 1°F and may induce a rise as a result of the shivering.

 Clinical Pearls: Do not give alcohol sponge baths. Do not give aspirin. Give sponge baths in conjunction with antifever medications.

Initiate pharmacologic measures to reduce fever. Alcohol may cause the fever to decrease too rapidly; the use of aspirin has been linked to Reye's syndrome. Dosages for acetaminophen and ibuprofen are given in Tables 3–5 and 3–6.

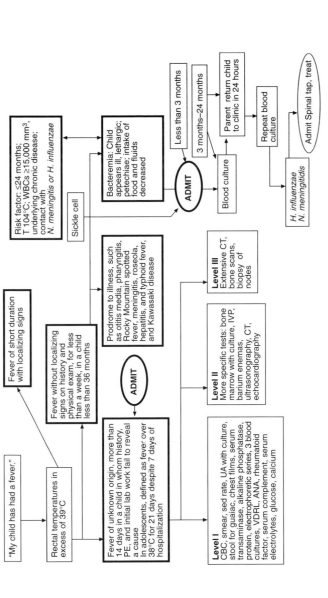

Figure 3–4. Evaluation of fever I. (ANA, antinuclear antibody; CBC, complete blood count; CT, computed tomography; IVP, intravenous pyelogram; PE, physical examination; T, temperature; UA, urinalysis.)

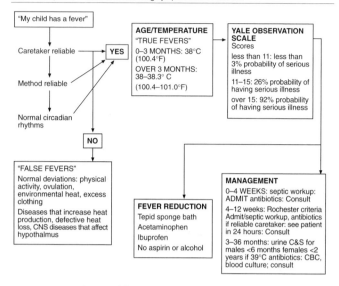

Figure 3–5. Evaluation of fever II. (C&S, culture and sensitivity.)

Table 3–7 Yale Observation Scale

Observation Item	1: Normal	2: Moderate Impairment	3: Severe Impairment
1. Quality of cry	Strong or none	Whimper or sob	Weak or moaning; has high-pitched, continuous cry or hardly responds
2. Reaction to parent stimulation	Cries briefly, or does not cry and is content	Cries off and on	Persistent cry with little response
3. State variation	If awake, stays awake; if asleep, awakens quickly	Eyes close briefly when awake or awakens with prolonged stimulation	No arousal and falls asleep
4. Color	Pink	Pale extremities or acrocyanosis	Pale, cyanotic, mottled, or ashen
5. Hydration	Skin and eyes normal; moist membranes	Skin and eyes normal and mouth slightly dry	Skin doughy or tented; dry mucous membranes and/or sunken eyes
6. Response to social overtures	Smiles or alert (consistently)	Brief smile or alert	No smile, anxious, dull; no alertness to social overtures

A total score of <11 signifies a <3% probability of serious illness
A total score of 11–15 signifies a 26% probability of serious illness
A total score of >15 signifies a >92% probability of serious illness
Reproduced with permission from *Pediatrics*, Vol. 70, page 804, Table 1, copyright 1982.

Table 3–8   Rochester Criteria

Previously healthy febrile infants <60 days of age are considered at low risk for serious bacterial infection if all of the following criteria are met:

1. Infant appears generally well and nontoxic
   Activity, hydration, and perfusion normal*

2. **Infant has been previously healthy:**
   Born at term (37 weeks' gestation)
   No antcnatal or perinatal antimicrobial therapy
   No treatment for unexplained hyperbilirubinemia
   Not hospitalized longer than mother
   Has not received and not currently receiving antimicrobial therapy
   No previous hospitalization
   No chronic or underlying illnesses

3. Infant has no evidence of skin, soft tissue, bone, joint, or ear infection on physical examination

4. **Infant meets the following laboratory parameters:**
   Peripheral white blood cell count of 5000–15,000 cells/mm^3 (5.0–15.0 $\times$ 10^9 L)
   Absolute band cell count of <1500 bands/mm^3
   <10 white blood cells per high-power field on microscopic examination of spun urine sediment† or gram-stained smear*
   <5 white blood cells per high-power field on microscopic examination of a stool smear (in infants with diarrhea)†

5. **Social situation:**
   Parents/caregiver mature and reliable
   Reliable transportation available
   Thermometer and telephone at child's home
   Travel time to care facility <30 minutes*

* Adapted from Baraff, L J, et al: Practice guidelines for the management of infants and children 0–36 months of age with fever without source. Pediatrics 92:1, 1993.

† From McCarthy et al: Predictive value of abnormal physical examination findings in ill appearing and well appearing febrile children. Pediatrics 76:167, 1985.

Management

   Infants aged 0 to 28 days: Order septic work-up and admit to hospital. Direct antibiotics at apparent focus; if none, give ampicillin and a third-generation cephalosporin.

   Infants aged 4 to 12 weeks: If Rochester criteria are met, order septic work-up and give ceftriaxone, 50 mg/kg intramuscularly, if spinal tap and blood culture were obtained; recheck in 12 to 24 hours (severe bacterial infection develops in only 1%).

   Toxic infants: If infant is toxic and fails Rochester criteria, order septic work-up, admit, and direct antibiotics at apparent focus; if none, give ampicillin and a third-generation cephalosporin pending culture results.

   Nontoxic child with temperature greater than 39.9°C (102.2°F): Order septic work-up, give empirical antibiotics, and instruct parents to return child to clinic in 24 hours.

Follow-up: Routine postinfection follow-up after the administration of antibiotics.

Sequelae: Depend on the underlying etiology and the appropriateness of the treatment; "false fevers" can be harmful if steps are not taken to recognize the basis of the "fever" and eliminate its cause (e.g., removing excess clothing).

Prevention/prophylaxis: Reduction of environmental risks and initiation and maintenance of appropriate immunization status.

Referral: Refer patient to pediatrician for admission in the following cases:

- Any infant younger than age 28 days
- Any child in whom the etiology cannot be determined
- Sickle cell anemia patients with fever
- Any level II or III evaluation

Education: When the child is sent home to be observed, instruct the parent or caregiver to assess the child every 4 hours for temperature, activity, and skin color. Have the parent call immediately if there are changes such as poor feeding, not taking fluids, little or no urinary output, the presence of a rash, cyanosis, jerky movements (including eye movements), bulging fontanels, and any difficulty in arousing or comforting. Teach parents the definition of fever and how to use and read a thermometer properly. Instruct parents in ways to reduce environmental factors and to avoid overreporting of false fevers. Provide for in-service education for day care center employees on the definition of fever and how to use and read a thermometer or other measurement device properly.

PAIN

SIGNAL SYMPTOMS▶   prime indicator of a traumatic event

| Pain | ICD-9 CM: 789.0 (with modifier) |

Description: Pain is the objective response to a traumatic event that occurs with varying degrees of severity.

Etiology: Trauma, infection, burns, lesions, and tumors.

Occurrence: Common.

Age: All age groups.

Ethnicity: Ethnicity is not significant.

Gender: Occurs equally in males and females.

Contributing factors: Individual responses to pain may be culturally determined, especially as related to appropriate gender responses. A person's pain threshold determines the reported severity of the pain as well as previous experience.

Signs and symptoms: Signs and symptoms may vary from stoicism to crying; from verbalization of the area of discomfort to guarding of the body part.

Diagnostic tests:

- Self-report (children aged ≥5 years old are considered reliable reporters) and physiologic changes, such as crying, changes in facial expression, and changes in observed behavior
- Changes in pulse rate, blood pressure, and skin color

Pain assessment tools include the following.

Simple descriptor scales: Severity rating is selected by words ranging from "very little" to "a whole lot." Words can be changed to fit the age of the child.

Numeric scales: Severity is rated using a scale from 0 to 10 or 100. The tool can be easily constructed using a ruler, using 1 inch per degree of severity of pain.

Visual analogue scales: Severity is rated on scale from 0 to 10. A rating of 10 is twice as severe as a rating of 5.

Color analogue scales: The colors used are either a gradation of one color or gradation of several colors, with the highest intensity of pain related to the most intense color. The clinician then matches this scale with a numerical scale.

Pain thermometer: Severity of pain is described by matching the perceived pain to the drawing of a thermometer.

Faces scales: Severity of pain is described by matching the perceived pain to the facial drawing that most matches the feeling.

Oucher: This is an adaptation of the Faces scale that allows children to select the photograph that most adequately describes the severity of pain.

Poker chip tool: The degree of severity is measured by the number of poker chips chosen from a group of 10.

Noncommunicating children's pain checklist: This is a checklist of behaviors for use by caregivers to assess pain in children that are unable to communicate verbally.

Pain observation pain tool for young children: This is a dichotomous pain scale of nine behavioral and physiologic categories for children 1 to 4 years old.

Neonatal Facial Coding System: This system uses facial grimaces, body movements, and reflex limb withdrawal and torso activity to assess response to pain.

Differential diagnosis: Assess the child for the degrees of fear and anxiety because these factors relate to the intensity of the pain.

Treatment: Specific pain management depends on the causative event. Refer to other chapters on each causal event. Table 3–9 lists recommended dosages of controlled substances (opiates) used to control pain.

Follow-up: Monitor the child to assess efficacy of treatment.

Sequelae: Unrelieved pain may result in increased anxiety, panic, or combativeness.

Table 3–9 Recommended Dosages for Selected Controlled Substances Used for Pain Management

| Drug | Persons Greater Than 50 kg Body Weight | | Persons Less Than 50 kg Body Weight (over age 6 months) | |
	Oral	Parenteral	Oral	Parenteral
Morphine	30 mg q 3–4 h	10 mg q 3–4 h	0.3 mg/kg q 3–4 h	0.1 mg/kg q 3–4 h
Codeine	60 mg q 3–4 h	60 mg q 2 h IM, SC	1 mg/kg q 3–4 h	Not recommended
Meperidine (Demerol)	Not recommended	100 mg q 3 h	Not recommended	0.75 mg/kg q 2–3 h
Hydrocodone (Lorcet, Lortab, Vicodan)	10 mg q 3–4 h	Not available	0.2 mg/kg q 3–4 h	Not available
Oxycodone (Percocet, Percodan, Tylox)	10 mg q 3–4 h	Not available	0.2 mg/kg q 3–4 h	Not available

Prevention/prophylaxis: Elicit from parent and child their expectations of the visit and a history of past painful experiences and the child's usual coping mechanisms.

Referral: Refer patient to a physician if it is necessary to administer opiates.

Education: Counsel parents to assist the child in approaching new experiences in a realistic manner and not to use scare tactics as related to health care provider visits, such as "Behave or they will give you a shot." Instruct parents in the proper administration of analgesics with a syringe or graduated dropper.

RASHES

SIGNAL SYMPTOMS lesions of the skin

Rashes	ICD-9CD (see specific diagnosis)

Etiology: Varied. May be primary or indicative of systemic diseases, such as allergies or childhood illnesses (Table 3–10).

Incidence: Common

Ethnicity: Note that areas of skin affected by hormones (genitalia, nipples, areolae) are darker in dark-skinned people compared with light-

Table 3–10   Categorizing Skin Lesions

Type	Description
Primary	
Macule	A flat hypopigmented or hyperpigmented lesion up to 1 cm in diameter, such as a freckle
Patch	A macule >1 cm in diameter
Papule	An elevated lesion up to 0.5 cm in diameter, such as an elevated nevus
Nodule	Large, elevated papule approximately 0.05–2 cm in diameter; may be in the epidermis, dermis, or subcutaneous tissue
Plaque	Elevated flat, circular lesions 0.3 cm or larger in diameter; it may have distinct edges or blend with the adjacent skin
Vesicle	Elevated lesion <0.3 cm in diameter, often transparent and filled with fluid
Pustule	A pus-filled vesicle that may indicate the presence of infection
Bulla	Large, translucent >0.3 cm in diameter, filled with fluid
Wheal	Firm, flat-topped, well-circumscribed elevation of skin from edema of the dermis
Secondary	
Scale	Dry, thin plaques of keratinized epidermal cells
Crust	Dried exudates on the surface of the skin
Lichenification	Shiny surface with exaggerated skin lines and induration from chronic rubbing of the skin

skinned people. Darker skinned groups include Native Americans, African-Americans, and Asians. Because these people have increased amounts of melanin, which protects the skin against ultraviolet rays, they have a lower incidence of skin cancer compared with whites.

Gender: Gender distribution often depends on specific diagnosis.

Age: All ages.

Contributing factors: Varied.

Signs and symptoms: Child presents with changes in skin.

Changes in Pigmentation

Butterfly distribution of face is suggestive of lupus erythematosus.

Absence of color in localized areas indicating decreased pigmentation is vitiligo.

Total absence of pigmentation is albinism.

Localized areas of skin color variation may indicate skin tumors (Table 3–11). Any skin tumor larger than 6 mm indicates malignant melanoma.

Pinkish yellow lesions are seen in pityriasis rosea and seborrheic dermatitis.

Dull red-silver lesions are seen in psoriasis.

Changes in Skin Texture

"Soft" indicates secondary hypothyroidism, hyperpituitarism, and eunuchoid states.

"Hard" indicates scleroderma, myxedema, and amyloidosis.

"Velvety" indicates Ehlers-Danlos syndrome.

Table 3–11   Skin Tumor Comparisons

Color	Texture	Probable Tumor Type
Normal	Corrugated	Warts
	Smooth	Cysts
	Irregular	Keloids
	Varied, flat, verrucoid, smooth	Nevi
Pink or red	Flat, rough, smooth	Hemangiomas
	Varied, flat, verrucoid, smooth	Nevi
Brown	Crumbly, "pasted on"	Seborrheic keratosis
	Varied, flat, verrucoid, smooth	Nevi
	Smooth, sharply marginated	Lentigines
	Indurated	Dermatofibromas
Tannish yellow	Hard	Xanthomas
	Plaques	Xanthelasmas
	Corrugated	Warts
	Irregular	Keloid
Dark blue or black	Crumbly, "pasted on"	Seborrheic keratosis
	Flat, rough, smooth	Hemangiomas
	Flat	Blue nevi
	Indurated	Dermatofibromas

Changes in Nails

Pallor of nail beds may indicate anemia.

Bluish discoloration (cyanosis) can indicate poor tissue oxygenation.

Clubbing often indicates cardiovascular problems or cystic fibrosis.

Pitting of nail beds may be seen in psoriasis.

Lines in the nail beds are often associated with renal or hepatic diseases.

Diagnostic tests: None.

Differential diagnosis: Pattern or distribution of lesions is an important clue to diagnosis (Fig. 3–6).

Treatment: See specific diagnosis.

Follow-up: See specific diagnosis.

Sequelae: See specific diagnosis.

Referral: See specific diagnosis.

Prevention/prophylaxis: See specific diagnosis.

Education: See specific diagnosis.

STRESS

SIGNAL SYMPTOMS a nonfunctional response to an event

Grief, brief	ICD-9 CM: 309.0
Grief, prolonged	ICD-9 CM: 309.1
Post-traumatic stress syndrome	ICD-9 CM 308.9

Description: Stress is a manifestation of forces that are being experienced by individuals that produce negative physical, psychosocial, and emotional changes.

Etiology: Any event that causes nonfunctional responses from the child.

Occurrence: Common.

Age: Usually children older than age 3 years.

Ethnicity: Not significant.

Gender: Occurs in males and females.

Contributing factors: May be due to natural causes (hurricanes, tornadoes), accidents (falls from bicycles, auto accidents), family events (separation, divorce, death in family, exposure to violence), or chronic illness.

Signs and symptoms: Wide range of somatic complaints; increased irritability or anger; reliving the event through play or dreams; regressive behavior such as thumb sucking, whining, or clinging. Symptoms may not occur until months after the event.

Diagnostic tests: None.

Differential diagnosis: Evaluate the somatic complaints.

Treatment: Treatment is age dependent.

Younger than age 3: Talk with the child; assure them of their safety.

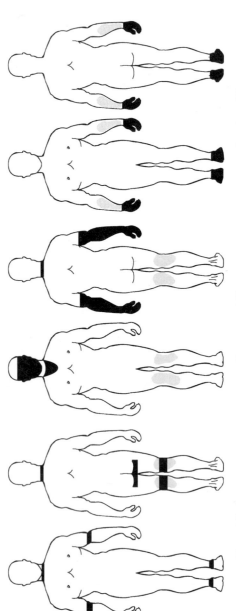

Flexural Rashes

Atopic dematitis (childhood)
Infantile seborrheic dermatitis
Vertrigo
Candidiasis
Tinea cruris
Epidermalytic hyperkeratosis (ichtyosis)
Inverse psoriasis

A

Sun-exposed Sites

Phototoxic reaction (sunburn)
Photocontact dermatitis
Lupus erythematosus
Polymorphous light eruption
Viral exanthem
Parphyria
Xeroderma pigmentosum

B

Acrodermatitis

Papular acrodermatitis (viral exanthem)
Acrodermatitis enteropathica
Atopic dermatitis (infantile)
Tinea pedis with "id" reaction
Dyshidrotic eczema
Poststreptococcal desquamation

C

Figure 3–6. Pattern diagnosis. (*A*) Flexural rashes. (*B*) Sun-exposed sites. (*C*) Acrodermatitis.

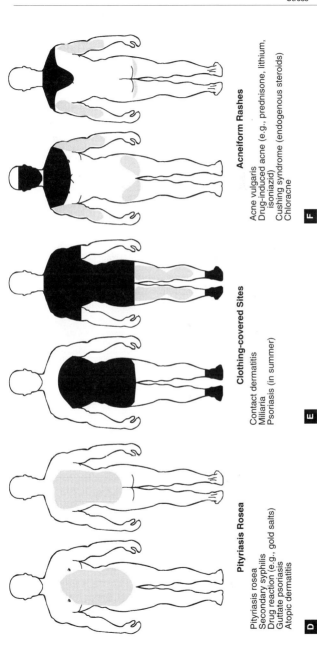

Pityriasis Rosea

Pityriasis rosea
Secondary syphilis
Drug reaction (e.g., gold salts)
Guttate psoriasis
Atopic dermatitis

D

Clothing-covered Sites

Contact dermatitis
Miliaria
Psoriasis (in summer)

E

Acneiform Rashes

Acne vulgaris
Drug-induced acne (e.g., prednisone, lithium, isoniazid)
Cushing syndrome (endogenous steroids)
Chloracne

F

Figure 3–6. (cont'd.) (*D*) Pityriasis rosea. (*E*) Clothing-covered sites. (*F*) Acneiform rashes. (Reprinted from Atlas of Pediatric Physical Diagnosis, Davis, B and Zittelli, B (eds.) p 213. Mosby-Year Book, St. Louis, copyright 1997, with permission from Elsevier.)

4–5 years of age: Talk with child; assure them of their safety. In cases of family events, the children often blame themselves for the loss or absence of the parent or loved one; reassure the child that they did not cause the event. Drawings by children often assist in diagnosis and treatment.

School-age child: This age group is capable of expressing their concerns and of expressing sadness. Counseling with the child and family is most helpful.

Adolescent: This age group often masks their true feelings under the cover of bravado or anger. Assist adolescents to express themselves and their feelings about the event.

All age groups may benefit from reading selected books with parents as a means of assisting in dealing with the problem. Selected books by age and topic are listed in the references.

Follow-up: May be as often as weekly until the health care provider believes the problem has been resolved.

Sequelae: Withdrawal, clinical depression, and suicide.

Prevention/prophylaxis: None.

Referral: Refer to mental health professional or to pastoral counseling if no progress or if the health care provider is not comfortable working with child and family.

Education: Educate families in what they may expect from their children in cases of traumatic events.

VOMITING

SIGNAL SYMPTOMS▶   forceful ejection of gastric contents

Vomiting	ICD-9 CM: 787.03

Description: Vomiting is a common symptom of many disease processes, gastrointestinal and nongastrointestinal, described as the forceful ejection of gastric contents often preceded by nausea. Vomiting is differentiated from regurgitation, which is a passive ejection of gastric contents caused by reflux.

Etiology: Caused by the coordination of gastric atony, relaxation of the gastroesophageal junction, and increased abdominal pressure; mediated by the medullary emesis center in the floor of the fourth ventricle and influenced by visceral afferent and chemoreceptive trigger zone stimuli. Less common causes are ear infections, brain tumor, hepatitis, and increased intracranial pressure.

Occurrence: Common.

Age: Any age.

Ethnicity: Ethnicity is not significant.

Gender: Occurs equally in males and females.

Contributing factors: Various stimuli, including drugs and motion, affect the emesis center.

Signs and symptoms: The child presents with a history of nausea, retching, and forceful ejection of gastric contents. Assessment of the child with vomiting includes a history of time (i.e., since last feeding and number of times vomited); character of vomiting (forceful, projectile); description of the vomitus (color and amount); and other associated symptoms, such as abdominal pain, fever, and headache (Fig. 3–7).

On palpation, there may be epigastric tenderness; auscultation may reveal increased bowel sounds. Nausea is assumed to be present in infants if after vomiting they do not want to feed but do drool. Obtain an accurate weight.

Diagnostic tests:

Test	Results Indicating Disorder	CPT Code
Complete blood count	Indicating viral or bacterial	85007
Urinalysis	Urinary tract infection or dehydration	81000
Blood urea nitrogen	Acidosis	84520
Sodium, calcium, magnesium	Metabolic disorders	84295/82310/83735
Amylase screen	Rule out pancreatitis	82150
Erythrocyte sedimentation rate	Presence of inflammatory bowel disease	85651

Differential diagnosis: Regurgitation differs from vomiting because there is no associated nausea or retching (Tables 3–12 and 3–13).

Treatment: Goal is to treat underlying etiology and to restore hydration.

Nonpharmacologic

No solid foods: only clear liquids for 24 hours. Use an oral rehydration solution, such as Pedialyte.

Pharmacologic

Promethazine (Phenergan) suppositories, 12.5 mg, 1/2 to 1 suppository every 6 hours for vomiting. Give intravenous fluid replacement if child is severely dehydrated.

Follow-up: Follow-up in the first 24 hours and again in 72 hours to evaluate progress.

Sequelae: Child may become dehydrated, depending on the underlying etiology.

Prevention/prophylaxis: None.

Referral: Consult with or refer patient to a primary physician in case of dehydration or suspicion of a complex underlying disorder. Refer to a surgeon if appendicitis is suspected.

Education: Reassure parents that most cases are self-limiting and that vomiting is a symptom, not a disease.

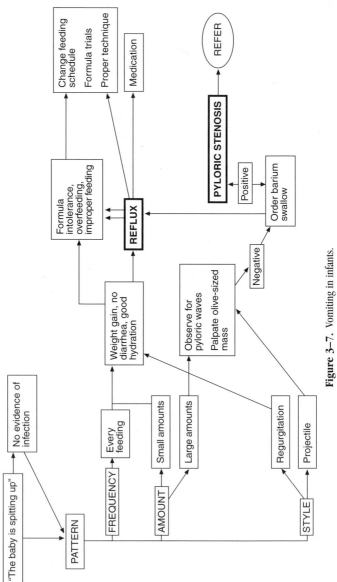

Figure 3–7. Vomiting in infants.

Table 3–12   Diagnostic Signs in Vomiting

Color	Quality	Suspect
Gastric contents	Passive	Reflux
	Forceful	Overfeeding
		CNS lesions
		Peptic ulcer
		Chronic UTIs
		Chronic otitis
	Projectile	Pyloric stenosis
Bile-colored		Obstruction
		Gastroenteritis
Mucus/blood		Intussusception
		Toxic colitis

CNS, central nervous system; UTIs, urinary tract infections.

Table 3–13   Common Age-Specific Causes of Vomiting

Disease or Symptom	Infancy Cause
Volvulus intussuception	Congenital malformations
Gastroenteritis	Bacterial or viral infection
Formula intolerance	Milk-protein intolerance
Overfeeding	Not true vomiting
Reflux	Not true vomiting

Disease or Symptom	Children/Adolescents Cause
Gastroenteritis	Bacterial or viral infection
Systemic diseases	Inflammatory bowel disease, ulcers, appendicitis
Signs of toxic ingestion	Ingestion of poisons, drugs, medications
Abdominal pain	Appendicitis
Bulimia	Self-induced vomiting immediately after meal

Less common causes of vomiting: ear infections, brain tumor, hepatitis, and increased intracranial pressure

REFERENCES

Constipation

Bishop, W: Miracle laxative? J Pediatr Gastroenterol Nutr 32:514, 2001.

Constipation in infants and children: Evaluation and treatment. J Pediatr Gastroentrol Nutr 29:12, 1999.

DiLorenzo, C: Childhood constipation: Finally some hard data about hard stools. J Pediatr 136:42, 2000.

DiPalma, J, Gremse, D: Chronic constipation in children: Rational management. Consult for Pediatricians 2(4):151,2003.

Felt, B, et al: Guideline for the management of pediatric idiopathic constipation and soiling. Arch Pediatr Adolesc Med 153:380, 1999.

Gold, DM, et al: Frequency of digital rectal examination in children with chronic constipation. Arch Pediatr Adolesc Med 153:377, 1999.

Nurko, S, et al: Managing constipation: Evidence put into practice. Contemp Pediatr 12:56, 2001.

Pashankar, D, and Bishop, W: Efficacy and optimal dose of daily polyethylene glycol 3350 for treatment of constipation and encopresis in children. J Pediatr 139:428, 2001.

Patel, H, et al: Predictive factors for short-term symptom persistence in children after emergency department evaluation for constipation. Arch Pediatr Adolesc Med 154:1204, 2000.

Van Ginkel, R, et al: Lack of benefit of laxatives as adjunctive therapy for functional nonretentive fecal soiling in children. J Pediatr 137:808, 2000.

Diarrhea

American Academy of Pediatrics, Committee on Nutrition: The use and misuse of fruit juice in pediatrics (RE0047). Pediatrics 107:1210, 2001.

Duggan, C, et al: Oral rehydration solution for acute diarrhea prevents subsequent unscheduled follow-up visits. Pediatrics 104:e29, 1999.

Kleiman, R, et al: Infant diarrhea: Management and comfort. J Pediatr Nutr Dev 91:16, 2000.

Lasche, J, and Duggan, C. Managing acute diarrhea: What every pediatrician needs to know. Contemp Pediatr 74, 1999.

Lifschitz, C. Carbohydrate absorption form fruit juices in infants. Pediatrics 105: e4, 2000.

Oral rehydration therapy for acute diarrhea. In Kleinman, R (ed): American Academy of Pediatrics: Pediatric Nutrition Handbook, 4th ed. American Academy of Pediatrics, Elk Grove, Ill., 1998, p 351.

Ribeiro, H, et al: Incomplete carbohydrate absorption from fruit juice consumption after acute diarrhea. J Pediatr 139:325, 2001.

Febrile Seizures

American Academy of Pediatrics Committee on Quality Improvement, Subcommittee on Febrile Seizures: Practice parameter: Long term treatment of the child with simple febrile seizures (AC9859). Pediatrics 103:1307, 1999.

American Academy of Pediatrics Provisional Committee on Quality Improvement, Subcommittee on Febrile Seizures: The neurodiagnostic evaluation of the child with a first simple febrile seizure. Pediatrics 97:769, 1996.

Fever

Bachur, R, et al: Occult pneumonias: Empiric chest radiographs in febrile children with leukocytosis. Ann Emerg Med 33:166, 1999.

Baker, MD, and Bell LM: Unpredictability of serious bacterial illness in febrile infants from birth to one month of age. Arch Pediatr Adolesc Med 153:5508, 1999.

Brower, J, and Powell, K: Unexplained fever in infants and young children: When is it serious? Consultant April 15:693, 2001.

Finkelstein, J: Fever in pediatric primary care: Occurrence, management, and outcomes. Pediatrics 105:260, 2000.

First, L, and Rideout, M: Fever: Measuring and managing a sizzling symptom. Contemp Pediatr 5:42, 2001.

Herr, S, et al: Enhanced urinalysis improves identification of febrile infants ages 60 days and younger at low risk for serious bacterial illness. Pediatrics 108:866, 2001.

Huffman, G: Alternating antipyretics: Is this an alternative? Pediatrics 105:1009, 2000.

Park, J: Fever without source in children: Recommendations for outpatient care in those up to 3. Postgrad Med 107:259, 2000.

Prober, C: No golden rules for managing fever in infants. Patient Care Jan 15:69, 2000.

Pain

American Academy of Pediatrics Committee on Psychosocial Aspects of Child and Family Health, Task Force on Pain in Infants, Children, and Adolescents: The assessment and management of acute pain infants, children, and adolescents. Pediatrics 108:793, 2001.

Bieri, D, et al: The Faces Pain Scale for the self-assessment of the severity of pain experienced by children: Development, initial validation, and preliminary investigation for ratio scale properties. Pain 41:139, 1990.

Breau, L, et al: Measuring pain accurately in children with cognitive impairments: Refinement of a caregiver scale. J Pediatr 138:721, 2000.

Buchholz, M, et al: Pain scores in infants: A modified infant pain scale vs. visual analogue. J Pain Symptom Manage 15:117, 1998.

Hicks, CL, et al: The Faces Pain Scale–Revised: Toward a common metric in pediatric pain measurement. Pain 93:173, 2001.

Lynn, A, et al: Pain control in very young infants: An update. Contemp Pediatr 11:39, 1999.

McGrath, PA, et al. A new analogue scale for assessing children's pain: An initial validation study. Pain 64:435, 1996.

McGrath, PA, et al: A survey of children's acute, recurrent, and chronic pain: Validation of the pain experience interview. Pain 87:59, 2000.

Rashes

Corder, R, and Weston, W: Atypical viral exanthems: New rashes and variations on old themes. Contemp Pediatr 2:11, 2002.

Gali, F, et al: Location, location, location! Contemp Pediatr August, 1998.

Pride, H: When a rash is more than a rash: Skin signs of systemic disease. Contemp Pediatr 11:104, 2000.

Stress

American Academy of Child and Adolescent Psychiatry: Children and grief. Fact Sheet for Families #8, 1998.

American Academy of Child and Adolescent Psychiatry: Helping children after a disaster. Fact Sheet for Families #36, 2000.

American Academy of Child and Adolescent Psychiatry: Helping teenagers with stress. Fact Sheet for Families #66, 1999.

American Academy of Child and Adolescent Psychiatry: Posttraumatic stress disorder (PTSD). Fact Sheet for Families, #70, 1997.

American Academy of Pediatrics: Pediatrician's role in helping children and families deal with separation and divorce (RE9419). Pediatrics 94:119, 1994.

American Academy of Pediatrics Committee on Environmental Health and Committee on Infectious Disease: Chemical-biological terrorism and its impact on children: A subject review (RE9959). Pediatrics 105:662, 2000.

American Academy of Pediatrics, Committee on Psychosocial Aspects of Child and Family Health: How pediatricians can respond to the psychosocial implications of disasters (RE9813). Pediatrics 103:521, 1999.

American Academy of Pediatrics Committee on Psychosocial Aspects of Child and Family Health: The pediatrician and childhood bereavement (RE9917). Pediatrics 105:445, 2000.

Hurt, H, et al: Exposure to violence: Psychological and academic correlates in child witnesses. Arch Pediatr Adolesc Med 155:1351, 2001.

Olness, K. How humanitarian disasters affect children. Contemp Pediatr 4:79, 2000.

Rivlin, D: Books for children whose pet has died. Contemp Pediatr 4:179, 2000.

Rivlin, D: Books for children when a friend dies. Contemp Pediatr10:134, 2001.

Rivlin, D: Books for children whose parents are divorced. Contemp Pediatr 9:134, 1999.

Rivlin, D: Books for children with chronic illness. Contemp Pediatr 9:134, 1999.

Rivlin, D: Stories for children who have lost a parent. Contemp Pediatr 8:169, 1998.

Sammons, W, and Lewis, J: Helping children survive divorce. Contemp Pediatr 3:103, 2001.

Stein, M: The use of family drawings by children in pediatric practice. J Dev Behav Pediatr 4, 2001.

Tellerman, K, et al: When a parent dies. Contemp Pediatr 9, 1998.

Vernema, T, and Schroeder-Bruce, K: The aftermath of violence: Children, disaster, and post-traumatic stress disorder. J Pediatr Health Care 16:235, 2002.

Vomiting

Acker, M: Vomiting in children: A comprehensive review. ADVANCE for NP 10:59, 2002.

Kimura, K, and Loening-Baucke, V: Bilious vomiting in the newborn: Rapid diagnosis of intestinal obstruction. Am Fam Physician 6:2791, 2000.

Murray, K, and Christie, D: Vomiting in infancy: When should you worry. Contemp Pediatr 9:81, 2000.

Chapter 4

SKIN DISORDERS

ABSCESS

SIGNAL SYMPTOMS▶   pus-filled red nodule at wound site

Abscess	ICD–9 CM: 682 (use additional codes to identify site and organism)
Furuncles/Carbuncles	ICD-9-CM: 680.9
Hidradenitis suppurative (apocrine glands)	ICD-9-CM: 705.83
Paronychia (nailbeds)	ICD-9-CM: 681.9

Description: An abscess is a firm, tender, erythematous pus-filled nodule in the dermis; it is usually self-limiting with effective treatment. Furuncles (boils) develop around hair follicles; carbuncles are a cluster of furuncles.

Etiology: The entrance of bacteria into a superficial skin wound as a result of laceration or puncture wound of a pathogen, usually *Staphylococcus aureus*.

Occurrence: Furuncles are more common in males and in children with diabetes, malnutrition, or human immunodeficiency virus (HIV). Apocrine gland lesions are more common in females (3:1).

Age: Occurs at any age.

Ethnicity: Apocrine gland involvement is more common in African-Americans.

Gender: Occurs in males and females.

Contributing factors: Any alteration in the integrity of the skin, such as soft tissue trauma or insect bite, and conditions such as malnutrition and immune system deficiencies.

Signs and symptoms: Patient may give a history of superficial skin trauma and may have a fever. Examination of the lesion reveals swelling, erythema, and a fluctuant mass with or without drainage. Pain is increased if lesion is present in area where skin is taut.

Diagnostic tests:

Test	Results Indicating Disorder	CPT Code
Culture of abscess	Identifies organism	87070

Differential diagnosis: Abscesses are rarely confused with other entities.

Treatment:

Furuncles/Carbuncles

Nonpharmacologic
- Warm moist compresses facilitate drainage; large lesions may require surgical incision and drainage

Pharmacologic
- Erythromycin or dicloxacillin, 30 to 50 mg/kg per day in divided doses for 1 week
- Cefadroxil, 30 mg/kg twice a day for 10 days

Hidradenitis Suppurativa (Apocrine Glands)

Nonpharmacologic
- Avoidance of tight-fitting clothes because these tend to exacerbate the condition

Pharmacologic
- Antibiotics chosen on basis of culture and sensitivity

Paronychia (Nail Beds)

Nonpharmacologic
- Warm moist compresses facilitate drainage; large lesions may require incision and drainage

Pharmacologic
- Amoxicillin plus clavulanic acid preferred for empirical treatment
- Dicloxacillin preferred if organism is known to be *S. aureus.*

Follow-up: Return to clinic for evaluation of treatment efficacy in 7 days.
Sequelae: If not treated promptly and appropriately, bacteremia may occur.
Prevention/prophylaxis: Keep fingernails short and avoid scratching sites of insect bites and other minor trauma. Practice good hand-washing techniques.
Referral: Refer when child has recurrent abscesses, severe infection with *S. aureus* or *Candida albicans,* or an infection caused by an organism not usually associated with abscesses.

Education: Instruct parents in hygienic measures, such as keeping fingernails short and avoiding scratching lesions, and in the ways of keeping cross-contamination at a minimum.

ACNE

variety of coexisting skin lesions primarily on face and shoulders of adolescents

Acne	ICD-9 CM: 706.
Cystic Acne	ICD-9 CM: 706.1

Description: Acne is a disorder of the pilosebaceous follicles. Lesions present as:

- Closed comedones (whiteheads)—follicular openings are small and contents trapped
- Open comedones (blackheads)—follicular openings are filled with keratin and lipids and contents are easily extruded
- Papules, pustules—form when closed comedones rupture
- Cysts—an intense nodular inflammatory process, may yield deep, pitted scars

Acne is classified as:

- Grade I: Presence of closed and open comedones
- Grade II: Presence of erythematous papules
- Grade III: Presence of papules and pustules
- Grade IV: Presence of cysts

Etiology: Increase in the sebaceous glands owing to androgen stimulation, blockage of the follicular canal, and growth of the skin bacterium *Propionibacterium acnes*.

Occurrence: Common.

Age: Neonatal acne, as a response to maternal androgen, appears at ages 2 to 4 weeks and subsides by ages 4 to 6 months. Acne vulgaris eruptions begin in preadolescence (50% of boys, ages 9–11); 85% of adolescents have the lesions. Peak incidence occurs at ages 16 to 19 for males and 14 to 17 for females.

Ethnicity: Not significant.

Gender: Occurs in males more frequently, but the lesions are more persistent in females.

Contributing factors: Increase in sebaceous gland stimulation as a result of hormonal changes (female exacerbations increase at time of menses). There may be a seasonal variation noted, with worsening during the winter and improvement during the summer. Tension, fatigue, and individual foods may trigger an acne flare-up. Washing and drying the skin roughly and squeezing and picking at the lesions irritate the skin and promote an inflammatory reaction. Medications such as cortiocosteroids and lithium may contribute to appearance of skin lesions.

Signs and symptoms: The child presents with a history of skin lesions on the face, neck, chest, upper back, and shoulders, which have been increasing in number. The child usually gives a history of trying over-the-counter (OTC) preparations without any benefit.

Inspection reveals mild-to-severe skin lesions present as noninflamed comedones, inflammatory papules, pustules, nodules, and cysts, which may exist concomitantly.

Diagnostic tests: None.

For females with cystic acne who are being considered for treatment with isotretinoin (Accutane), the following blood tests should be done before initiating treatment.

Test	Results Indicating Disorder	CPT Code
CBC		85007
High- and low-density lipoproteins	If level is 350 mg/dL, repeat in 2 weeks, and discontinue if levels are >700 mg/dL	83716/83721
Liver enzymes	If become elevated, reduce dosage by 50% or discontinue	80076
Pregnancy test	Positive: not recommended for pregnant women	84702

CBC, complete blood count.

 Clinical pearl: If treatment with isotretinoin is initiated, pregnancy test results should be obtained monthly. Treatment should be initiated only by a physician.

If abscess formation occurs, a culture of drainage from lesions may be done.

Differential diagnosis:

Flat warts of the face may be confused with the comedones, but the warts are small, flesh-colored, flat-topped papules with a finely textured surface.

Bacterial folliculitis, the presence of visible hairs in the pustules, is noted. If cultured, *S. aureus* is present.

Rosacea occurs in middle-aged, fair-skinned persons. Does not present with comedones.

Treatment:

Grade I

Nonpharmacologic

The patient should use only gentle facial soap, such as Dove or Neutrogena, and pat—not rub—the skin dry.

Pharmacologic

For patients with oily skins, gels, solutions, and lotions are the best vehicles; for dry skin, creams and lotions are best. Gels and lotions may cause a burning-type sensation.

> Topical benzoyl peroxide gel (5%, 10%) should be applied to the entire face every morning (may increase to twice-daily application if tolerated). Usually treatment is begun with the 5% gel; benzoyl peroxide may cause skin irritation that disappears after the first 2 weeks of use.

> Topical tretinoin (Retin-A), 0.025%, 0.05%, and 0.1% cream or 0.01% and 0.025% gel, is applied nightly a half hour after cleansing skin. Tretinoin may cause skin irritation that disappears after the first 2 weeks of use. If there is no response after 6 weeks, the concentration should be increased to 0.25% of the gel or 0.05% to 0.1% of the cream. Improvement should be evident in 5 to 6 weeks.

Azelaic acid cream (Azelex), 20% cream, is applied twice a day.

 Clinical Pearl: Irritation is increased with sun exposure; apply only at bedtime. This is a pregnancy category C drug.

 Clinical Pearl: Decreases pigmentation, so use with caution in patients with darker complexions.

> α-Hydroxy acids have been added to OTC preparations such as Oil-of Olay, Ponds, and Neutrogena. These may be used as a daily cleanser or moisturizer.

Grade II

Treatment is begun in accordance with the above-outlined regimen. If there is no response to the benzoyl peroxide and topical tretinoin or the medication causes significant irritation, a topical antibiotic solution should be substituted for the benzoyl peroxide.

- Clindamycin 1% gel, once a day
- Erythromycin 2% gel or solution, twice a day
- Sodium sulfacetamide, 10% lotion, once or twice a day

Topical and oral antibiotics usually are not combined.

Grade III

Benzol peroxide and topical antibiotic are used. If these are unsatisfactory, consider course of oral antibiotics.

- Tetracycline, 500 mg twice a day for 1 to 2 months; maintenance dose 250 to 500 mg daily. If no response, a trial of erythromycin, 250 to 300 mg twice a day

- Minocycline, initially 4 mg/kg twice daily, then 2 mg/kg twice daily as a maintenance dose
- Doxycycline, 100 mg twice a day, maintenance dose 50 to 100 mg daily

Grade IV

Oral antibiotics are used alone and combined with benzoyl peroxide. If results are unsatisfactory, consider isotretinoin, 0.5 to 1 mg/kg, twice a day, orally for 4 months (initiated by physician only). A Patient Information and Consent to Treatment form is recommended.

Follow-up: After initiating therapy, evaluate response at 2 weeks, 1 month, then every 2 months.

Sequelae: In severe cases, scarring may occur.

Prevention/prophylaxis:

Adolescents should avoid oil-based cosmetics and face creams, oily hair products, and hair spray.

Avoid use of harsh soaps and vigorous scrubbing of face.

Keep hair off the forehead (i.e., no bangs), hands off face, and shampoo frequently.

Avoid tanning beds.

Referral: In cases of severe acne and for recommendation or consideration for the use of isotretinoin, refer to a physician.

Education: The adolescent should be instructed to eat a balanced diet; not to restrict diet, unless he or she notices that certain foods seem to make the problem worse; to use water-based cosmetics sparingly; not to pick at the lesions; and to have patience because improvement does not occur overnight. Patients who use tretinoin and isotretinoin may experience redness, peeling, and itching for several weeks as the skin adjusts to the medication. Females taking antibiotics need to be aware of the risk of vaginal candidiasis. Oral antibiotics may interfere with oral contraceptives, requiring additional precautions. Patients taking tretinoin or tetracycline should be instructed to avoid excessive skin exposure, particularly during the hours of 10 AM and 2 PM.

ALOPECIA

SIGNAL SYMPTOMS hair loss in excess of normal breakage

Alopecia	ICD-9 CM: 704

Description: Alopecia describes the loss of hair, partial or complete, usually from the scalp, but the condition may affect other areas of the body. The term does not include the loss of hair because of breakage. Normal hair growth progresses in two cycles: the anagen cycle, or growth phase, and the telogen cycle, or resting phase (20% of hair follicles are in this stage). Normal loss of hair during the telogen phase is 50 hairs per day. The forms of alopecia include:

- Androgenetic alopecia (male pattern baldness)
- Alopecia areata (noncicatricial alopecia)
- Alopecia universalis (loss of all body hair)
- Follicular mucinosis or alopecia mucinosa (unknown cause; benign eruptions of lesions on face or scalp)
- Telogen effluvium (diffuse hair loss)
- Trichotillomania (compulsive, subconscious manipulation of the hair)
- Traction alopecia (owing to hairstyle)
- Toxic alopecia (a result of ingestion of certain medications or exposure to radiation or chemotherapeutic agents)

Alopecia is classified further as scarring or nonscarring. Nonscarring alopecias are reversible, whereas scarring alopecias result in permanent hair loss.

Etiology: The specific mechanism cannot always be determined but may be a result of intrinsic factors in growth or an indication of an underlying disorder (Fig. 4–1). Genetic links to HLA class II alleles (DQB1*03 and DQB1*1104) are being suggested. Family incidence may be a factor.

Occurrence: Fairly common.

Age: All age groups.

Ethnicity: Ethnicity is not significant.

Gender: Occurs equally in males and females.

Contributory factors:

- Genetic factors, such as progeria
- Metabolic defects, such as homocystinuria, endocrine-related illnesses (e.g., involving the thyroid, adrenals, pituitary glands), and celiac disease
- Infections, tinea, high fevers, seborrheic dermatitis
- Radiation and certain chemotherapeutic agents
- Behavioral patterns

Signs and symptoms: The child may present in the clinic with the complaint of hair loss when shampooing or when brushing the hair, or the condition may be discovered during the course of the physical examination. A careful history of drug use, behavior, grooming patterns, and recent illness is helpful. Inspection reveals a specific pattern of hair loss, the presence of lesions (inflammatory or tumorous), and the presence of scarring.

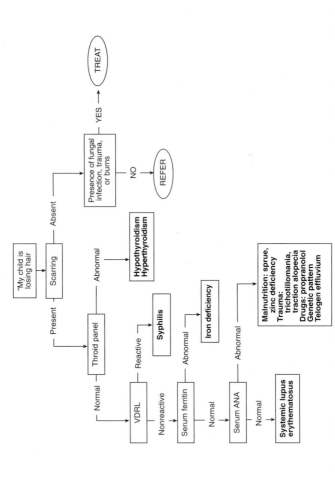

Figure 4–1. Evaluating the etiology of alopecia. (VDRL, Venereal Disease Research Laboratories [test]; ANA, antinuclear antibodies.)

Diagnostic tests:

Test	Results Indicating Disorder	CPT Code
Culture and sensitivity if infection is suspected	Identify organism	87070
Examination under Wood's lamp	Identify presence of fungal infections	87220
Microscopic examination of hair follicle	Presence of "exclamation-point" hairs*	96902
Biopsy of site	Confirmation of scarring of the follicles	11100

* Hairs located toward periphery of patch and extend above the skin surface.

Differential diagnosis:

- Telogen effluvium: Occurs in children ages 2 to 4 months, children with a history of severe febrile illness, or adolescents in the postpartum period
- Toxic alopecia: History of exposure to radiation or chemotherapeutic agents; also heparin and coumarin may induce shedding of hair
- Trichotillomania: History of habitual twisting or pulling at the hair. Consider alopecia areata and tinea capitis in the differential diagnosis
- Alopecia areata: Round or oval scalp patches and rapid hair loss; usually affects other body sites. Nails should be examined for signs of dystrophy

Review history for the presence of stress and systemic diseases, such as thyroiditis, anemias, and vitiligo, and family history of hair loss. Assess the child for tinea capitis and seborrheic dermatitis.

Treatment: If an underlying illness is found, usually treatment of the illness is sufficient to achieve regrowth.

For traction alopecia, an alteration in hairstyle is sufficient. Satisfactory regrowth depends on the degree to which the hair follicles have been scarred. If extensive scarring has occurred, regrowth of hair does not occur.

For trichotillomania, behavioral management techniques are useful for adolescents.

For alopecia areata, topical steroids may be applied to the scalp (topical minoxidil 1–5 %, 1 mL twice daily applied to scalp). Six months of treatment is usually considered reasonable.

Follow-up: Follow-up in 10 days to 2 weeks for evaluation of progress.

Sequelae: Long-term trauma to the follicles results in scarring and permanent loss of hair.

Prevention/prophylaxis: In cases of traction alopecia, teach client to reduce severe pulling of the hair resulting in structural damage to the follicles. Teach parents early identification of the pattern of trichotillomania.

Referral: Refer to dermatologist for suspected cases of skin tumors and to a mental health facility for counseling in cases of severe trichotillomania.

Education: Instruct parents that in most cases the condition is reversible. Instruct parents to change the child's hairstyle in cases of traction alopecia as well as regarding the importance of treating any underlying inflammatory processes. In severe cases, such as cases resulting from radiation or chemotherapeutic agents, the purchase of a wig improves the self-image of the child (most insurance companies cover the cost of the wig if prescribed as a "cranial prosthesis").

ATOPIC DERMATITIS

SIGNAL SYMPTOMS ▶ intermittent or chronic pruritic eczematous skin lesions

Atopic dermatitis	ICD-9 CM: 691

Description: Atopic dermatitis (AD) is characterized as a chronic, relapsing, pruritic, and eczematous skin condition. It is part of the "allergic triad" that includes allergic rhinitis and asthma. AD is characterized by three phases:

- Acute—erythematous, excoriated skin with papules and vesicles; may have serous exudates and crusting
- Subacute—excoriated papules, mild lichenification, and fine scaling
- Chronic—thickened skin, hypopigmentation or hyperpigmentation

Etiology: It is unknown whether there is a genetic predisposition, but it is highly possible: 66% of children have a family history of atopy. An immunologic basis has been proposed because 80% of children with AD have elevated IgE concentrations; food hypersensitivity needs to be considered as a causative factor. Structural differences in the skin also have been proposed (i.e., that the water content of the stratum corneum may have a reduced water-binding capacity and reduced water content).

Occurrence: Estimated that 5% of children have AD.

Age: Between 2 months and 5 years.

Ethnicity: Ethnicity is not significant.

Gender: Slightly higher in males (20% in males, 19% in females).

Contributing factors: Family history of AD, asthma, allergic rhinitis, food allergy, skin infection, irritation from clothing or chemicals, and stress have been considered.

Signs and symptoms: Parent gives history of lesion distributed in the following manner:

- Infants: Head, diaper area, and extensor surfaces of the extremities
- Older children: Neck, face, upper chest, and antecubital and popliteal fossa

In older children, the lesions are mildly to severely pruritic. There is often a family history of asthma, allergic rhinitis, or AD

Physical findings depend on age. Infants present with vesicles and juicy papules, whereas older children present with lichenified plaques on the head, neck, and antecubital and popliteal fossa. Depending on the degree of excoriation, secondary infection may be present.

Diagnostic tests:

Test	Results Indicating Disorder	CPT Code
IgE levels	Elevated	86003/86005

Differential diagnosis:

Scabies: The characteristic distribution of scabies on the hands and feet and the absence of linear burrows facilitate differentiation.

Seborrheic dermatitis: Yellow, greasy patches and areas of distribution—the scalp, face, and chest—are exclusionary.

Treatment:

Nonpharmacologic

Adequate skin hydration should be maintained, including measures such as nightly baths of 15 to 20 minutes and avoiding the use of abrasive materials. Only gentle soaps (e.g., Dove, Neutrogena) or nonsoap cleansing agents (e.g., Aveeno, liquid cleansers such as Dove, Moisturel, Neutrogena) should be used. A wet dressing may be applied (e.g., tube socks or pajamas applied to body part, using another pair of socks or pajamas to cover the wet dressing). Do not allow the child to become chilled. To prevent loss of moisture, moisturizers such as Vaseline, Crisco, Eucerin cream, or Aquaphor should be used during the day, as needed, for itching or dryness. In cases in which moisturizers do not help, the patient should be instructed to use special preparations such as Lac-Hydrin or LactiCare, which contain lactic acid, or urea creams, such as Carmol or Aquacare Cream. The patient should avoid using perfumed products and bath oils and should keep fingernails short.

Pharmacologic

Topical steroids are often used in acute situations. As a general guideline, prescribe the right vehicle and the right potency. Ointments are considered best for use on lichenified or thickened skin but are unacceptable for hairy or moist areas. For moist areas, prescribe creams; for the scalp, prescribe lotions or gels. For lichenified or thickened skin, a moderate-potency steroid ointment should be applied twice daily for 2 weeks. The following areas should be given special attention.

Scalp: Moderate-potency steroid gel or solution is applied daily for 2 weeks. Examples of moderate-potency steroid ointments are mometasone furoate 0.1% cream or ointment (Elocon), hydrocortisone valerate 0.2% cream or ointment (Westcort), and triamcinolone acetonide 0.01% cream or 0.1% ointment (Kenalog, Aristocort).

Moist dermatoses: Low-potency cream is applied twice daily for 7 to 10 days.

Face, groin, axillae, scrotum, or eyelids: Low-potency cream is applied three times daily for 7 to 10 days. Examples of low-potency steroid ointments are hydrocortisone 0.25%, 0.50%, 1%, 2.5% (Hytone, Nutracort, and OTC preparations) and methylprednisolone 1% (Medrol). Tar products such as Estar gel and T-Gel may be used for minor symptoms. These products may cause burning or skin irritation. Antihistamines may be used at night for their sedative and antipruritic effect. Oral antibiotics should be prescribed if there is further skin breakdown with impetiginization.

Nonsteroidal agent: Pimecrolimus (ASM 981) cream 1% is applied twice daily to lesions. Tacrolimus 0.03% or 0.1% ointment is applied twice daily (for children age 2–15 years, use 0.03%).

Follow-up: The patient should return to the clinic in 1 to 2 weeks for evaluation of healing process.

Sequelae: In cases of widespread skin breakdown, a secondary infection may develop with vesicles, honey-colored drainage, pain, and increased oozing. Asthma may develop in 50% of children.

Prevention/prophylaxis: Modification of the diet has been suggested as a preventive measure in infants; this entails avoiding milk, eggs, and wheat for first 6 months of life, although this has not been proved effective. Identify and avoid environmental and stress factors that may act as triggers to exacerbations. Maintaining increased moisture through the use of creams or ointment and avoidance of harsh soaps, perfumes, or additives may be helpful.

Referral: Refer to allergist for a radioallergosorbent test if food allergy is being considered as an underlying cause.

Education: Reassure parents that most children outgrow AD by adolescence. Teach parents to observe child for identification of trigger factors. Stress to parents the importance of good skin care and not allowing the child to get sunburned. Increased compliance may result if parents and child are provided with written instructions related to the therapeutic regimen.

BURNS

SIGNAL SYMPTOMS▶ thermal injuries to the epidermis and dermis

Burns	ICD-9 CM: 948 (add subclassification to indicate percentage of body surface with third-degree burns)
Sunburn	ICD-9: 692.71

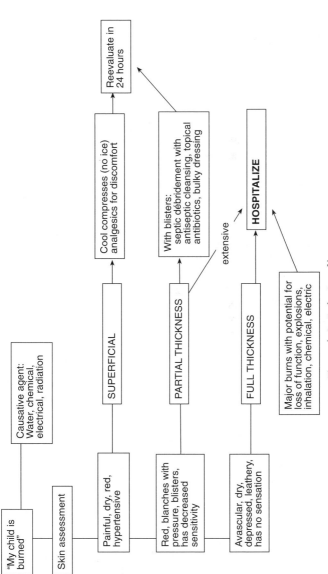

Figure 4–2. Evaluation of burns.

Description: Reddened areas of skin after exposure to thermal source; severity depends of source and degree and extent of exposure.

Burns are classified as:

- Superficial (first-degree)—involving the epidermis
- Partial-thickness (second-degree)—involving the epidermis and dermis
- Full-thickness (third-degree)—all epidermal and dermal levels (Fig. 4–2)

Etiology: The destruction of the skin by excessively hot liquids, chemicals, electricity, or radiation; accidents.

Occurrence: Each year, 1% of the population is burned or scalded; 2.3 in 10,000 die of burn injuries. The upper extremities are involved in 71% of cases; 52% of cases involve the head and neck.

Age: All age groups.

Ethnicity: African-American children are more at risk (3:1).

Gender: Occurs equally in males and females.

Contributing factors: Lack of knowledge related to proper safety and storage of hazardous substances, a lack of regard for known dangers, possibility of child abuse, minorities and lower socioeconomic status.

Signs and symptoms: Patient provides history of exposure of the skin to a hazardous substance that resulted in injury to the skin. Need to query as to the causative agent, circumstances related to the injury, time elapsed since injury, and tetanus immunization status. In cases of chemical burn, the nurse practitioner needs to know the type and concentration of the solution and any other pertinent past history.

An examination of the skin reveals the following.

Superficial: Skin is painful, dry, red, and hypersensitive.

Partial-thickness: Skin is red, may blister or turn white, is dry, blanches with pressure, and has decreased sensitivity.

Full-thickness: Skin is avascular, dry, depressed, and leathery, without sensation.

The percentage of body surface involved must be estimated adequately. The palm of a child's hand is approximately 1% of his or her body surface area. Burns on the face, eyes, ears, hands, feet, and perineum are always considered severe, as are those associated with major trauma, inhalation burns, and electrical burns. Children younger than age 10 have variations of body surface area on the Lund and Browder modification of the Berkow scale (Table 4–1).

Diagnostic tests: None.

Differential diagnosis: None.

Treatment: Minor partial-thickness burns of less than 10% total body surface usually can be treated in the office. Treatment is based on the type and degree of burn.

Superficial: Apply cool compresses (not ice). Analgesia may be given for minor discomfort.

Table 4–1 Variations from Adult Distribution in Infants and Children (in Percent)

	Newborn	1 yr	5 yr	10 yr
Head	19	17	13	11
Both thighs	11	13	16	17
Both lower legs	10	10	11	12
Neck	2			
Anterior trunk	13			
Posterior trunk	13			
Both upper arms	5			
Both lower arms	6	These percentages remain constant at all ages		
Both hands	5			
Both buttocks	5			
Both feet	5			
Genitalia	1			

Source: After Berkow, as cited in Hay, W, et al: Current Pediatric Diagnosis and Treatment, ed 12. Appleton & Lange, Norwalk, Conn, 1995, p 355, with permission.

Partial-thickness with blisters: Initially, do a septic débridement with antiseptic cleansing using 1% to 5% povidone-iodine, and rinse with normal saline. Apply topical antibiotic (silver sulfadiazine or mupirocin 2% [cream or ointment] twice daily for 10 days) and protect with bulky dressing.

Full-thickness: Refer for hospitalization.

Follow-up: The patient should return in 24 hours for evaluation, change of dressing, and further débridement, as required.

Sequelae: Secondary infection is a potential complication of burns. The risk for disability depends on the location of the burn. Burns to the face, eyes, ears, feet, perineum, or hands pose the greatest risk for disability. Superficial and partial-thickness burns do not cause permanent disability; however, full-thickness burns usually leave some impairment. Inhalation injuries can cause permanent respiratory compromise. Development of skin cancer is a concern because 2% of cases diagnosed yearly occur in children.

Prevention/prophylaxis: Proper use and storage of chemicals, appropriate safety measures for electrical current, covering electrical outlets, keeping cords and hand-held appliances out of reach of children, setting water heater thermostat at 120°F, not leaving child unattended in bathtub, care in preparing foods on surface units and in microwave, and proper sunbathing methods are all areas of prevention to be considered. Small children should have sun exposure restricted. Start sunscreens after 6 months of age. Sunscreen should be liberally applied to exposed areas of the skin before sun exposure and reapplied every 3 to 4 hours. Wearing protective clothing, hats with brims, and sunglasses is important for children.

Referral: Refer for hospitalization in the following cases: full-thickness, inhalation, chemical, and electrical burns, as well as explosions. Refer any patient with a burn that is suspicious of abuse, that has a potential for loss of function or scarring (e.g., hands, fingers), or if there are prior medical conditions that could complicate treatment or recovery.

Education: Instruct parents regarding safe practice in the use and storage of chemicals and safety measures for avoiding exposure to electrical current. Instruct parents in ways to monitor substances or elements that are potentially harmful. Instruct parents and children about the dangers of exposure to the sun especially between 11 AM and 1 PM, appropriate sunbathing methods, proper use of sunscreen lotions, and avoidance of tanning beds. Work with local schools to implement the "Guidelineas for School Programs to Prevent Skin Cancer." Sources of sun-protective clothing for children include Alex and Me (480) 425-8705, www.alexandme.com; Me No Fry (877) MeN-oFry, www.menofry.com; and Solumbra (800) 882-7860, www.sunprecautions.com. Teach young children the dangers of fire and develop a fire-escape plan for the family.

CANDIDIASIS

SIGNAL SYMPTOMS▶ beefy-red, erythematous area with satellite lesions

Candidiasis	ICD-9 CM: 112

Description: Candidiasis is an inflammatory skin reaction resulting from infection with *C. albicans.*

Etiology: The yeast organism *C. albicans* is the offending agent.

Occurrence: Common.

Age: Usually observed in infants; can be seen in other age groups.

Ethnicity: Ethnicity is not significant.

Gender: Occurs equally in males and females.

Contributing factors: Improper cleansing of the genital area, use of cornstarch as a diaper powder, and occlusion of the genital area by plastic pants or absorbent diapers that are too tight. Patients taking antibiotics or birth control pills or who have diabetes or HIV are at higher risk for the development of yeast infections.

Signs and symptoms: Presenting complaint is the presence of a red rash with accompanying itching and burning of the skin. Inquire as to the area of the body, for although the usual site is the genital area, candidal infections can occur in other moist areas, such as under the breasts, in the axillae, and in skin folds. Important clinical factors are past medical history; current medical regimen; and, in young children, a family history of diabetes. Physical findings are a beefy-red, erythematous area with satellite lesions (papules and pustules).

Diagnostic tests:

Test	Results Indicating Disorder	CPT Code
KOH preparation of scales or pustules	Presence of hyphae	87220
Blood glucose levels (in recalcitrant cases)	Elevated levels indicating diabetes	82947

KOH, Potassium hydroxide.

Differential diagnosis:

Contact dermatitis resulting from chemical irritants is a possibility, but it does not produce the characteristic satellite lesions of candidal infection.

Tinea cruris may be considered, but the lesions in tinea are much better demarcated.

Treatment:

Nonpharmacologic

General instructions for infants include encouraging frequent diaper changes, allowing the infant's bottom to air-dry during the day, and eliminating plastic pants.

Pharmacologic

Topical applications, such as nystatin (Mycostatin), are applied every 3 to 4 hours. Alternatives are clotrimazole (Lotrisone), miconazole (Micatin), or ketoconazole (Nizoral) applied twice daily.

Follow-up: The patient should return in 1 to 2 weeks for evaluation of healing process. In recalcitrant cases, order tests to check for diabetes.

Sequelae: Systemic infection may occur in persons who are immunosuppressed. There may be renal, hepatic, pulmonary, or cerebral abscesses, or "cotton-wool" retinal lesions.

Prevention/prophylaxis: Adjusting the factors that keep the person at risk, such as keeping the diaper area dry, or treating concomitant medical problems such as diabetes.

Referral: Refer if systemic infection or diabetes mellitus is suspected.

Education: Instruct parent regarding proper application of topical cream and general hygienic measures.

CELLULITIS

SIGNAL SYMPTOMS▶ red indurated area at site of wound

Cellulitis	ICD-9 CM: 682

Description: Cellulitis is a deep infection of the skin resulting in a localized area of erythema.

Etiology: Entrance into a superficial skin wound as a result of laceration or puncture wound of a pathogen, usually group A streptococci. In children younger than age 3 with facial cellulitis, the causative organism is usually *Haemophilus influenzae,* and the infection is associated with otitis media.

Occurrence: Common.

Age: Occurs at any age.

Ethnicity: Ethnicity is not significant.

Gender: Occurs in males and females.

Contributing factors: Any past alteration in the integrity of the skin, such as soft tissue trauma or insect bite.

Signs and symptoms: The child may give a history of superficial skin trauma and usually has a fever. In cases of buccal cellulitis, a history of otitis media or complaints of ear pain may be elicited. In cases of perianal infections, there is usually a prior streptococcal infection—pharyngitis or impetigo.

Physical examination: Examination of the lesion reveals swelling, erythema, local induration and discoloration, tenderness and pain, and minimal drainage and involvement of local lymph nodes. In perianal cellulitis, there is a bright red perianal rash that may involve the penis and the vulva. The child may have been treated for diaper rash without positive results.

Diagnostic tests: Obtaining a culture of the affected area in cellulitis is not usually possible, but a blood culture or culture of skin aspirate may show group A streptococci.

Differential diagnosis:

- Contact dermatitis; however, contact dermatitis is pruritic and there is absence of fever

Treatment:

Nonpharmacologic

Application of warm, wet compresses.

Pharmacologic

Treatment is with antibiotics. Erythromycin, 30 to 50 mg/kg per day (maximum dose 100 mg/kg per day), or dicloxacillin, 125 mg every 6 hours in children weighing more than 40 kg or 12.5 mg/kg in four divided doses in children weighing less than 40 kg, is given for 10 days. In cases of facial involvement, prescribe parenteral coverage for *H. influenzae*: ampicillin with chloramphenicol or a third-generation cephalosporin, such as cefadroxil (Duricef), 30 mg/kg twice a day for 7 to 10 days.

For perianal cellulitis, give amoxicillin, 40 mg/kg per day divided into three doses for 7 days, or topical application 3 times a day of mupirocin 2% (Bactroban) for 10 days.

Follow-up: The patient should return to the clinic in 24 to 48 hours and again in 10 days for evaluation of therapeutic response. The fever should respond in 24 to 48 hours, but the tissue swelling does not resolve for 1 to 2 weeks.

Sequelae: If the infection is treated promptly and appropriately, the patient will not develop bacteremia, local abscesses, or osteomyelitis (currently rare complications).

Prevention/prophylaxis: Appropriate cleansing of superficial skin lacerations.

Referral: Refer to consulting physician for cases of facial cellulitis and cases requiring incision and drainage.

Education: Instruct parents in practicing proper hygiene, keeping fingernails short, and avoiding scratching lesions.

CONTACT DERMATITIS

SIGNAL SYMPTOMS▶   red itchy skin reaction to external source

Contact dermatitis	ICD-9-CM: 692 (add additional codes to identify offending agent further)
Plants:	ICD-9-CM: 692.6
Diaper:	ICD-9-CM: 691

Description: Contact dermatitis is the inflammatory, pruritic reaction of the skin to an exogenous chemical. There are two types:

- Irritant—the result of a substance that has a direct, toxic effect on the skin
- Allergic—the immunologic reaction that causes tissue inflammation

Etiology: Examples of some agents:

- Irritant: Acids, alkalis, solvents, and detergents
- Allergic: Metals, plants (e.g., poison ivy and poison oak), medicines, and rubber compounds (Table 4–2)

Occurrence: Common.

Age: All age groups.

Ethnicity: Ethnicity is not significant.

Gender: Occurs equally in males and females.

Contributing factors: Exposure to offending substances.

Signs and symptoms: Patient usually presents with an itchy rash (Fig. 4–3). Allergic reactions usually take 24 to 48 hours, occasionally 8 to 12 hours, or as long as 7 days to manifest after exposure. Elicit history of exposures, hobbies, and changes in hygienic agents (e.g., soaps, detergents, laundry softeners), makeup, or perfumes. Query as to exposure to plants, animals, and metals.

Clinical presentation varies from acute vesicles to chronic, lichenified, eczematous reactions.

- Poison ivy, poison oak, or poison sumac: Linear streaks of papules and vesicles

- Rubber compounds: Eczematous reaction limited to hands, feet, and diaper area
- Chemical irritation (e.g., feces, urine): Extreme redness

Diagnostic tests: None.
Differential diagnosis:

In cellulitis, the skin is painful rather than pruritic.
With eczema and fungal infections, the distribution and history help in the differential diagnosis.

Treatment:

Generalized Contact Dermatitis (Poison Ivy, Poison Oak, Poison Sumac)

Nonpharmacologic
Astringent dressings (Domeboro) and soothing oatmeal baths (Aveeno) may relieve itching.

Table 4–2   Allergens Associated with Contact Dermatitis

Location	Possible Allergen
Scalp	Hair dyes Shampoos Tonics
Eyelids	Eye makeup Hair sprays
Neck	Aftershave lotions Perfumes Soaps Washing agents Nickel jewelry
Trunk	Clothing Washing agents
Axillae	Deodorants Soaps
Genitalia	Soaps Contraceptives Deodorants Washing agents
Feet	Shoes Sneakers Deodorants Socks Washing agents
Hands	Nickel jewelry Soaps Dyes Plants

Source: Swartz, M: Textbook of Physical Diagnosis: History and Examination, ed 2. WB Saunders, Philadelphia, 1994, p 95, with permission.

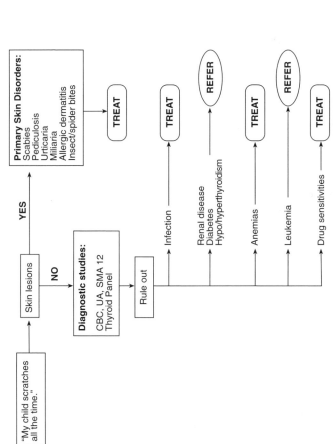

Figure 4–3. Differentiating pruritus. (CBC, complete blood count; UA, urinalysis; SMA, Sequential Multiple Analyzer.)

Pharmacologic

For an acute, severe response, give a short course of steroids (methyl-prednisolone [Medrol], 4 mg, 21-day Dosepak, or prednisone [Sterapred], 5 mg Unipack) for a minimum of 5 days, then taper for a total of 10 days. In cases of a milder response, topical steroids may be applied to lesions. Antihistamines may be given to relieve itching (hydroxyzine [Atarax], 10–25 mg four times a day, or diphenhydramine [Benadryl], 25–50 mg four times a day).

Clinical Pearl: Do not coadminister diphenhydramine lotion when giving the drug systemically because the lotion is absorbed systemically, and an overdose of medicine can occur.

Diaper Dermatitis

For mild diaper dermatitis, encourage the mother to make frequent diaper changes, not to use plastic pants, and to clean the diaper area thoroughly after each diaper change. Some time during the day, allow the infant's bottom to air-dry. Trying a different type of diaper might assist in healing. Use powder sparingly.

Clinical Pearl: Do not use talc because of danger of aspiration pneumonia.

For more severe cases, apply a barrier of zinc oxide to the area (Fig. 4–4).

Follow-up: The patient should return in 1 to 2 weeks for evaluation of the healing process.

Sequelae: Excoriations as a result of the intense pruritus can result in impetiginization. Autosensitization is a generalized subacute dermatitis following a localized dermatitis. It is considered a hypersensitivity reaction to the substance produced by the acute dermatitis.

Prevention/prophylaxis:

Generalized Contact Dermatitis

Recognition, avoidance, and removal of the offending plant are important. Poison ivy (*Rhus radicans*) is a perennial woody climbing vine. There are three leaves that are ovate, thin, bright green, and shiny. Poison oak (*Rhus toxicodendron*) is a low shrub similar to poison ivy; lobate leaves are thicker, dull green, and hairy on both sides. Poison sumac (*Rhus vernix*) is a deciduous shrub with 7 to 13 leaves that are elliptical to oblong (Fig. 4–5).

Apply barrier lotion (bentoquatam [IvyBlock]) 15 minutes before possible exposure.

Washing of the exposed skin with soap and water within 10 minutes of exposure may reduce chance of dermatitis, scrubbing especially under the fingernails.

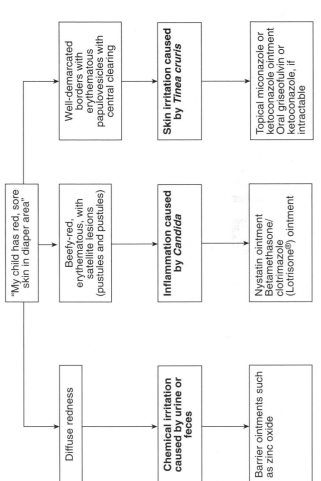

Figure 4—4. Differential diagnosis and treatment of diaper rash.

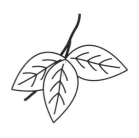

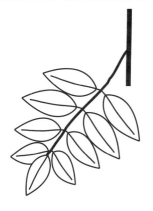

Rhus radicans
Rhus toxicodendron

Rhus vernix

Figure 4–5. Leaves of poison ivy, poison oak, and poison sumac.

When working in the garden, use vinyl gloves, and rinse tools when finished.

Caution children not to rub other areas of skin after exposure, especially around the eyes.

Wash clothes immediately and separately after exposure to the sap of the offending plant.

Wash pets that have been playing in the affected areas because pet fur can carry the sap.

Take precautions when handling firewood.

Diaper Dermatitis

Expose child's bottom to air at sometime during the day and avoid the use of rubber or plastic pants.

Use water-impermeable barriers (zinc oxide).

Keep child clean; change diapers frequently.

Change type of diaper; disposable diapers with polyacrylase gel, petroleum on top sheets of diaper, and a breathable nonocclusive outer covering seem to be the best.

Referral: None.
Education:

Contact Dermatitis (Poison Ivy, Poison Oak)

Teach parents and children to recognize poison ivy and poison oak. Poison ivy leaves, stems, and roots are still toxic in winter. The reaction may be worse because the plant is dehydrated and the toxic substance is enhanced. Instruct parents and children to wear protective clothing, gloves, and long sleeves, even in winter, when handling the plant.

Diaper Dermatitis

Teach parents that they need to keep the child's genital area as dry as possible. Teach parents and children to recognize substances that irritate.

DRUG ERUPTIONS

SIGNAL SYMPTOMS▶ varied skin reactions resulting from administration of a drug

Drug eruptions	ICD-9-CM: 692.3

Description: There are varied skin eruptions resulting from administration of a drug. Some eruptions occur immediately, whereas others occur 7 to 14 days after administration of the drug; the reaction may occur 2 weeks after the drug is administered. The reaction arises from immunologic or nonimmunologic mechanisms.

Etiology: Immune reactions are of four major types.

Type I (IgE-dependent) reactions, which produce histamine and other vasoactive amines, occur within minutes of administration. These reactions constitute "true" drug allergy; the most common offenders are penicillin, cephalosporin, and insulin.

Type II (cytotoxic) reactions are tissue-reactant. Haptenic groups are introduced onto a cell surface, making the tissue susceptible to antibody-mediated or lymphocyte-mediated cytotoxicity. These groups bind to cell surfaces, damaging the cells and inducing antibodies against specific human tissue antigens.

Type III (immune complex) reactions develop when the drug acts as an antigen, producing an immune complex vasculitis leading to serum sickness. The most common offenders are penicillin, sulfonamides, and cephalosporins.

Type IV (cell-mediated) reactions occur when the drug antigen comes in contact with T cells, producing acute allergic dermatitis usually after 3 days. Common offenders are topical antihistamines and neomycin sulfate/polymixin B sulfate.

Nonimmunologic drug reaction, the most common type, results from overdose, cumulative toxicity, drug interactions, and metabolic changes.

Occurrence: Fairly common.

Age: Any age group.

Ethnicity: Not significant.

Gender: Occurs equally in males and females.

Contributing factors: A family history of drug reactions, previous inoculation by the substance, and the individual's unique response to medication.

Signs and symptoms: Parent complains, "my child has a rash." There may or may not be a history of itching. History should include a general medical history; a drug history, including dosage and duration of therapy; history of past drug reactions; and family history of drug allergies. Findings reveal a rash that may have the following characteristics.

Urticaria (type I): Pruritic, erythematous wheals or hives, varied in size and location. They change shape and location and rarely last longer than 24 hours. Onset is minutes to days after exposure to the drug. Common drugs that precipitate a reaction by an immunologically mediated mechanism are acetylsalicylic acid, cephalosporins, griseofulvin, penicillins, sulfonamides, tetracyclines, and barbiturates. Nonimmunologic reactions that produce urticaria are reactions to alcohol, aspirin, codeine, estrogens, meperidine, and vancomycin.

Angioedema (type I): Large, deep areas of swelling. Swelling is manifested by abdominal colic, hoarseness, stridor, and urticaria. Examples of responsible drugs are the above-mentioned ones that produce urticaria (type I).

Morbilliform eruptions: Symmetrically distributed, small macular or papular red spots, often confluent, starting at the head and neck and progressing downward. These reactions are not medication specific and are the most common of the reactions listed. Drugs most often associated with this eruption are barbiturates, carbamazepine, penicillins, phenothiazines, and streptomycins; less commonly associated are chloramphenicol, erythromycin, sulfonamides, and tetracylines.

Fixed drug eruptions: A solitary or a few sharply demarcated erythematous plaques, often tender and bulbous; often occur on the lips and genitalia. Common drugs are barbiturates, metronidazole, naproxen, nystatin, oral contraceptives, phenacetin, salicylates, sulfonamides, and tetracyclines. One study found the most common etiology was trimethoprim/sulfamethoxazole.

Photosensitivity eruptions: Usually confined to the sun-exposed areas of the skin. Eruptions occur with the first exposure to the drug and are dose-related. Phototoxic reactions resemble sunburn, whereas photoallergic reactions resemble eczema. Medications leading to a photosensitivity reaction are griseofulvin, nonsteroidal anti-inflammatory drugs, sulfonamides, and tetracycline.

Erythema multiforme minor: An acute, self-limited inflammatory disorder of the skin and one mucous membrane with distinctive target lesions. The most frequent causative agents are aminopenicillins, barbiturates, carbamazepine, sulfadiazine, sulfadoxine, and trimethoprim/sulfamethoxazole. Less commonly associated are cephalosporins, ibuprofen, rifampin, and vancomycin. Herpes simplex virus is often associated with erythema multiforme minor.

Stevens-Johnson syndrome (erythema multiforme major): Characterized by fever, headache, malaise, and severe involvement of the skin and at least two mucous membranes. Sulfonamides, barbiturates, aminopenicillins, and trimethoprim/sulfamethoxazole are examples of drugs that can cause this reaction. *Mycoplasma pneumoniae* may be associated with this syndrome.

Toxic epidermal necrolysis: Characterized by sudden onset of generalized, tender erythema, with areas of flaccid blistering, widespread denudation, and severe mucosal erosions. Nikolsky's sign, a sloughing of the skin when lateral pressure is applied, is usually present. Drugs that have been implicated are sulfonamides, barbiturates, aminopenicillins, and trimethoprim/sulfamethoxazole.

Leukocytoclastic vasculitis: Patients present with palpable purpuric lesions involving the lower extremities and other codependent areas. They may also have hemorrhagic blisters, urticaria, ulcers, nodules, and digital necrosis. Widespread organic and musculoskeletal responses may be noted. This reaction usually occurs 7 to 14 days after exposure. Common drugs implicated are ketoconazole, nonsteroidal anti-inflammatory drugs, penicillin and aminopenicillin, sulfonamides, and tetracyclines.

Erythema nodosum: An inflammation of the subcutaneous fat. This reaction appears as erythematous, tender, subcutaneous nodules on the anterior lower extremities. Oral contraceptives, penicillins, sulfonamides, and tetracyclines have been implicated.

Unique eruptions: Caused by certain drugs. Some drugs, such as the tetracyclines, often permanently stain the teeth of children if given to children younger than age 6 or to pregnant women. Patients taking steroids may present with acne-like lesions, striae, and delayed wound healing. Phenytoin reactions consist of erythematous eruptions that become purpuric over time. Patients may present with fever, edema of the face, and tender, generalized lymphadenopathy. The reaction usually occurs 1 to 3 weeks after initial administration of the drug.

Diagnostic tests: None.

Differential diagnosis: Viral exanthems are indistinguishable from morbilliform eruptions except by biopsy. A careful history is necessary.

Treatment:

 Clinical Pearl: Discontinue suspected drug immediately.

For photosensitivity reactions, discontinue the drug and avoid ultraviolet (UV) light.

For pruritic lesions, diphenhydramine, 12.5 to 25 mg three times a day, or hydroxyzine, 10 to 25 mg three times a day may be given; prednisone, 1 to 2 mg/kg per day, is often given. Premeasured steroidal packaging, such as methylprednisolone (Medrol), 4 mg, 21-day Dosepak, or prednisone (Sterapred), 5 mg Unipack, may be used to prevent recurrent or prolonged symptoms.

Follow-up: Monitor closely for complications. Consider telephone contact in 24 hours to assess therapeutic response.

Sequelae: Toxic epidermal necrolysis patients are at significant risk for pneumonia, pulmonary embolism, and fluid electrolyte disturbance. Of patients with these complications, 30% die. Steroid use can put the patient at risk for yeast, fungal, and viral infections and can precipitate contact dermatitis.

Prevention/prophylaxis: Taking a careful history of known allergies and considering a prior history of reactions when prescribing medications.

Referral: None for minor reactions. Refer to a primary physician for any major drug reactions for definitive treatment.

Education: Instruct patient or caregiver about the dangers related to continued or recurrent use of the offending agent. If the patient is currently having a photosensitivity reaction, instruct the patient to avoid UV light, including riding in a car on a sunny day (UV light passes through glass).

IMPETIGO

SIGNAL SYMPTOMS ▶ yellow-crusted itchy skin lesions at site of minor skin trauma

| Impetigo | ICD-9 CM: 684 |

Description: Impetigo is a superficial skin infection caused by gram-positive bacteria. There are two types.

Nonbullous is characterized by pustular lesions that rupture early and form honey-colored crusts.

Bullous usually occurs on normal skin. The crust has a lacquered appearance as opposed to the thick appearance that is seen in the nonbullous type.

Impetigo has several local folk names, such as "Indian fire."

Etiology: Most common agent is the gram-positive organism *Staphylococcus aureus*.

Occurrence: Common.

Age: All age groups.

Ethnicity: Not significant.

Gender: Occurs equally in males and females.

Contributing factors: Minor skin trauma, such as an insect bite, that allows penetration by the causative organism. Participation in contact sports and the wearing of occlusive equipment places athletes at risk.

Signs and symptoms: Patients present with concerns about their "sores." Parents may have treated the child at home with OTC preparations without success. They often provide a history of an insect bite or other sore that the child has scratched, but the child may have no memory of trauma. There may be a history of contact with other children who have had similar lesions, such as other children in the family, day care center, or school.

Physical findings include the presence of pustules with honey-colored crusts. These lesions may be on any body part but are most common on the face and extremities. There may be a single or multiple lesions. Usually there is more than one lesion because of the delay in seeking services. Bullous lesions occur more commonly in the diaper area, axilla, and neck folds.

Diagnostic tests: Culture and sensitivity testing of the drainage from the lesion would be confirmatory, but this is not usually done.

Differential diagnosis:

Ecthyma, caused by group A streptococci, is differentiated by the depth of the infection. When the crust is removed, an ulcer formation is present rather than the shallow erosion as seen in impetigo.

Herpes simplex also forms crusts, but on questioning, the patient reports noticing a clear vesicle before crust formation.

Cigarette burns, caused by abuse, may be mistaken for the circular erosions seen after the bulla vesicles rupture.

Treatment:

Topical

- Mupirocin 2% (Bactroban), applied to the affected area three times daily for 7–10 days.

Systemic

- Cefadroxil (Duracef, Ultracef), infants and children, 30 mg/kg per day in divided doses every 12 hours for 10 days
- Cephalexin (Keflex), infants and children, 25 to 50 mg/kg per day in divided doses every 12 hours
- Cefaclor (Ceclor), infants and children, 20 mg/kg per day in divided doses every 8 hours for 10 days
- Cloxacillin, 50 to 100 mg/kg per day in two to four divided doses
- Dicloxicillin, 25 to 50 mg/kg per day in four divided doses

Follow-up: Reassess in 3 to 5 days for clinical response.

Sequelae: Usually none; however, a scar may result, especially in darker skinned people. Cellulitis occurs in about 10% of cases.

Prevention/prophylaxis: Not scratching insect bites and not using washcloths or other personal items that belong to an infected child. For athletes, showering with antibacterial soap after workouts, using a topical antibiotic on all cuts and abrasions, and sterilizing the athletic mats and equipment after use may help. Exclusion of athlete from competition while contagious (4–7 days) may prevent transmission.

Referral: None.

Education: Teach importance of good hand-washing techniques, keeping fingernails short, and isolating the child's personal items (e.g., washcloth, drinking glass, linens) from others until lesions are healed.

MOLLUSCUM CONTAGIOSUM

SIGNAL SYMPTOMS ▶ dome-shaped lesion with center indentation, may be flesh-colored, gray-white, yellow, or pink

Molluscum Contagiosum	ICD-9-CM: 078.0

Description: A flesh-colored, gray-white, yellow, or pink dome-shaped lesion with center indentation. In children, lesions usually occur on face, trunk, legs, and arms; in adults, the lesions are seen on thighs, buttocks, groin, and lower abdomen and occasionally on the external genital and anal region. Transmission is by direct contact.

Etiology: Skin disease caused by the molluscum contagiosum virus (a member of the DNA poxvirus family), usually benign and self-resolving. There is an incubation period of 1 week to 6 months (usually 2–3 months).

Occurrence: Usually occurs in children; in HIV-positive patients, prevalence may be 5% to 18%.

Age: Children and adults.

Ethnicity: All ethnic groups.

Gender: Occurs in males and females.

Contributing factors: Immunocompromised conditions such as acquired immunodeficiency syndrome, therapy with methotrexate and prednisone, malignancy, atopic dermatitis, sarcoidosis, and lymphocytic leukemia. Hot weather and high humidity seem to be factors.

Signs and symptoms: Parents or patients notice the appearance of the lesion, which sometimes is pruritic.

Diagnostic test: Diagnosis usually is made based on the appearance of the lesions.

Differential diagnosis:

Lichen planus consists of pin-headed red papules that coalesce into scaly patches that itch.

Milia are white, pin-headed, keratin-filled cysts.

Nongenital warts take a variety of forms and are caused by papillomavirus.

Varicella is an acute infectious process that erupts in stages: macules, papules, vesicles, and crusts.

Treatment: Lesions are self-limiting and usually heal after months or years.

Note: Common treatments have not been approved by the Food and Dug Administration.

- Cantharidin (Verr-Canth): single application once or twice every 3 to 4 weeks. Adult and pediatric dose the same. Do not use in patients with diabetes or on eyes, mucus membranes, moles, birthmarks, unusual warts with hair, or if surrounding tissue is irritated
- Trichloroacetic acid (Tri-Chlor): single application every 1 to 2 weeks. Not established for pediatric patients
- Podophyllin
- Tincture of iodine
- Cryotherapy with liquid nitrogen

Systemic Agents

Improvement has been seen in HIV patients who are taking zidovudine, ritonavir, or cidofovir.

Surgical Therapy

Curettage has been found to be effective.

Follow-up: None, unless surgical intervention for removal of lesions.

Sequelae: May develop irritation, inflammation, and secondary infections. Conjunctivitis may occur if lesions are on the eyelids.

Prevention/prophylaxis: Patients should be advised not to scratch lesions to avoid autoinoculation.

Referral: Usually none. Refer to dermatologist for surgical intervention for removal of lesions.

Education: Parents should be taught to avoid skin-to-skin contact for the child to prevent transmission. If sexually active, partners should be examined.

PEDICULOSIS (LICE)

SIGNAL SYMPTOMS ▶ itchy, excoriated lesions on the areas covered by body hair.

Pediculosis	ICD-9 CM: 132.9

Description: Pediculosis is the infestation of hairy body areas by lice. Common areas of infestation include the head, axillae, and pubic area.

Etiology: Human-to-human contact with *Pediculus humanus capitis* (head louse) or *Phthirus pubis* (pubic or crab louse).

Occurrence: Common.

Age: Pediculosis is endemic among school-age children (*Pediculus humanus capitis*) and sexually active adolescents and young adults (*Phthirus pubis*).

Ethnicity: Ethnicity is not significant.

Gender: Occurs more in females.

Contributing factors: Using infested combs and clothing (caps), hanging garments together in school lockers, and engaging in sexual activity all contribute to becoming infested.

Signs and symptoms: Child presents with complaint of "itchy" scalp or the presence of the adult louse or eggs in other hairy areas of the body, such as the pubic area and axillae. Children are most often referred by the school nurse. Findings reveal itchy, red, excoriated areas. The offending louse may be seen on the hair shafts; the eggs (nits), which are small, white, translucent, and 2 to 3 mm in diameter, may be seen adherent to the hair shafts. The lice and the nits may be found in the seams of clothing.

Diagnostic tests: Visualization of the adult lice or nits or both on the hair shafts.

Differential diagnosis: None.

Treatment: Topical application of lindane 1% (Kwell) shampoo or lotion, permethrin 1% (Nix) or pyrethrins (A-200, RID, R & C) shampoo, or malathion 0.5% (Ovide). It has been suggested that for multiple treatment failures combination therapy with 1% permethrin and oral trimethoprim/sulfamethoxazole be used or oral ivermectin.

> *Head:* Shampoo should be applied, left on for 5 minutes, then rinsed thoroughly, followed by combing with a fine-tooth comb to remove the nits. This procedure may be repeated in 7 days.
>
> *Body:* Lotion should be applied, left on for 4 hours, then rinsed.
>
> *Pubis:* Lotion should be applied, left on for 24 hours, then rinsed. Procedure may be repeated in 4 to 5 days.

 Clinical Pearl: Lindane is not indicated for infants or pregnant patients, and in others only after failure of other treatment.

Follow-up: Return in 1 week for evaluation of treatment efficacy.

Sequelae: None.

Prevention/prophylaxis: Treat all family members and sexual partners, if appropriate. Wash all linens and clothing in hot water and dry on hot cycle, iron the seams, and soak all the combs and brushes in hot water for 1 hour.

Do not use combs, brushes, and clothing belonging to another person or hang coats and jackets with the coats and jackets of others. In school, the child should be instructed to put coat in a plastic bag, rather than hanging it on a hook.

Clinical Pearl: Check with your local school nurse about the return to school policy.

Referral: None.

Education: Instruct parents about proper application of medication. Educate parents and children about not using combs and other personal items belonging to others.

PITYRIASIS ROSEA

SIGNAL SYMPTOMS ► itchy, tannish pink rash primarily on trunk or lower limbs

Pityriasis rosea	ICD-9 CM: 696.3

Description: Pityriasis rosea is an acute, self-limiting inflammatory pruritic dermatitis characterized by oval, slightly elevated, scaling patches and papules that are located mainly on the trunk. Days to several weeks before the generalized eruption, the patient notices a single lesion, called a *herald patch*.

Etiology: Unknown.

Occurrence: Increased incidence in the winter, fall, and spring; occurs less commonly in summer.

Age: Most common in children 10 years old and older.

Ethnicity: Ethnicity is not significant.

Gender: Occurs equally in males and females.

Contributing factors: The possibility of a preceding viral respiratory infection has been suggested but has not been proved.

Signs and symptoms: The child often presents with complaints of itchy rash. The child may give a history of a single lesion (herald patch), 2 to 10 cm in diameter, several weeks before the generalized rash, which was thought to be ringworm.

Inspection reveals a pattern of rash distribution that in whites is mainly on the trunk and in African-Americans is mainly on the extremities.

The clinical presentation of tannish pink or salmon-colored, oval, minimally elevated, scaling patches, papules, and plaques typically follows cleavage, giving rise to the characteristic "Christmas tree" configuration. Pruritus may be mild to moderate. Children may have oral lesions, which present with punctate hemorrhages, erythematous annular lesions, ulcerations, or plaques.

Diagnostic tests: None. When "atypical lesions" are noted, a serologic test for syphilis should be done.

Differential diagnosis:

With tinea corporis, there are usually a few lesions. If in doubt, complete a KOH preparation.

Lichen planus lesions are characteristically purple.

Secondary syphilis is the most important differential diagnosis to be considered. If there is no herald patch, there are lesions on the palms of the hands and soles of the feet, or the person appears ill, do a serologic test for syphilis.

Treatment: Moisturizing creams may be given for the dry skin and antihistamines, if needed, for the itching: diphenhydramine, 25 to 50 mg four times a day, or hydroxyzine, 10 to 25 mg four times a day.

UV light therapy (UVB) may accelerate resolution. Exposure to sunlight may help.

Follow-up: None. The rash usually disappears in 2 weeks to 2 months.

Sequelae: None.

Prevention/prophylaxis: None.

Referral: None.

Education: Reassure the patient that the lesions will disappear without specific treatment.

SCABIES

SIGNAL SYMPTOMS▶   itchy, small, linear rash

Scabies	ICD-9 CM: 133.0

Description: Scabies, a pruritic maculopapular rash, results from epidermal infestation by the itch mite (*Sarcoptes scabiens*) or from person to person. Incubation period is 1 month. Clinical variants include the following.

Scabies incognito occurs when treatment with topical or oral glucocorticoids masks the usual presentation.

Norwegian (crusted) scabies is seen in immunocompromised or debilitated patients and is highly contagious.

Nodular scabies are discrete, orange-red nodules usually in the groin or axilla. It has been suggested these are a reaction to retained mite parts or antigens.

Animal-acquired scabies has a similar skin presentation but no burrows.

Etiology: Human-to-human contact with the mite *Sarcoptes scabiei.*

Occurrence: Common.

Age: Occurs in any age, has been seen ats 3 weeks of age, but is endemic among school-age children.

Ethnicity: Ethnicity is not significant.

Gender: Occurs equally in males and females.

Contributing factors: Contact with other infected family members and pets.

Signs and symptoms: Child presents with an itchy rash. Elicit a history of related illness in other family members and association with pets within the last month. The itching may keep the child awake. Inspection reveals the classic distribution of burrows on the sides and webs of fingers, flexor surface of wrist, elbow, axillae, girdle area, and feet. The burrows are white and thread-like, with a black dot at the end of the burrow. The inflammatory papules are small and excoriated. In infants, the burrows are rarely seen, and the lesions produce a "flea-bitten" look. Distribution is atypical, and lesions are found on the face, neck, palms, and soles of the feet.

Diagnostic tests:

Test	Results Indicating Disorder	CPT Code
Skin scrapings of lesions (using a no. 15 blade) from either the burrow or the papule, mounted on a slide with saline	May reveal the adult mite or eggs	87220

Differential diagnosis:

Consider neurotoxic excoriations if only excoriated areas are observed.

Consider eczematous dermatitis if infestation is widespread.
Scrapings would be diagnostic.

Treatment:

Nonpharmacologic

Treatment should include the identified child and all other family members. All linen and clothing should be washed in hot water and dried on hot cycle.

Pharmacologic

The therapeutic agent (permethrin 5% [Elimite, Nix, Acticine] cream) is applied to the entire body at bedtime and washed away in the morning. Oral antihistamines may be given for intense itching: diphenhydramine, 12.5 to 25 mg three times a day, or hydroxyzine, 10 to 25 mg three times a day.

Lindane (1%), 1 ounce of lotion or 30 g of cream, is applied in a thin layer, neck down, and washed off in 8 hours. Lindane is *not* for children younger than 2 or pregnant and lactating women, and should be used only when other attempts at treatment have failed.

An alternative is ivermectin, 200 µg/kg orally; repeat in 2 weeks. Ivermectin is *not* for pregnant or lactating women or children who weigh less than 15 kg.

Follow-up: Patients should return in 1 week. Some require a second treatment. Do not treat more than two times.

Sequelae: Secondary infection arising from the excoriated lesions.

Prevention/prophylaxis: Treatment of family members and washing of clothing and linens is needed; scabies is contagious, and treatment of the environment is crucial to stop the spread.

Referral: None.

Education: Educate parents regarding the proper application of the therapeutic agent. Instruct parents to wash items such as clothing, bed linens, and favorite toys and stuffed animals. To prevent reinfection, care should be taken to treat the environment, including rugs, blankets, sofa, and chairs.

SEBORRHEIC DERMATITIS

SIGNAL SYMPTOMS yellowish, greasy scaling process in areas of sebaceous glands

Seborrheic dermatitis	ICD-9 CM: 691.10

Description: Seborrheic dermatitis, also called *cradle cap*, is a chronic, superficial inflammatory process involving the areas where there are sebaceous glands, particularly in the scalp, the eyebrows, and the face. It may also be seen in the groin and on the chest. Pruritus is variable. The mildest form is dandruff.

Etiology: It has been suggested that seborrheic dermatitis is an inflammatory reaction to *Pityrosporum* (a yeast).

Occurrence: Common.

Age: Occurs in all pediatric age groups. If seen in infancy, it is usually outgrown by 6 to 8 months.

Ethnicity: Ethnicity is not significant.

Gender: Occurs equally in males and females.

Contributing factors: Possible hormonal stimulation of sebum has been suggested by the incidence in infants and after puberty.

Signs and symptoms: Parent may bring child in because of cradle cap; adolescents may present with the complaint of itchy scalp or facial scaling. Inspection reveals lesions with indistinct margins; mild-to-moderate erythema; and yellowish, greasy scaling. The lesions are bilateral and symmetrically distributed.

Diagnostic tests: None.

Differential diagnosis:

In atopic dermatitis, the presence of lesions on the arms is a distinguishing characteristic.

Psoriasis may be distinguished by the involvement of the elbows and knees.

Treatment: In infants, application of mineral oil or white petroleum jelly followed in 2 hours by a mild baby shampoo may resolve the problem. In older children, shampoo daily with mild soap or antiseborrheic shampoo containing 2% ketoconazole or selenium sulfide 2.5% (Selsun Rx 2.5%, selenium sulfide lotion, Exsel shampoo). Use OTC antiseborrheic shampoos. Low-potency topical steroid (hydrocortisone 1%) can be applied three times per day to facial lesions, if present. The patient may use ketoconazole ointment on the scalp if shampoos do not seem to be effective.

Follow-up: Reassess in 1 to 2 weeks for progress.

Sequelae: None.

Prevention/prophylaxis: None.

Referral: None.

Education: Reassure parents of infants that the seborrheic dermatitis will resolve by age 6 to 8 months. Instruct parents on proper application of ointments and shampooing techniques.

TINEA

SIGNAL SYMPTOMS ▶ patchy scaly lesions at a variety of anatomic sites

Tinea capitis	ICD-9 CM: 110.0
Tinea corporis	ICD-9 CM: 110.5
Tinea cruris	ICD-9 CM: 110.3
Tinea pedis	ICD-9 CM: 110.4
Tinea versicolor	ICD-9-CM: 111.0

Description: Tinea is a fungal infection of the epidermis found on many anatomic sites.

- Tinea capitis—scalp
- Tinea corporis (tinea circinata, ringworm)—glabrous skin
- Tinea cruris (jock itch)—groin, genitalia, pubic area
- Tinea pedis (athlete's foot)—feet
- Tinea versicolor—area on body with sebaceous glands, upper trunk, neck, and arms

The organisms depend on keratin for nutrition and do not invade deeper dermal layers. Tinea capitis, tinea pedis, and tinea corporis are contagious.

Etiology: The infection originates from contact with a pet or an infected person. The specific causative organisms are:

- Tinea capitis—*Trichophyton tonsurans, Microsporum canis*
- Tinea corporis—*Trichophyton rubrum, M. canis*
- Tinea cruris—*T. rubrum* or *Epidermus floccosum*
- Tinea pedis—*Trichophyton mentagrophytes*
- Tinea versicolor—*Pityrosporum orbiculare*

Occurrence: Common.

Age: Occurs across all pediatric age groups. Tinea capitis occurs most frequently in prepubertal children.

Ethnicity: Of asymptomatic inner-city children, 40% carry *Trichophyton tonsurans*. Most cases are seen in crowded inner cities, particularly among African-Americans (e.g., 12% of African-American females have tinea capitis) and Latinos.

Gender: Tinea capitis and tinea pedis are more common among males than females.

Contributing factors: Susceptibility increases with exposure to infected animals; living in hot, humid areas; minor skin trauma that allows for penetration of the organism; tight hair braiding; and the use of hair pomades.

Signs and symptoms: Child presents with a history of the presence of patchy, scaly lesions on a variety of anatomic sites.

Tinea capitis: Noninflammatory; small, erythematous papules; hairs are gray, lusterless and broken off; inflammatory, pustular folliculitis to kerion formation. Erythematous, papular eruptions are on scalp, possibly accompanied by itching and fever. In the black-dot type, the brittle hair breaks off and is left in the infected follicle, giving the appearance of a black dot; there is minimal hair loss or inflammation. Kerion is a boggy, erythematous nodule with perifollicular pustules. The presence of enlarged cervical lymph nodes is often noted.

Tinea corporis: An elevated, scaling border with central clearing is noted.

Tinea cruris: There are well-demarcated borders with erythematous papulovesicles and central clearing.

Tinea pedis: Chronic type involves fissuring, scaling, and macerations; hyperkeratonic type has moccasin distribution on soles of feet. Acute type involves ulceration, maceration, oozing, and denudation.

Tinea versicolor: Changes in pigmentation (hypopigmentation or hyperpigmentation or both) are noted as well as macules and scaly patches, especially on the trunk, neck, and shoulders.

Diagnostic tests:

Test	Results Indicating Disorder	CPT Code
Fluorescence of lesions with Wood's light	Identify infections of scalp but not of skin	87220
KOH preparation or scrapings of follicles	Positive for fungal elements: spores and hyphae	87220
Mycologic cultures	Distinguish between tinea and infection with Candida	87220

Differential diagnosis:

Tinea Capitis

   Trichotillomania has irregular patches of alopecia containing stubble of broken hairs.

   Alopecia areata has well-circumscribed, round patches of hair loss with smooth scalp. KOH preparation would be confirmatory for tinea.

Tinea Corporis

   Impetigo has vesicles, pustules, and crusts as distinguishing features.

Tinea Cruris

   In intertrigio, KOH preparation is negative.

   In *Candida* infection, KOH preparation is negative; *Candida* also affects the scrotum.

Tinea Pedis

   In hyperhidrosis, KOH preparation is negative.

Treatment:

Tinea Capitis

Griseofulvin, 15 to 20 mg/kg per day; ultramicronized griseofulvin (Gris-PEG), 10 mg/kg per day with a fatty meal for 6 weeks. *Note:* Griseofulvin may inactivate birth control pills. Patients resistant to griseofulvin should be given itraconazole, 5 mg/kg per day for 4 to 6 weeks, or terbinafine, 10 mg/kg per day for 4 weeks. For severe inflammatory kerion, prednisone (1 mg/kg per day) for 5 to 7 days and erythromycin (30 to 50 mg/kg per day) may be given for 10 days.

Tinea Corporis

Topical imidazole (clotrimazole [Lotrimin], miconazole [Micatin]), ciclopirox (Loprox), or an allylamine agent may be given twice daily for 14 days, or oral griseofulvin may be given, 15 to 20 mg/kg per day for 4 to 8 weeks.

Tinea Cruris

Topical antifungals may be administered. In recalcitrant cases, give oral griseofulvin or ketoconazole.

Tinea Pedis

Administer topical agents, such as econazole nitrate (Spectazole), ketoconazole (Nizoral), or terbinafine hydrochloride (Lamisil).

Tinea Versicolor

As *primary* treatment, selenium sulfide (2.5% lotion or shampoo; leave on 10–15 minutes, then shower off; use daily for 1 week); ketoconazole shampoo or cream, one or two times per day for 1 week; oral ketoconazole, 400-mg single dose; or itraconazole, 200 mg daily for 5 days, can be given.

As *secondary* treatment, selenium sulfide (2.5%) shampoo or lotion; benzoyl peroxide soaps; propylene glycol (50%) solution; or oral keto-conazole, 400-mg single dose, can be given.

Follow-up: Re-evaluate at 2-week and monthly intervals for treatment efficacy. Monitor complete blood count monthly for leukocytosis in children receiving long-term griseofulvin. Also obtain liver function studies before starting drug and at 4 weeks. If serum glutamic oxaloacetic transaminase (SGOT) and serum glutamic pyruvic transaminase (SGPT) are elevated, stop drug.

Sequelae: Hair loss may be a permanent feature in kerion, or may take 6 months to regrow. Bacterial and yeast overgrowth may be seen in tinea pedis.

Prevention/prophylaxis:

Tinea capitis: Recommendations include not sharing combs, brushes, or headgear with others; evaluation and treatment of infected family members; washing linens; vacuuming and mopping floor with strong disinfectant; and not using oil on hair or scalp.

Tinea corporis: Keep intertriginous areas dry, use absorbent powders, and avoid tight clothing.

Tinea cruris: Keep area dry, and avoid tight-fitting clothing.

Tinea pedis: Maintain good foot hygiene, wear light footwear, and either throw away or wash infected shoes.

Referral: Refer to a physician in cases of chronic infection or lack of response to treatment.

Education: Instruct patients regarding good foot hygiene; drying of feet; not sharing combs, brushes, or headgear; and inspection and treatment of infected animals. Teach medication administration, dosage, and side effects.

VERRUCA

SIGNAL SYMPTOMS▶   proliferation of epidermal cells in a variety of shapes and at a variety of anatomic sites

Verruca vulgaris	ICD-9 CM: 078.10
Verruca plantaris	ICD-9 CM: 078.19
Verruca acuminata	ICD-9 CM: 078.11

Description: Verruca is a proliferation of epidermal cells resulting in a warty growth. There are three common types.

Verruca vulgaris (human papillomavirus [HPV] 2, 4, 7, 26, 27, 29) has firm, discrete gray or brownish gray papules with a diameter up to 1 cm; surface may be flat and smooth, but may become rough and fissured. These are found primarily on the hands and feet but may occur anywhere on the body.

Verruca plantaris (plantar wart) (HPV 1, 2, 4) has thick, firm, and flat, sometimes painful, lesions on soles of feet and sometimes palmar surfaces.

Verruca acuminata (condyloma acuminatum) (HPV 1–6, 10, 11, 16, 18, 31, 33, 35, 39, 41, 42) has filiform, papular lesions in the perineal and genital areas.

Etiology: Infection with HPV.

Occurrence: Common.

Age: All age groups; 10% of teenagers have warts.

Ethnicity: Ethnicity is not significant.

Gender: Occurs equally in males and females.

Contributing factors: Chemotherapy and steroids may contribute to verruca vulgaris; verruca acuminata is sexually transmitted.

Signs and symptoms: Patient presents with a complaint of a wart. Further history depends on the site of the wart. In genital warts, there is a history of sexual activity; in the common wart, there is a history of chemotherapy or steroid use. There may be multiple or single lesions.

Diagnostic tests: None.

Differential diagnosis:

Molluscum contagiosum is differentiated from warts by its umbilicated center.

Calluses can resemble warts but do not have the thrombosed punctate capillaries.

Treatment:

Verruca vulgaris: May disappear in 6 to 9 months. The following may be effective, however: application of 40% salicylic acid plasters, cut to fit the wart and left on for 5 days (reapply every 5 days; sometimes effective in 2–4 weeks), or cryosurgery with liquid nitrogen or prescription wart preparations (e.g., DuoFilm, Occlusal-HP, or Trans-Ver-Sal).

Verruca plantaris: Usually excision is the treatment of choice.

Verruca acuminata: Apply topical 25% podophyllin in alcohol, and wash off in 4 hours. Retreat in 7 to 10 days if necessary. If the wart is not on the mucosa, it may be treated as a common wart and cryosurgically removed. Newer medications for home use are not recommended for children.

Follow-up: The patient should return to the clinic in 2 weeks for evaluation of treatment. If the area becomes red or sore or shows signs of infection, the patient should contact the office. If verruca acuminata is diagnosed, sexual abuse should be suspected.

Sequelae: Recurrences are often reported in 20% to 30% of treated cases.

Prevention/prophylaxis: For verruca plantaris, cleaning the inside of shoes with alcohol, using shower shoes in public showers (e.g., after gym classes), and using clean towels and bath mats.

Referral: Refer patient to primary physician for cryosurgery.

Education: Instruct patients not to pick at lesions.

REFERENCES

Abscess

Darmstadt, G: A guide to abcesses in the skin. Contemp Pediatr 4, 1999.

Acne

Alagheband, M: Update on acne vulgaris. Clin Advisor 4:33, 2001.

American Academy of Dermatology: Guidelines of care for acne vulgaris. J Am Acad Dermatol 22:676, 1990.

Buck, M: Improving patient education and reducing risk. Pediatr Pharm 7, 2001.

Johnson, B, and Nunley, J: Topical therapy for acne vulgaris: How do you choose the best drug for each patient. Postgrad Med 107:69, 2000.

Johnson, B, and Nunley, J: Use of systemic agents in the treatment of acne vulgaris. Am Fam Physician 62:1823, 2000.

Mancini, A: Acne vulgaris: A treatment update. Contemp Pediatr 17:122, 2000.

Russell, J: Topical therapy for acne. Am Fam Physician 61:357, 2000.

Sidbury, R, and Paller, A: The diagnosis and management of acne. Pediatr Ann 29:17, 2000.

Alopecia

Bertolino, A: (2000) Alopecia areata: A clinical review. Postgrad Med 107:81, 2000.

Hilton, L: Alopecia areata common in children. Derm Times April, 2001.

Price, V: Treatment of hair loss. N Engl J Med 3341:964, 1999.

Whitaker, H., et al: Chronic hair pulling. Recognizing trichotillomania. Clinical Reviews 13(3):37, 2003.

Atopic Dermatitis

Eichenfield, LF, et al: Safety and efficiacy of Pimercronlinuci (ASM 981) cream 1% in the treatment of mild and moderate atopic dermatitis in children and adolescents. J Am Acad Dermatol 46:495, 2002.

Ellison, J, et al: Hypothalamic-pituitary-adrenal function and glucocorticoid sensitivity in atopic dermatitis. Pediatrics 105:794, 2000.

Ghidorzi, A: Dermatitis: Atopic. EMedicine J 2, June 28, 2001.

Hill, D, et al: The association of atopic dermatitis in infancy with immunoglobulin E food sensitization. J Pediatr 137:475, 2000.

Nicol, N: Managing atopic dermatitis in children and adults. Nurse Practit 25:58, 2000.

Burns

American Academy of Pediatrics, Committee on Environmental Health: Ultraviolet light: A hazard to children (RE9913). Pediatrics 104:328, 1999.

Bell, E: Using sunscreens on infants and children. Infect Dis Child August, 2001.

Boyette, T, et al: The value of sunscreens. Patient Care NP 3:17, 2000.

Glanz, K, et al: Guidelines for school programs to prevent skin cancer. MMWR Morb Mortal Wkly Rep 51:1, 2002.

Rodgers, G: Reducing the toll of childhood burns. Contemp Pediatr 4:152, 2000.

Smith, M: Pediatric burns: Management of thermal, electrical, and chemical burns and burn-like dermatologic conditions. Pediatr Ann 29:367, 2000.

Starr, NB: Sun Smarts: The essentials of sun protection. J Pediatr Health Care 13:136, 1999.

Cellulitis

Brilliant, L: Perianal streptococcal dermatitis. Am Fam Physician 61:391, 2000.

Givner, L, et al: Pneumonococcal facial cellulitis in children. Pediatrics 106:e61, 2000.

Contact Dermatitis

Boiko, S: Making rash decisions in the diaper area. Pediatr Ann 29:50, 2000.

Brodell, R, and Williams, L: Taking the itch out of poison ivy: Are you prescribing the right medication? Postgrad Med 106:69, 1999.

Bruckner, A, and Weston, W: Beyond poison ivy: Understanding allergic contact dermatitis in children. Pediatr Ann 30:203, 2001.

Guin, J, et al: Poison ivy update. Contemp Pediatr 4:54, 2000.

Lee, N, and Arriola, R: Poison ivy, oak, and sumac dermatitis. West J Med 177:354, 1999.

Spraker, M: Diaper rash: Prevention and treatment. J Pediatr Nutr Dev 91:20, 2000.

Ward, D, et al: Characterization of diaper dermatitis in the United States. Arch Pediatr Adolesc Med 154:943, 2000.

Drug Eruptions

Huang, S: Drug allergy in children. Pediatr Ann 29:760, 2000.

Morelli, J, et al: Fixed drug eruptions in children. J Pediatr 134:365, 1999.

Impetigo

Basler, R, and Seraly, M: Common dermatological problems in athletes. Patient Care for the NP 4:55, 2001.

McEvoy, M: Pediatric impetigo: A challenging etiologic scene. ADVANCE for Nurse Practitioners Feb:69, 2000.

Pediculosis (Lice)

American Academy of Pediatrics, Committee on School Health and Committee on Infectious Diseases: Head lice. Pediatrics 110:638, 2002.

Hipolito, R, et al: Head lice infestation: Single drug versus combination therapy with one percent permethrin and trimethoprim/sulfamethoxazole. Pediatrics 107:e30, 2001.

Korioth, T: AAP supports treat-and-return policy for children with lice: No-nit policies needless. AAP News 21:113, 2002.

Meinking, T, et al: Comparative efficacy of treatments for pediculosis capitis infestations: Update 2000. Arch Dermatol 137:287, 2001.

Pierzchalski, J, et al: Phthirus pubis as a predictor for Chlamydia infection in adolescents. Sex Transm Dis 29:331, 2002.

Stevens, M: Controlling head lice. Patient Care for the NP 3:37, 2000.

United States Food and Drug Administration Center for Drug Evaluation and Research. FDA Public Health Advisory: Safety of topical Lindane products for the treatment of scabies and lice. April 10, 2003.

Williams, L, et al: Lice, nits, and school policy. Pediatrics 107:1011, 2001.

Pityriasis Rosea

Hsu, S, et al: (2001) Differential diagnosis of annular lesions. Am Fam Physician 64:289, 2001.

Scabies

Chouela, E, et al: Equivalent therapeutic efficacy and safety of ivermectin and lindane in the treatment of human scabies. Arch Dermatol 135:651, 1999.

Marlière, V, et al: Crusted (Norwegian) scabies induced by use of topical corticosteroids and treated successfully with ivermectin. J Pediatr 135:122, 1999.

Metry, D, and Hebert, A: Insect and arachnid stings, bites, infestations, and repellents. Pediatr Ann 29:39, 2000.

Tanphaichitr, A, and Brodell, R. How to spot scabies in infants. Postgrad Med 105, 1999.

United States Food and Drug Administration Center for Drug Evaluation and Research. FDA Public Health Advisory: Safety of topical lindane products for the treatment of scabies and lice. April 10, 2003.

Seborrheic Dermatitis

McDonald, L, and Smith, M: Diagnostic dilemmas in pediatric/adolescent dermatology: Scaly scalp. J Pediatr Health Care 12:80, 1998.

Tinea

Elewski, B: Tinea capitis: A current perspective. J Am Acad Dermatol 42:1, 2000.

Friedlander, S, et al: Use of the cotton swab method in diagnosing tinea capitis. Pediatrics 104:276, 1999.

Temple, M, et al: Pharmacotherapy of tinea capitis. J Am Board Fam Pract 12:236, 1999.

Zuber, T, and Baddam, K: Superficial fungal infection of the skin: Where and how it appears help determine therapy. Postgrad Med 109:117, 2001.

Verruca

Medical Society for the Study of Venereal Diseases (MSSVD): National guideline for the management of anogenital warts. Sex Transm Infect 75(Suppl 1):S71, 1999.

Chapter 5

HEAD, NECK, AND FACE ASSESSMENT

CONCUSSION

SIGNAL SYMPTOMS▶ loss of consciousness after trauma

Concussion	ICD-9 CM: 850.9

Description: A concussion is a brief period of unconsciousness, lasting seconds or minutes, occurring immediately after trauma and followed by normal arousal. Coaches, to determine a player's eligibility for continued play, use a concussion grading scale:

Grade I concussion (ICD-9 CM: 850.9): No loss of consciousness occurs, or there is a brief state of confusion; amnesia lasts less than 30 minutes. Player may return to the game when fully recovered but must be carefully observed.

Grade II concussion (ICD-9 CM: 850.1): Loss of consciousness lasts less than 5 minutes; amnesia lasts more than 30 minutes but less than 24 hours. Player may return in 1 week if asymptomatic. After a second grade II episode, player may return if asymptomatic for 1 month. After a third grade II episode, player must end the season.

Grade III concussion (ICD-9 CM: 850.3): Loss of consciousness lasts more than 5 minutes; amnesia lasts longer than 24 hours. Player may return in 1 month if asymptomatic for 1 week. After the second grade III episode, player must end the season.

Etiology: A shearing lesion of white matter as the brain is shaken within the cranium, causing failure of axon conduction.

Occurrence: Common.

Age: All age groups.

Ethnicity: Not significant.

Gender: Occurs equally in males and females.

Contributing factors: Falls and sports injuries are contributing factors.

Signs and symptoms: The child comes to the clinic with history of an impact head injury. History should include a description of the event. Evaluate the episode using the concussion scale as a guide. Perform a physical examination, including a neurologic examination. Usually the examination is negative for any abnormal findings.

Diagnostic tests: None. A computed tomography (CT) scan may be indicated when there is prolonged unconsciousness.

Differential diagnosis:

Increased intracranial pressure (ICP) would be manifested by increasing irritability, lethargy, vomiting, and altered mental status.

Treatment: Observe level of consciousness and degree of amnesia.

Follow-up: The client should return to the clinic in 1 week for assessment of resolution of symptoms.

Sequelae: Retrograde or antegrade amnesia may occur. Retrograde amnesia is the inability to remember events immediately before the trauma. Antegrade amnesia is the inability to form new memories. The period of amnesia is related to the degree of the trauma. Focal or generalized brain swelling may occur if contusion or laceration has occurred. The athlete who returns to play while still experiencing symptoms and sustains a second head injury is at increased risk for experiencing a loss of autoregulation of cerebral blood flow, leading to increased ICP. This second-impact syndrome results in progressive cerebral edema and is associated with a high mortality rate.

Prevention/prophylaxis: Increased safety measures to reduce risk of head injury, such as seat belts, car seats, gates at top of stairs, safe schoolyard equipment, and safety equipment for sports.

Referral: If parent is not capable of observing the child, refer for admission to the hospital for observation.

Education: Teach parents how to observe for alertness, orientation, neurologic functioning, increase in headaches, or vomiting. Teach parents how to test extraocular motions, pupillary reactions, and gait every 2 to 4 hours for 24 hours. Teach environmental safety, such as use of car seats, seat belts, and gates at top of stairs, and the importance of wearing protective headgear when participating in sports such as skateboarding and bicycling.

CRANIOSYNOSTOSIS

SIGNAL SYMPTOMS▶   abnormal head "molding" and circumference

Craniosynostosis   ICD-9 CM: 756

Description: Craniosynostosis, or premature closure of suture lines of the skull (usually involving sagittal, coronal, and lambdoid), may be associated with other disorders, such as Apert's disease, Crouzon's disease, or metabolic disease (e.g., hyperthyroidism). Despite fusion of the skull bones, normal brain growth continues; any resultant disability (e.g., craniostenosis) depends on the duration of the process and the ability of the other sutures to compensate for brain growth. The clinical picture depends on which suture is affected.

Etiology: Unknown.

Occurrence: Occurs in 1 to 2.5 per 1000 children.

Age: Infancy.

Ethnicity: Not significant.

Gender: Occurs equally in males and females.

Contributing factors: Metabolic disorders, such as hyperthyroidism and hypercalcemia, increase the incidence of craniosynostosis.

Signs and symptoms: Abnormal or unusual shape of the head may be first noticed during a well-baby visit. Inspection reveals an elongation of the head anterior to posterior (most common because the sagittal suture is most often affected), an increase in cranial diameter from left to right (when the coronal sutures are affected), and fontanels smaller than expected for age. Palpation reveals a suture ridge.

Diagnostic tests:

Test	Results Indicating Disorder	CPT Code
Skull radiographs	Fusion of cranial sutures	70260
Thyroid panel	Hyperthyroidism	84481/84482
Serum calcium	Elevated	82310

Differential diagnosis:

Children with Down's syndrome have brachycephaly.

Head molding is due to sleeping prone.

Treatment: Surgery is done to reopen the suture lines that have prematurely closed. Often a Teflon-type barrier is applied to keep suture line from prematurely closing again. Surgery is performed within the first 6 months of life to preserve normal skull shape and to prevent compression and brain damage.

Follow-up: Monitor for appropriate growth and development and achievement of developmental milestones.

Sequelae: None, unless many or all of the sutures are involved and the brain is compromised.

Prevention/prophylaxis: None.

Referral: Refer immediately to a pediatric neurologist for confirmation and surgical intervention, if needed.

Education: Reassure parents that they were not responsible for the defect.

Table 5–1   Clinical Classification of Head-Injured Patients

Mild	No loss of consciousness or amnesia. Alert and oriented. Asymptomatic or with only slight headache and dizziness
Moderate	Possible findings: history of loss of consciousness, amnesia; post-traumatic seizures, vomiting, more than slight headache, listlessness, lethargy
Severe	Possible findings: disoriented, unable to follow commands, decreasing level of consciousness, focal neurologic signs, penetrating skull injury or depressed skull fracture

Source: Rosenthal, BW, and Begman, I: Intracranial injury after moderate head trauma in children. J Pediatr 115:346, 1989.

HEAD TRAUMA

SIGNAL SYMPTOMS   head trauma with or without overt signs of injury

Injury, head NEC   ICD-9 CM: 959.01

Description: Head trauma, an injury of accidental or intentional origin to the head, causes the brain to move within the cranium. The injury may cause damage at the site of the trauma (coup), on the opposite side of the site of trauma (contrecoup), or in some cases, bilaterally. Head injury is the leading cause of morbidity and mortality in pediatric trauma patients. Head injuries are classified as mild, moderate, or severe (Table 5–1 and Fig. 5–1).

Common head trauma injuries occurring in children include cerebral edema, skull fractures, and acute subdural or epidural hematomas. Cerebral edema is a focal bruising or shearing of brain tissue. A skull fracture is a crack or fracture in the skull. It may be depressed or non-depressed. All patients with depressed fractures should be referred immediately. Acute subdural or epidural hematoma, which is associated with significant brain contusion, results in a collection of blood below the dura.

Etiology: Head trauma may be the result of a fall, a vehicular accident, or a sports-related injury. Severe head trauma in very young children is often caused by abuse. Typically the causes of head trauma vary by age group: young children fall, school-age children have pedestrian or bicycle accidents, and adolescents are victims of assault or motor vehicle accidents.

Occurrence: Annually, about 250,000 children per year sustain head trauma. Of those, about 150,000 sustain injury to the brain tissue, with 20% resulting in permanent neurologic damage. Mortality range is 6% to 35%.

Age: All ages.

Ethnicity: Not significant.

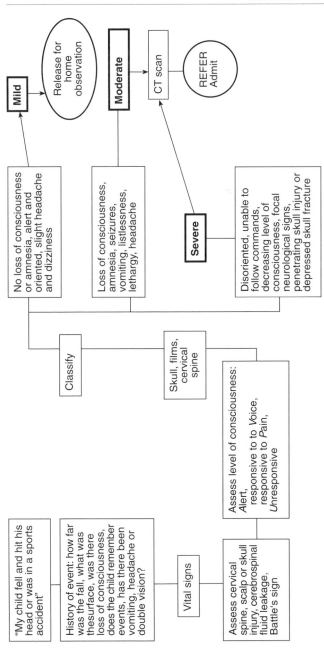

Figure 5–1. Evaluation of head injury.

Gender: Boys have a slightly higher incidence of traumatic injuries.
Contributing factors:

- Lack of safety helmets or precautions, such as child restraints in cars
- Child abuse
- Poor parental supervision
- Drug or alcohol use, which can alter one's perceptions
- Risk-taking behaviors, which can increase the incidence of injuries
- Unsafe home and school environments

Signs and symptoms: The child is brought to the clinic or emergency department with a history of a fall or other type of closed head trauma. Obtain a detailed history related to the injury: where it occurred; length of time since the injury; if a fall, the distance and type of surface; whether safety equipment was worn; whether the child lost consciousness; whether the child could remember events before, during, and after the accident; and whether there has been vomiting, headache, or complaints of diplopia.

A complete physical examination with a focus on the neurologic examination is essential.

Note vital signs; alterations may include irregular breathing, hypertension, and bradycardia.

Assess pupil size, equality, reaction to light; perform a funduscopic examination.

Examine the face for signs of associated facial injuries, such as mandibular fracture.

Note the presence or absence of cerebrospinal fluid (CSF) in the ears.

Assess the level of consciousness using the *AVPU* system. Is the child: *A*lert, responsive to *V*oice, responsive to *P*ain, or *U*nresponsive? The Glasgow Coma Scale (Table 5–2) is particularly beneficial in assessing children older than 3 years. The Pediatric Trauma Scale is also useful (Table 5–3).

When a head injury has occurred, there may be a history of a preceding event, such as a fall or an automobile accident. There may be accompanying injuries and apparent bruising. If there is cerebral edema, there may be changes in strength and sensation, altered senses, altered level of consciousness, and increased ICP.

With a skull fracture, there is swelling or depression of the skull, "raccoon eyes," altered level of consciousness, altered or normal neurologic examination, and altered reaction to stimuli. If a subdural or epidural hematoma is present, there may be altered level of consciousness, vomiting, lethargy, irritability, sluggish pupillary response, and seizures.

Vital signs are altered and may include irregular breathing, hypertension, and bradycardia.

Table 5–2 Glasgow Coma Scale

Activity	Response	Score
Opens eyes	Spontaneously	4
	To sound	3
	To pain	2
	No response	1
Motor response	Obeys commands	6
	Localizes painful stimulus	5
	Responds to pain with:	
	Normal flexion	4
	Abnormal flexion	3
	Extension	2
	No response	1
Verbal response	Oriented	5
	Confused	4
	Inappropriate	3
	Incomprehensible	2
	No response	1
		Maximum score 15

Scoring: 13–15, mild impairment; 9–12, moderate impairment; 3–8, severe impairment.
Source: Adapted from Burns, C, et al: A Handbook for Nurse Practitioners. Philadelphia: WB
   Saunders, 1996.

Table 5–3 Pediatric Trauma Scale

Score	+2	+1	−1
Weight	>44 lb	22–44 lb	<22 lb
Airway	Normal	Oral/nasal airway	Intubated
BP	>90 mm Hg	50–90 mm Hg	<50 mm Hg
LOC	Awake	Drowsy, but *no* history of LOC	Unresponsive
Open wound	—	Minor	Major or penetrating
Fracture	—	Minor	Open or multiple

Score of
<2 = 100% mortality
<6 = Increased risk for preventable mortality or morbidity
<8 = Immediate transfer

BP, blood pressure; LOC, loss of consciousness.

Diagnostic tests:

Test	Results Indicating Disorder	CPT Code
Radiograph of skull	Evidence of fracture	73050–73260
MRI	Evidence of fracture Increased ICP	70551
CT scan	Evidence of bleeding	70470
Hemoglobin and hematocrit	Decreased values if bleeding	83051 85104
EEG	Evidence of seizure activity	95816
Drug screen	Evidence of type and amount of drug use	80100–80101, 82486
Radiograph of neck (two views)	Evidence of fracture	73060

MRI, magnetic resonance imaging; EEG, electroencephalogram

ICP levels are increased in cases of severe injury.

Assess weight, blood pressure, open wounds, fracture, and level of consciousness.

Evaluate severity of situation with the Glasgow Coma Scale (see Table 5–2).

Evaluate severity using the Pediatric Trauma Scale (see Table 5–3).

Differential diagnosis:

Drug/alcohol intoxication is indicated by positive tests.

Meningitis is manifested by elevated white blood count (WBC), fever, and positive culture of fluid obtained by lumbar puncture.

Shaken baby syndrome is evidenced by the presence of retinal hemorrhage.

Treatment:

Nonpharmacologic

The airway should be maintained. Children should be hyperventilated to reduce ICP. Circulation should be evaluated and maintained. Hyperthermia should be avoided. Prompt consultation with a neurosurgeon should be done. If trauma is mild, observe behavior for 24 hours for signs of neurologic impairment, nausea, or vomiting.

Observe ears and nose for clear fluid, a sign of CSF leakage and basilar skull fracture. Evidence of intracranial hemorrhage may necessitate surgical intervention.

Pharmacologic

Analgesia can be given for headache.

Follow-up: Follow-up interval depends on the injury sustained. Initially at 2 weeks post-trauma, the child should be seen by a neurologist and should maintain a regular schedule of visits with a health care provider.

Sequelae: Death or permanent brain damage is possible. Although some children do recover, even mild head traumas may have cumulative effects.

Prevention/prophylaxis: Maintain a safe environment at home and school. Instill safety measures for children, including safety helmets, car seats, and restraints. Ensure adult supervision. Maintain awareness of possible abuse or the potential for abuse.

Referral: A pediatric neurologist should be consulted for all cases of head trauma. Social services or child protective services should be called when abuse is suspected.

Education: Safety measures, including the use of helmets for bike riding, rollerblading, and skateboarding, should be stressed. Convey the importance of proper side rails on cribs and proper use of car seats and restraints. Assess house and schoolyard for the presence of hazardous equipment and surfaces. Warning signs of late sequelae, such as seizures, should be taught to parents.

MACROCEPHALY

SIGNAL SYMPTOMS head circumference in excess of normal limits for age

Macrocephaly	ICD-9 CM: 742.4

Description: Macrocephaly or megalocephaly is an abnormal head size more than 2 standard deviations greater than the mean for age and sex.

Etiology: It may be caused by metabolic disease, leukodystrophies, or bone disease or genetically transmitted as an autosomal dominant trait.

Occurrence: Uncommon.

Age: Usually at birth.

Ethnicity: Not significant.

Gender: Occurs equally in males and females.

Contributing factors: Genetic factors are related.

Signs and symptoms: The child presents with normal birth weight and height but later develops obesity. There are variable developmental delays. The typical clinical picture is square facies with frontal bossing, dished-out midface with parietal narrowing, long philtrum, broad hands, and hypotonia.

Diagnostic tests:

Test	Results Indicating Disorder	CPT Scan
MRI or CT scan	Evidence of structural causes	70661–70553, 70470, 70496
Skull ultrasound (if anterior fontanel is open)	Evidence of structural causes	76506, 76536
Metabolic screen	Rule out inborn errors of metabolism	80048

Differential diagnosis:

Tumors are evident on the imaging studies.

Hydrocephalus, enlargement of the ventricles, (ICD-9 CM: 331.4): The child may be brought to the clinic because of vomiting, a problem with gait, or a headache. Findings may include impairment of upward gaze, setting-sun sign, growth failure, enlarged head circumference (compared with national standards), small anterior fontanels, or prematurely closed anterior fontanels. Transillumination may show subdural effusion or presence of large cysts.

Treatment: None for true megalocephaly.

If megalocephaly is secondary to hydrocephalus, continue monitoring growth and development; measure head circumference at each clinic visit until age 18 months, noting the size of the anterior fontanel and comparing data with national standards for age. Surgical intervention for the placement of a shunt, which bypasses the obstruction and diverts the CSF to other sites, is done when macrocephaly is secondary to hydrocephaly.

Follow-up: Regular childhood visits.

Sequelae: For megalocephaly secondary to hydrocephalus, acute manifestations of increased ICP. The etiology of hydrocephalus is increased production, blockage of the flow, or impaired absorption of CSF, resulting in an increase in the size of the ventricles. If child has a shunt, watch for infection and "outgrowing" of the shunt.

Prevention/prophylaxis: Prenatal care that includes assessment of rubella titer, treatment for maternal syphilis, avoidance of alcohol, and exposure to radiation during the prenatal period.

Referral: Referral to a pediatric neurologist for definitive diagnosis and care plan.

Education: Support for the parents as they deal with having a child with a chronic disability is important. In cases involving children who have had this condition for some time, assist the parents in obtaining occasional respite care for their children.

MICROCEPHALY

SIGNAL SYMPTOMS ▶ head circumference less than normal for age

Microcephaly	ICD-9 CM: 742.1

Description: Microcephaly, abnormal head size 2 standard deviations less than the mean for age, sex, height, and weight, may be congenital or acquired. In this disorder, the skull remains small because the brain does not grow. Primary microcephaly may be inherited through a familial autosomal dominant or recessive trait.

Etiology: Among the causes are transplacental transfer of toxins (alcohol, maternal phenylketonuria [PKU]), chromosomal disorders (trisomy 13, 18, or 21), and metabolic disorders (hypoglycemia, PKU).

Occurrence: Uncommon.

Age: Infancy.

Ethnicity: Ethnicity is not significant.

Gender: Occurs equally in males and females.

Contributing factors: Maternal radiation during the first and second trimesters, maternal and perinatal infections, and genetics may be factors.

Signs and symptoms: Parents may not notice the subtle changes in head size but may bring the child to the clinic because of seizures or developmental delay. Up to 6 months of age, chest circumference exceeds head circumference. There may be a backward slope to the forehead with narrowing of the bitemporal diameter. Progressive lack of growth in head circumference with advancing age may occur; fontanels may close early.

Diagnostic tests:

Test	Results Indicating Disorder	CPT Code
MRI or CT scan	Evidence of intracranial calcifications, malformations, or atrophic patterns of brain growth	70661–70553, 70470, 70496
If warranted by history, antibody titers for:	Evidence of maternal or perinatal infection	86777–86778
Toxoplasmosis		86644–86645
Cytomegalovirus		86762
Rubella		86694–86696
Herpes simplex virus		86781
Syphilis		86592–86593

Regular skull films are of little value.

Differential diagnosis:

Craniosynostosis, defined as premature closure of the skull suture lines, is differentiated by CT or MRI and shows that the brain is growing normally.

In Rett's syndrome mental ability and head circumference are normal until age 6 months. Between 5 and 30 months, there is a decline in language and development of mental retardation; between 2 and 4 years, head circumference decreases, and there is loss of purposeful hand skills.

Poor head growth may precede other clinical signs of celiac disease. Head growth resumes after placing the child on a gluten-free diet.

Treatment: Supportive, directed at management of neurologic and sensory deficits that may occur.

Follow-up: Regular monitoring of growth and development.

Sequelae: Mental retardation resulting from diminished brain growth.

Prevention/prophylaxis: Good prenatal care that treats maternal infections promptly can decrease the incidence of microcephaly. Protection of the maternal pelvis from radiation during the first and second trimesters is essential to avoid affecting the fetus' skull.

Referral: Immediate referral to a pediatric neurologist for definitive diagnosis and plan of care.

Education: Provide genetic counseling for parents of children with significant microcephaly.

CERVICAL LYMPHADENITIS

SIGNAL SYMPTOMS▶   swelling and erythema of lymph glands in neck

Cervical lymphadenitis	ICD-9 CM: 289.3

Description: Cervical lymphadenitis is an acute, unilateral cervical adenitis accompanied by local pain, fever, and tenderness. Any node may be involved, but the cervical node is the most common. The size of the node ranges from that of a walnut to an egg; it is firm, tender, and associated with local erythema. The condition is a sequela to infections of the ear, nose, and throat.

Etiology: Most common infectious agents are group A β-hemolytic streptococcus (70%), staphylococci (20%), and viruses (10%).

Occurrence: Common.

Age: All pediatric age groups.

Ethnicity: Not significant.

Gender: Occurs equally in males and females.

Contributing factors: Breaks in the mucous membrane that occur during teeth eruption, allowing inoculation by mycobacteria; exposure to cats plus a minor skin lesion allowing entrance of the causative organism.

Signs and symptoms: The child is brought to the clinic with the complaint of "swollen glands" and fever. History should include which nodes are involved and past medical history, particularly any past infections. Palpation reveals a large, swollen, taut, firm, or tender mass in any lymph node, usually cervical or inguinal (Fig. 5–2). Record the measurements of the nodes for future comparison. Observe the neck for protective torticollis. Examine each tooth for the presence of a periapical abscess.

Diagnostic tests:

Test	Results Indicating Disorder	CPT codes
Complete blood count	WBC >20,000/mm^3 with a shift to left	85007
Throat culture	Evidence of pathogen	87070
Streptococcal screen	Evidence of streptococcal infection	87430
Culture aspirate of node	Evidence of specific organism	87070

Obtain a tuberculin skin test because early tuberculosis of the cervical nodes may be confused with lymphadenitis.

Differential diagnosis:

Thyroglossal duct cyst is often mistaken for submandibular lymph node, but the cyst moves upward in the neck when the patient protrudes the tongue.

Cystic hygroma may be associated with a large tongue.

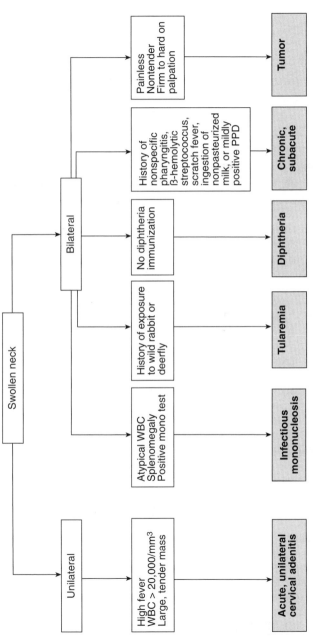

Figure 5–2. Differential diagnosis of neck masses. (WBC, white blood cell; PPD, purified protein derivatives.)

Mumps affects the parotid glands, usually bilaterally and crossing the angle of the jaw.

Ranula is a bluish retention cyst of the sublingual gland on one side of the frenulum under the tongue.

Brachial cleft cyst occurs along the anterior border of the sternocleidomastoid muscle. Although rarely seen, drainage is clear and mucoid, when present.

Malignancies include neuroblastomas in young children and Hodgkin's disease or non-Hodgkin's lymphoma, usually painless adenopathy in posterior or lower cervical chains, in older children.

Treatment:

Nonpharmacologic

Apply warm moist dressings.

Pharmacologic

During the first few days, give analgesics for pain.

If a periapical abscess is suspected, begin prophylactic penicillin V, 50 mg/kg every 6 hours for 10 days, to prevent facial cellulitis, and refer patient to a dentist.

Other regimens include the following:

Cefadroxil (Duricef, Ultracef), infants and childrens, 25 to 50 mg/kg per day in divided doses every 12 hours or once daily, if tolerated, for 7 to 10 days or

Dicloxacillin, 15 or 20 mg/kg in divided doses every 6 hours for 10 days or

Erythromycin, 250 mg every 6 hours for 10 days (EryPed, 30–50 mg/kg per day in four divided doses for 10 days) or

Amoxicillin/clavulanate (Augmentin), 90 mg/kg per day in divided doses every 12 hours in children weighing less than 40 kg or usually 500 mg every 12 hours or 875 mg every 12 hours in children weighing more than 40 kg for 10 days

Follow-up: The patient should return to the clinic daily. There is usually a good response after 48 hours of treatment.

Sequelae: If untreated, illness may progress to suppuration of the node, a poststreptococcal glomerulonephritis, and bacteremia.

Prevention/prophylaxis: Adequate treatment of streptococcal infections.

Referral: Refer patient to primary care physician in cases of acute bilateral adenitis; if periapical abscess is suspected, refer to a dentist. Refer to primary care physician if no improvement in 24 hours, for aspiration of node for identification of infective agent; if there is no marked improvement after 10 days of antibiotics, refer for incision and drainage. Refer to primary care physician for admission to the hospital if child is less than 6 months old or is toxic, dehydrated, dysphagic, or dyspneic.

Education: Stress the importance of completing the therapeutic regimen to avoid complications. Use good hand-washing technique to lessen cross-contamination if there is drainage from the node.

TORTICOLLIS

SIGNAL SYMPTOMS pain in neck with limited muscular movement; head tilted to one side

Torticollis	ICD-9 CM: 754.1

Description: Torticollis is a contracture of the sternocleidomastoid muscle secondary to muscle or bone pathology. Clinically there is a shortened muscle, a rotation of the head toward the opposite side, and a tilting of the head toward the involved side.

Etiology: In infancy, torticollis occurs as a result of an injury during delivery particularly breech presentations, congenital deformities of the cervical spine, spinal cord or cerebellar tumors, syringomyelia, rheumatoid arthritis, or shortening of the muscle. In older children, it may occur as a sequela of an upper respiratory infection.

Occurrence: Unknown.

Age: Any pediatric age group.

Ethnicity: Not significant.

Gender: Occurs equally in males and females.

Contributing factors: In older children, infectious agents are implicated as contributing to the problem.

Signs and symptoms: The parent brings the child to the clinic with a complaint such as, "My child isn't holding his head right." Inspection reveals a muscular deformity characterized by chin rotation to the side opposite the affected muscle contracture. On palpation, there may be a mass in the midportion of the muscle.

Diagnostic tests:

Test	Results Indicating Disorder	CPT Code
Radiograph of cervical spine	Normal; evidence of tumors or cervical spine defects	72240
Radiograph of hips	Evidence of hip dysplasia	73525

 Clinical Pearl: In infants, there is a 20% incidence of concomitant hip dysplasia, and hip radiographs should be obtained.

Differential diagnosis:

Tumors and cervical spine defects are visible on radiographs.

Treatment: Torticollis usually resolves after passive stretching (congenital) but may require the use of traction or a cervical collar (acquired).

Follow-up: In infancy, follow the regular well-baby visits. Monitor the status of the muscle after the stretching exercises are implemented. In the acquired form, re-evaluate in 7 to 10 days.

Sequelae: If untreated, the child may have unsightly asymmetry of the face and cranial vertebrae.

Prevention/prophylaxis: None.

Referral: If the etiology is congenital and treatment is not effective within the first year, obtain surgical consultation and intervention to release the contracture. In the acquired form, obtain an immediate referral for consultation and possible surgical intervention.

Education: Instruct parents in methods of passive exercise. Reassure parents that they are not at fault for either the congenital or the acquired forms of the condition.

APHTHOUS STOMATITIS

SIGNAL SYMPTOMS▶   small painful ulcerations of mouth with yellowish covering

Aphthous stomatitis	ICD-9 CM: 528.2

Description: Aphthous stomatitis is the painful recurrence of ulcerations of the buccal mucosa and lips, also known as *canker sores*.

Etiology: Unknown; may be an autoimmune or allergic response.

Occurrence: Common.

Age: Any pediatric age group (peak onset, 10–19 years).

Ethnicity: Not significant.

Gender: Occurs equally in males and females.

Contributing factors: Chocolate, nuts, and tomatoes have been suggested as offending agents. Hereditary factors have been implicated, as has increased stress.

Signs and symptoms: Patient complains of painful sores in mouth. Inspection reveals two to five painful, pin-sized vesicles covered with a yellowish gray membrane inside lips and mouth. If the membrane is removed, there is a raw area. There is no fever and no lymphadenopathy.

Diagnostic tests: None.

Differential diagnosis: See Figure 5–3.

Herpangina is an acute viral infection accompanied by fever. Oral lesions are papulovesicular with a zone of erythema and ulcers ranging from grayish yellow to white. Ulcers appear on the soft palate and tonsillar pillars, not on the buccal mucosa or gingivae.

Herpetic stomatitis causes small, irregular vesicles that leave ulcers when they rupture. These ulcers are characteristically red at the edge with a gray center. The patient is febrile and has enlarged cervical lymph nodes.

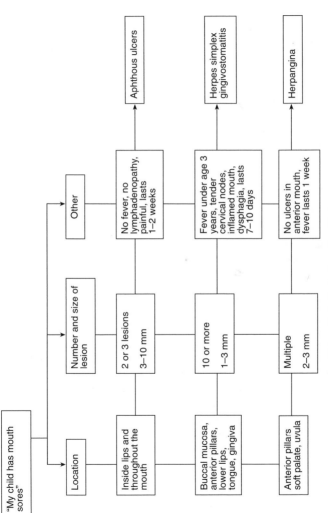

Figure 5–3. Evaluation of oral lesions.

Treatment: Treatment is supportive. Apply topical antacids to lesions four times per day or steroidal mouthwash (0.1%). ("Miracle mouthwash": Rinse with equal parts of Maalox, diphenhydramine [Benadryl], and viscous lidocaine, or apply to single lesion with a cotton applicator.) Apply Zilactin, an over-the-counter preparation, four times a day. In severe cases, use mouth rinse of tetracycline, 250 mg in 50 mL of water, three to four times a day for 5 to 7 days. Recommend a bland diet, avoiding salty food, to reduce pain during eating.

 Clinical Pearl: Do not use smallpox vaccine, antibiotics, chemical cautery, and products containing *Lactobacillus*.)

Follow-up: None, if lesions heal.
Sequelae: None.
Prevention/prophylaxis: Avoid food that may trigger the reaction.
Referral: None.
Education: None.

GLOSSITIS

SIGNAL SYMPTOMS sore tongue with circular smooth areas

Glossitis	ICD-9 CM: 529.0

Description: Glossitis is an inflammation of the tongue characterized by painless, circular or elliptical, smooth areas devoid of papillae and surrounded by a narrow ring of hyperkeratosis; pattern may change daily. This is also known as "geographic tongue" or benign migratory glossitis.
Etiology: Glossitis may be due to presence of infection; local trauma or irritants; or systemic causes, such as iron-deficiency anemia or vitamin deficiencies, particularly the B vitamins.
Occurrence: Occurs in 3% of general population.
Age: Usually before age 6 years but more prevalent in adults.
Ethnicity: Ethnicity is not significant.
Gender: Occurs equally in males and females.
Contributing factors: Unknown.
Signs and symptoms: The parent complains that the child's tongue "looks funny." Inspection reveals characteristic lesions.
Diagnostic tests: None.
Differential diagnosis:

Fissured tongue (scrotal tongue) is characterized by numerous irregular fissures on dorsum. It occurs in 1% of persons and is usually a dominant trait. It may be seen in persons who chew on their protruded tongues (e.g., patients with trisomy 21).
Coated tongue (furry tongue) occurs as a result of impaired mastication and when the patient is on a liquid or soft diet.

Treatment: None.
Follow-up: None.
Sequelae: None.
Prevention/prophylaxis: None.
Referral: None.
Education: Reassure parents that the condition is benign and will resolve in several months.

HERPES SIMPLEX STOMATITIS

SIGNAL SYMPTOMS▶ thin-walled vesicular lesions on oral mucus membrane

Herpes simplex stomatitis	ICD-9 CM: 529.0

Description: Herpes simplex stomatitis is a viral infection of the oral mucosa and oropharynx.
Etiology: Herpes simplex virus, type 1.
Occurrence: Common.
Age: Any age, but predominantly in children aged 1 to 3.
Ethnicity: Not significant.
Gender: Occurs equally in males and females.
Contributing factors: Immune deficiencies and increased stress are suggested factors.
Signs and symptoms: Children may complain of a burning sensation in the mouth 26 to 48 hours before lesions appear. In infants, there is a history of irritability, drooling, and feeding problems. Inspection reveals multiple, grouped lesions on an erythematous base on the tongue and the buccal and gingival mucosa, along with friable, red gums; lesions may extend to the pharynx. There may be swollen cervical nodes and fever (see Fig. 5–3).
Diagnostic tests: None.
Differential diagnosis:

In aphthous stomatitis, painful ulcers are present throughout the mouth; there is no fever or adenopathy.

In Vincent's angina, crater-like ulcers are present on the gingival margins, covered with a whitish gray membrane. Gums are tender and bleed easily. The patient may have submaxillary adenopathy.

Herpangina is an acute illness in which the patient is febrile. Oral lesions are papulovesicular lesions. The lesions are on the palate and tonsillar pillars, not on the buccal mucosa.

Thrush is white, raised patches on the oral mucosa, lips, tongue, and pharynx that are difficult to remove; usually there is no fever or adenopathy.

Treatment:

Nonpharmacologic:
Treatment is supportive; the condition usually lasts 7 to 14 days. Suggest a bland diet and increased liquids for sore mouth.

Pharmacologic
Do not prescribe steroids because they may cause spread of the infection. For severe cases, may give acyclovir suspension, 200 mg/5 mL, 20 mg/kg per dose, four times a day for 5 days.

Follow-up: None, if lesions heal.

Sequelae: Immunosuppressed patients may have severe chronic disease and esophageal involvement. Some patients have episodic recurrences; recurrent lesions (fever blisters) are usually perinasal or perioral, at the mucocutaneous junction, with a tingling sensation in the prodromal phase. The vesicles and subsequent crusts resemble impetigo.

Prevention/prophylaxis: None.

Referral: None.

Education: Instruct parents and children not to share drinking glasses or toothbrushes.

THRUSH

SIGNAL SYMPTOMS ➤   adherent, painful, white, curd-like plaques with oral mucosal ulceration.

Thrush	ICD-9 CM: 112.0

Description: Thrush is an infection of the oral mucosa with the yeast *Candida albicans*.

Etiology: Hand-to-mouth contact with the causative organism, *C. albicans*.

Occurrence: Common.

Age: Any pediatric age group, but predominantly in infants.

Ethnicity: Ethnicity is not significant.

Gender: Occurs equally in males and females.

Contributing factors: Factors include long-term antibiotic use and immune disorders.

Signs and symptoms: The parent complains that the child is a "problem feeder" and may report having noted lesions. The child may refuse to eat because mouth is painful.

Inspection of the mouth reveals adherent, painful, white, curd-like plaques with mucosal ulceration. Assess the diaper area for evidence of a candidal diaper rash.

Diagnostic tests: None.

Differential diagnosis:

Herpetic lesions are small, irregular vesicles that leave ulcers when they rupture. The lesions are characteristically red at the edge with a gray center.

Aphthous ulcers (canker sores) are pin-sized vesicles that leave grayish yellow ulcers covered with a similarly colored membrane. If the membrane is removed, there is a raw area.

Treatment:

Infants

- Nystatin, oral suspension, 1 million units, 2 mL onto lesions four times per day for 1 week. If breast-feeding, nystatin cream applied to the mother's breast as well as prescribing oral fluconazole

Older Children

- Nystatin, oral suspension, 200,000 to 500,000 units, 4 to 6 mL four times per day for 1 week as a mouthwash
- Fluconazole (Diflucan, 10 mg/mL), 6 mg/kg first day, then 3 mg/kg for 6 more days
- Clotrimazole troches, 10 mg four times per day
- For refractory lesions, gentian violet 0.5% to 1.0% to paint the lesions (messy and colorful, but often effective)

Follow-up: Re-evaluate in 1 week for efficacy of treatment.

Sequelae: Left untreated, condition may develop into disseminated candidiasis.

Prevention/prophylaxis: Wash all toys, synthetic nipples, pacifiers, and if child is breast-fed, mother's nipples to prevent reinfection. Stop antibiotics and steroids if possible.

Referral: None.

Education: Instruct parents about washing toys, nipples, and pacifiers.

CHALAZION

SIGNAL SYMPTOMS ▶ tender pustule under conjunctiva of inner eyelid

Chalazion	ICD-9 CM: 373.2

Description: A chalazion is a granulomatous inflammation and obstruction of the meibomian glands.

Etiology: Unknown.

Occurrence: Common.

Age: All age groups.

Ethnicity: Not significant.

Gender: Occurs equally in males and females.

Contributing factors: Retention of the secretions of the meibomian glands.

Signs and symptoms: The child comes to the clinic with the complaint of a "red, scratchy eyelid." Inspection reveals edema of the lid, swelling, and irritation. Swelling may be seen in the tarsus of the lid, generally appearing subconjunctivally as a red or gray mass.

Diagnostic tests: None.

Differential diagnosis: None.

Treatment:

Nonpharmacologic

Apply warm compresses to the eyelid four to five times per day. The chalazion often resolves spontaneously after application of compresses.

Pharmacologic

Local incision may be required if the chalazion is refractory to treatment. Apply an antibiotic ointment four to five times per day to the eyelid. Continue the antibiotic for several days after the lesion has subsided. Apply sulfacetamide sodium (Sodium Sulamyd) ophthalmic ointment 10%, in 0.5- to 1-cm thin ribbon, along the lower lid four times daily for 7 days.

Follow-up: None.

Sequelae: None.

Prevention/prophylaxis: None.

Referral: Refer to primary care physician for incision and drainage if necessary.

Education: Instruct parent or caregiver in the application of the "ribbon" of antibiotic ointment from the tube.

CONJUNCTIVITIS

SIGNAL SYMPTOMS▶   red eye

Conjunctivitis	ICD-9 CM: 372
Noninfectious:	
Infantile glaucoma	ICD-9 CM: 743.70

Description: Conjunctivitis is an inflammation or infection of the conjunctivae with a rupture of small vessels, causing bleeding into the sclera. When noninfectious, it is due to other ophthalmic conditions.

Etiology:

- Inflammatory/infectious—bacterial (*Staphylococcus, Streptococcus pneumoniae, Haemophilus influenzae, Neisseria gonorrhoeae, Chlamydia*), viral (adenoviruses 3, 4, or 7 [30–40%]), allergic processes,and chemicals or other irritants
- Noninfectious—congenital conditions such as glaucoma, entropion, epiblepharon, corneal abrasion, or nasolacrimal duct obstruction

Occurrence:

- Inflammatory/infectious—common

- Noninfectious—infantile glaucoma: 1:12,500 infants

Age:

- Inflammatory/infectious—any age
- Infectious—infantile glaucoma: during the first year of life.

Ethnicity: Not significant.

Gender:

- Inflammatory/infectious—occurs equally in males and females
- Noninfectious—infantile glaucoma: more prevalent in males

Contributing factors:

- Inflammatory/infectious—silver nitrate administered at time of delivery, allergies, colds, and the wearing of contact lenses
- Noninfectious—infantile glaucoma: tends to occur in families.

Signs and symptoms:

Inflammatory/Infectious

The child presents to the clinic with complaint of "pink eye"; older children describe an itchy sensation. Caregivers give history of sticky eyelids on awakening, swelling of lid, and photophobia (Figs. 5–4 and 5–5).

Physical findings vary depending on the underlying etiology: (1) watery discharge (viral or allergic) and (2) purulent discharge (usually bacterial; if associated with otitis media, suggestive of *H. influenzae* as causative agent). Other distinguishing characteristics are erythema of conjunctivae; preauricular adenopathy (viral agents); cobblestone papillae beneath upper lid; stringy, thick, mucoid discharge (vernal conjunctivitis); primary skin lesion of single or grouped vesicles or crusted ulcers (primary herpes infection) and micro and giant papillae on the tarsal conjunctiva; and stringy white discharge (allergic reaction to contact lenses). Vision is normal.

Noninfectious

Infantile glaucoma (ICD-9 CM: 743.70): The child is brought to the clinic because of "red eye." The child is extremely photophobic. A corneal haze and a dulled "red reflex" indicative of corneal edema may be observed.

Diagnostic tests:

Test	Results Indicating Disorder	CPT Code
Culture drainage on all infants <1 month of age	Evidence of specific organism	87070

Differential diagnosis:

- Keratitis—severe pain and corneal swelling
- Endophthalmitis—acute onset, pain, and loss of vision
- Anterior uveitis—irregular pupils, pain, and poor vision
- Kawasaki syndrome—usually no drainage; acute illness accompanied by erythematous rash

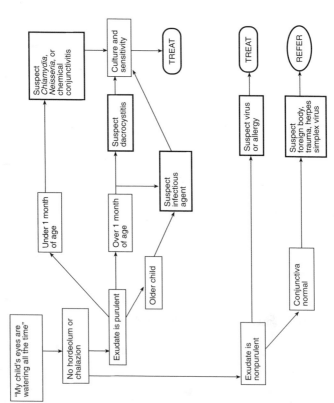

Figure 5–4. Conjunctivitis.

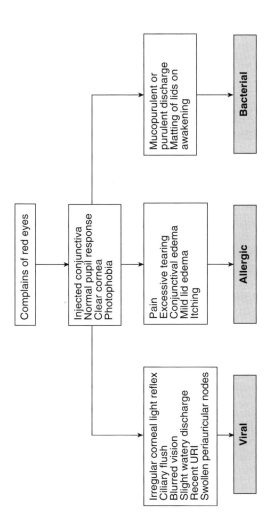

Figure 5–5. Evaluating red eye (URI, upper respiratory infection.)

- Stevens-Johnson syndrome—follows a viral illness or drug reaction; mucosal lesions in the mouth are characterized by three areas of color (target lesions)
- Measles—erythematous maculopapular rash, coryza, and Koplik spots
- Juvenile rheumatoid arthritis—usually a fever, rash, and arthralgia
- Vitamin A deficiency—usually the presence of a malabsorption syndrome, as seen in persons with cystic fibrosis or persons who are on fad diets

Treatment:

Nonpharmacologic

Inflammatory/Infectious
Apply cool compresses.

Pharmacologic

Inflammatory/Infectious
BACTERIAL

- Trimethoprim sulfate 0.1% plus polymyxin B sulfate, 10,000 U/mL (Polytrim ophthalmic solution), 1 drop every 3 hours with maximum of six doses daily (children >2 months) or
- Sulfacetamide sodium ophthalmic ointment or solution, 1%, four times daily for 7 to 10 days or
- Tobramycin 0.3% plus dexamethasone 0.3% (TobraDex ophthalmic ointment or solution), 2 drops four times per day or $^1/_2$ inch two to three times per day

VIRAL

Viral conjunctivitis is self-limiting (usually associated with upper respiratory infection). To prevent secondary infection, apply sulfacetamide solution 1% five times daily.

ALLERGIC

Treat underlying problem.
Prescribe ketorolac tromethamine (Acular 0.5%) solution, 1 drop per affected eye, four times a day up to 3 days
Levocabastine hydrochloride (Livostin), 1 drop per affected eye, four times a day (children >12 years) or
Cromolyn sodium (Opticrom), 1 to 2 drops per affected eye four to six times a day

 Clinical Pearl: Eye drops should be administered 1 hour before inserting contact lenses.

CHEMICAL

Flush eye with a copious amount of tepid water or normal saline.

Noninfectious

Infantile glaucoma requires surgical intervention.

Follow-up: The child should return to the clinic in 2 to 3 days if there is no improvement; parent should call back immediately if condition becomes worse, child complains of pain, or child initially gets better then gets worse.

Sequelae: A secondary bacterial infection may develop. If untreated, the long-term effects may be blepharitis, corneal ulcers (bacterial infection), sloughing of the cornea, or corneal ulcer (chemical irritation). Untreated infantile glaucoma can result in optic nerve damage.

Prevention/prophylaxis: Proper hand-washing techniques and proper disposal of compresses. Instruct parents to avoid cross-contamination by keeping the child's washcloth and towels separate from those of other family members. Instruct parent and youth to clean contact lenses well daily or use daily wear disposable contacts.

Referral: Consult with ophthalmologist for prompt referral for corneal ulcer, chemical conjunctivitis, complaints of pain, photophobia, and any irregularities in pupil size, as well as for infants younger than 1 month old.

Education: Instruct parents in proper eye care.

Wipe eyes gently from inner canthus to avoid spreading infection to the other eye. Clean eye before instilling medication.

To instill ointment or drops, pull down inner canthus of lower eyelid toward center of eye; apply a thin ribbon of ointment or drops to the "pocket."

Rubbing of eyes can cause the infection to spread to the other eye. Instruct parents to teach child not to rub his or her eyes.

EYE INJURIES

SIGNAL SYMPTOMS ▶ pain in eye with or without loss of vision

Eye injuries	ICD-9 CM: 921.9

Description: Eye injuries include any trauma, accidental or nonaccidental, to the eye or its structures.

Etiology: Foreign body, lacerations, abrasions, burns, fractures, contusions, and child abuse (shaken-baby syndrome).

Occurrence: Fairly common.

Age: All age groups.

Ethnicity: Not significant.

Gender: Occurs equally in males and females.

Contributing factors: Lack of knowledge about safety when using hammers, firearms, or chemicals; fireworks; and exposure to ultraviolet

(UV) light are contributing factors. Baseball and basketball have the highest incidence of eye injuries.

Signs and symptoms: The child is brought to the clinic with a complaint such as, "I have something in my eye." Obtain a history of the event, the activity engaged in, where the activity took place, time elapsed before seeking health care, any home remedy used, and the presence of pain or bleeding.

> Foreign body: Evert the upper lid; inspection usually reveals the foreign body in the furrow immediately behind the margin of the upper lid.
> Corneal foreign body: Refer immediately to primary care physician or ophthalmologist.
> Intraocular foreign body: Refer immediately to ophthalmologist.
> Injuries to the eyelids (ecchymosis and lacerations): Refer to primary care physician or ophthalmologist.
> Corneal injuries: Refer to primary care physician or ophthalmologist.
> Burns: Refer to primary care physician or ophthalmologist.

Diagnostic tests:

Test	Results Indicating Disorder	CPT Code
Radiographic studies of the orbit	Evidence of presence of fracture of the orbit	70030
Vision testing appropriate to age of child (Snellen or a count of upheld fingers)	Diminished visual acuity	99172–99173

Differential diagnosis: None.

Treatment:

> *Conjunctival foreign body:* After visualizing the foreign body, gently remove with a moist cotton applicator.
> *Corneal and intraocular foreign bodies:* Refer immediately to primary care physician or ophthalmologist.

Follow-up: For minor injuries, the patient should return in 24 hours; patients with major injuries should return to the clinic after hospitalization.

Sequelae: If not treated promptly and appropriately, there could be loss of vision or loss of the entire eye.

Prevention/prophylaxis: Wear safety goggles when working with tools or hazardous chemicals or when exposed to UV light. Do not allow children to play with firearms, fireworks, or other harmful items. Appropriate sports-related eyewear should be worn. Children with a history of eye injury or surgery should not participate in boxing, wrestling, and full-contact martial arts.

Referral: After initial assessment, refer all ocular injuries to the primary care physician or ophthalmologist.

Education:

- Safety rules related to tools and hazardous substances
- Dangers and safety measures related to UV rays
- Firearm safety

HORDEOLUM

SIGNAL SYMPTOMS▶ painful foreign-body sensation, tearing

Hordeolum	ICD-9 CM: 373.11

Description: Hordeolum is an abscess of the sebaceous glands of the lid margin. External hordeolum is commonly called a *sty*. Internal hordeolum is an acute infection of the meibomian glands.

Etiology: The infectious agent is a staphylococcal organism, usually *Staphylococcus aureus*.

Occurrence: Common.

Age: All age groups.

Ethnicity: Not significant.

Gender: Occurs equally in males and females.

Contributing factors: Hand-to-eye contact with the infectious agent.

Signs and symptoms: Parent complains, "My child has a sty." Obtain history of duration of illness, other persons at home with the problem, and what they have done at home in an attempt to cure the sty. Findings include localized tenderness, redness, and swelling.

Diagnostic tests: None.

Differential diagnosis: None.

Treatment:

Nonpharmacologic

Apply warm, moist compresses to the eyelid four times per day.

Pharmacologic

Apply an antibiotic ointment to the eyelid four to five times per day. Continue the antibiotic for several days after the lesion has subsided.

Apply sulfacetamide sodium ophthalmic ointment 10%, in a 0.5- to 1-cm thin ribbon, along lower lid four times per day for 7 days.

Follow-up: None.

Sequelae: None.

Prevention/prophylaxis: Employ good hand-washing techniques. Purchase new eye makeup, throwing out the old makeup and the old applicators. Keep child's washcloth and towels separate from those of other family members. Dispose of warm compresses properly to prevent reinfection.

Referral: None, unless treatment is ineffective or the lesion needs to be incised and drained.

Education: Instruct parent and patient in good hand-washing techniques and to take care not to cross-contaminate the eyes. Older children and adolescents should not wear eye makeup until the infection has cleared.

NASOLACRIMAL DUCT OBSTRUCTION

SIGNAL SYMPTOMS▶   excessive tearing

| Dacryocystitis | ICD-9 CM: 375.30 |

Description: This condition is defined as obstruction of the nasolacrimal duct with or without an infectious process. There may also be a concomitant infection of the lacrimal sac, termed *dacryocystitis*.

Etiology: Failure of nasolacrimal duct to canalize completely.

Occurrence: Common.

Age: Infancy.

Ethnicity: Not significant.

Gender: Occurs equally in males and females.

Contributing factors: Failure of tears to drain or stasis of tears in the tear sac predisposes infants to infection, usually with *S. aureus*.

Signs and symptoms: The child presents with a history of persistent tearing and mucoid discharge in the inner corner of the eye; the child may have matting of the eyelashes during sleep. Inspection reveals watering of the eye, with tears spilling over onto the cheek. If dacryocystitis is present, there is swelling and erythema medial and inferior to the inner canthus, and purulent material may be expressed from the duct opening.

Diagnostic tests: None; may do culture of exudate to assess for infective organisms.

Differential diagnosis: Excessive lacrimation is an early sign of congenital glaucoma, as are photophobia and a cloudy cornea.

Treatment: Gently massage the lacrimal sac, expressing exudate toward the nose to clear the passage. Instill antibiotic ointment or drops, as indicated.

Follow-up: Evaluate monthly; if no improvement by 6 months of age, refer patient to the ophthalmologist.

Sequelae: May be secondary inflammation owing to the obstruction.

Prevention/prophylaxis: None except for proper eye care to prevent secondary infection.

Referral: If no improvement in 6 months, refer patient to ophthalmologist for surgical intervention.

Education: Instruct parents in lacrimal massage and in the proper manner of instillation of medications.

NYSTAGMUS

Nystagmus	ICD-9 CM: 379.50

Description: The involuntary ocular movements are classified as follows:

- Pendular (undulatory)—equal in each direction of gaze
- Jerking (rhythmic)—slow component followed by quick, corrective component
- Congenital—jerky movements, present in all directions of gaze, usually decrease when eyes converge
- Latent—occurring when one eye is covered

Etiology: Varies by classification: poor vision (pendular), congenital (jerky), inner ear disease, secondary to central nervous system disease (jerky).

Occurrence: Fairly uncommon ($<2\%$).

Age: All age groups.

Ethnicity: Ethnicity is not significant.

Gender: Occurs equally in males and females.

Contributing factors: Physiologic disease, central nervous system disease, drug or alcohol toxicity.

Signs and symptoms: The child presents with a history of spontaneous, involuntary movements of one or both eyes. Family history, drug and chemical history, illnesses, and duration of symptoms are all avenues of investigation.

Inspection reveals rapid eye movements. Notations of the plane and the rate of movement assist in the classification: equal in all directions, pendular; quicker movements in one direction, jerky.

Diagnostic tests: A funduscopic examination may reveal cataracts, retrolental fibroplasia, decreased visual acuity, and weakness of the ocular muscles.

A neurologic examination is indicated because premature infants with persistent or horizontal nystagmus are predisposed to intracranial hemorrhage. Horizontal nystagmus is often associated with a brain tumor.

Problems related to cranial nerve VIII (vestibular branch of auditory nerve) may also be a source of nystagmus. The rotational test is done (if nystagmus does not occur after rotation, there is labyrinth damage). The caloric test is done to determine which labyrinth is affected. Screening for vestibular abnormalities may be done using the past pointing test, in which the arm moves to the side of the disorder. In the Romberg test, the child falls toward the side of the vestibular lesion.

Differential diagnosis: None. Nystagmus is a symptom of an underlying disorder. Clarification of the type of nystagmus provides some diagnostic clues for identifying the cause. End-point nystagmus, which occurs when the child looks out of the far corner of the eye, is not true nystagmus.

Treatment: To treat nystagmus, the underlying cause must be treated.

Follow-up: Follow-up is done with respect to the underlying cause and in concert with the consulting physician.

Sequelae: Later outcomes include extreme vertigo, oscillopsia, and permanent nystagmus. Permanent disability and death can occur if underlying causes are not found and treated.

Prevention/prophylaxis: None.

Referral: Immediate referral to a primary care physician, ophthalmologist, and neurologist.

Education: Explain possible causative factors to parents and the need for referral to a specialist.

STRABISMUS

SIGNAL SYMPTOMS abnormal ocular alignment

Esotropia	ICD-9 CM: 378
Exotropia	ICD-9 CM: 378.10
Exophoria	ICD-9 CM: 378.50

Description: Strabismus, or abnormal ocular alignment, is nonparallelism of the visual axes in the various fields of gaze. It is usual in infants up to age 6 months, may be transitory in infants age 6 to 18 months, and is abnormal after age 18 months. Nonparalytic strabismus is characterized by a constant angle of deviation in all fields. Strabismus may be classified as follows:

- Esotropia (convergent strabismus)—eye turns medially
- Exotropia (divergent strabismus)—eye turns laterally
- Hypertropia—upward deviation of the eye
- Hypotropia—downward deviation of the eye
- Esophoria—tendency of eyes to converge
- Exophoria—tendency of eyes to diverge

Etiology: In paralytic strabismus, a motor imbalance caused by paresis of an extraocular muscle causes the condition. In nonparalytic strabismus, muscle weakness, visual defects, intracranial hemorrhage, lead poisoning, and infection have been implicated.

Occurrence: Occurs in 2% to 3% of children.

Age: Occurrences past age 6 months require further investigation.

Ethnicity: Not significant.

Gender: Occurs equally in males and females.

Contributing factors: There is often a family pattern of strabismus. Febrile illness, head injury, fatigue, or stress may precipitate concomitant (nonparalytic) strabismus.

Signs and symptoms: In infants and young children, strabismus is usually identified at the time of the well-baby visit. Parents of an older child may bring the child to the clinic because an abnormal look to the eyes is apparent. The onset and duration should be investigated. Examination of the eye reveals ocular deviation.

Diagnostic tests: Visual accuracy tests can identify any defect causing the problem.

Hirshburg test (corneal light reflection test): When a light is shined into the eyes, the light should fall nearly in the center of each pupil. Lateral displacement indicates esotropia; nasal displacement indicates extropia.

Alternate cover test: The movement of the covered eye is observed when the cover is removed. If the eye remains in the deviated position, atropia is present; if it returns to center, it is normal.

Cardinal positions of gaze: There is limited movement in one direction of gaze if strabismus is present. Testing each eye separately assists in determining the presence of true paralysis of an extraocular muscle.

Differential diagnosis:

Sudden onset indicates intracranial hemorrhage, encephalitis, lead poisoning, or intraorbital tumors.

Hypoglycemic patients may have transient strabismus.

Pseudostrabismus, usually seen in Asian children, can be differentiated by comparing the position of the light reflex in each eye.

Treatment: Surgery is done to correct strabismus resulting from muscular problems. In cases of strabismus resulting from other physical problems, underlying causes should be treated.

Follow-up: Follow-up depends on the cause and treatment. Care should be provided in conjunction with the referring physician.

Sequelae: Monocular strabismus may develop in persons with amblyopia.

Prevention/prophylaxis: Prompt identification and treatment of underlying cause prevents further complications.

Referral: Refer to ophthalmologist any child older than age 6 months with presenting history and physical examination indicating the presence of strabismus. Refer to ophthalmologist any child younger than age 6 months if strabismus is fixed or constant.

Education: None.

COMMON COLD

SIGNAL SYMPTOMS ▶ congestion of nasal mucosa with watery discharge, sneezing, lacimation

| Common cold | ICD-9 CM: 460 |

Description: The common cold, a viral infection of the upper respiratory tract, is limited to the nasopharynx and nasal mucosa. A cold is a highly communicable disease, extremely common in the pediatric population; it is the second most commonly diagnosed illness seen in the primary health care setting.

Etiology: Viruses of many different types (approximately 100) cause the common cold or upper respiratory infection. Rhinovirus is responsible for about one third of all colds. Parainfluenza virus, respiratory syncytial virus (RSV), and coronavirus are the other most common viral agents that cause colds.

Occurrence: Fall, winter, and early spring, or during a community outbreak. In children, winter is the most likely time during which most colds are seen.

Age: Preschoolers get colds more frequently (between three and nine per year) than any other age group of children.

Ethnicity: Not significant.

Gender: Occurs equally in males and females.

Contributing factors: Exposure to second-hand smoke, smoking, environmental pollutants, crowded areas, and day care settings increases the incidence of colds.

Signs and symptoms: The child or parent may report that rhinorrhea, nasal stuffiness, and a thin, watery discharge from the nose have been present for 1 to 4 days. Mouth breathing and frequent sneezing also is reported. For infants, the temperature ranges from normal to 102°F, whereas older children rarely are febrile. A decreased appetite, poor feeding, and a mildly upset stomach are reported. The child appears ill and fussy. Postnasal drip and swollen, erythematous nasal mucosa are noted. Auscultation reveals some referred nasal sounds, with occasional coarse breath sounds in the upper lobes.

Diagnostic tests: None are indicated; however, if a complete blood count is performed, there may be slight leukopenia followed by leukocytosis.

Differential diagnosis:

Pertussis, measles, and diphtheria in the early stages are differentiated by their clinical courses, which quickly become more serious. Auscultation in these diseases reveals findings that suggest lower respiratory infections.

Sinusitis, which causes a persistent fever and an accompanying cough and headache, is differentiated by symptoms.

Allergic rhinitis is differentiated by history, seasonality of the disease, and other allergic symptoms.

Cocaine use, which can produce chronic congestion and watery rhinorrhea, is differentiated by a drug screen.

Treatment:

Nonpharmacologic

Symptomatic treatment is the most appropriate regimen for the common cold or upper respiratory infections. Comfort measures such as elevating the head of the bed, using saline nasal spray up to four times a day, and taking acetaminophen for fever are all effective modes of treatment. Increasing the child's fluid intake helps to liquefy secretions. A cool-mist humidifier is also helpful for infants and toddlers, but it must be cleaned daily.

Pharmacologic

Oral antihistamines have not been shown to cause a significant reduction in the symptoms or discomfort of a cold.

Follow-up: Regular childhood visits, unless the cold fails to resolve within 2 weeks or symptoms worsen.

Sequelae: No serious sequelae have been documented.

Prevention/prophylaxis: Although many have suggested administering vitamin C for colds, most studies have shown that it has no impact on the incidence or severity of colds. Some risk does exist, however, with taking vitamin C in high doses because vitaminosis has been frequently documented. Good nutrition, avoidance of crowds when a community outbreak has been noted, adequate rest, and good hygiene are the best ways to decrease the spread of colds.

Referral: Referral is rarely needed, but if the cold does not resolve within 1 to 2 weeks or symptoms worsen, the patient should be referred to a pediatrician.

Education: Parents and children should be taught that this self-limiting disease has few, if any, serious consequences. Although parents often request antibiotics at the health care visit, antibiotics are of little value in the treatment of a cold. Parents should be made aware that if their child has school-age siblings, has a large family, or attends a day care center, he or she is more likely to get colds.

Nasal secretions, which contain the virus, can be on the skin, clothing, or toys; hand washing can decrease the spread of the cold. The importance of hand washing should be stressed to the child and the caregiver because the disease spreads by hand-to-mouth contact.

CROUP

SIGNAL SYMPTOMS▶ resonate barking cough with difficulty breathing

Croup	ICD-9 CM: 464.4

Description: Croup or laryngotracheobronchitis, an acute viral respiratory illness of short course (3–7 days), generally follows an upper respiratory infection. It is characterized by a barky cough, variable respiratory distress, and biphasic or inspiratory stridor. Croup may be categorized as:

- Mild—stridor with excitement or at rest without retractions
- Moderate—stridor at rest with retractions
- Severe—severe respiratory distress

Etiology: Parainfluenza, RSV, adenovirus, and influenza A are all thought to be the causative agents.

Occurrence: Usually during the fall and winter.

Age: Children ages 6 months to 5 years with 2 years seeing the highest incidence.

Ethnicity: Not significant.

Gender: Males affected more than females.

Contributing factors: Exposure to affected persons.

Signs and symptoms: Parent usually reports that the child had a mild cold or rhinitis and was awakened by a "barking cough." The child appeared frightened and at times unable to catch his or her breath. Chest retractions and nasal flaring are usually seen. There may or may not be a fever. Between episodes of cough, the child appears well. Inspection shows the child to have occasional nasal flaring during the coughing episode. The child may seem irritable and restless. Substernal retractions are noted. Palpation may reveal displacement of the cardiac apical beat toward an area of atelectasis. Percussion reveals dullness, which may indicate consolidation or atelectasis of the lung. Auscultation reveals tachycardia, bronchial breathing, and rales.

Diagnostic tests: Laboratory tests are usually not helpful or indicated. If indicated:

Test	Results Indicating Disorder	CPT Code
Radiograph of neck	Subglottic narrowing (the steeple sign)	703360
RSV titer	If positive, then diagnosis not croup	86756
Arterial blood gases	Monitoring $PCO_2 > 45$ mm Hg, PO_2 < 70 mm Hg Indicate need for supplemental oxygen	82803
Complete blood count	Assessment of infection	85007
Urinalysis	Determine dehydration	81000

Differential diagnosis:

Foreign body aspiration can affect all ages and is differentiated by a sudden onset, no fever, normal WBC count, and no growth in blood culture. It usually occurs after play or eating.

Epiglottitis affects children aged 1 to 8 years, onset is over several hours, the patient usually is febrile, blood culture is positive for *H. influenzae,* and swollen epiglottis is apparent on x-ray.

Peritonsillar abscess is a febrile process. It affects children age 1 and older, blood culture is positive, and tonsils are swollen and covered with exudate.

Gastrointestinal reflux should be considered if the child has recurrent episodes.

Treatment: The risk of obstruction increases when intubation is attempted, so care should be taken. A tracheostomy setup should be available in the room. The treatment of choice for croup is as follows: (1) cool-mist humidifiers, with or without additional oxygen (not recommended for children who are also wheezing); (2) racemic epinephrine, 0.25 mg in 2.5 mL normal saline nebulization, every 2 to 4 hours for the hospitalized patient; and (3) steroid, either intravenously (IV) or orally (PO) (methylprednisolone [Solu-Medrol] IV, 1 mg/kg every 6 hours, or dexamethasone PO, every 6 hours). Use of nebulized budesonide (2 mg) with oral dexamethasone has been found to be effective.

A child may be treated as an outpatient if there are no signs of dehydration or if PCO_2 and PO_2 are normal. If PCO_2 is greater than 45 mm Hg or PO_2 is less than 70 mm Hg, the child should be hospitalized. Hospitalization is suggested for children who have unreliable caregivers, live far from emergency department facilities, or have persistent symptoms (stridor) after observation for 3 hours.

 Clinical Pearl: Do not use any sedation or respiratory-depressing agents on the child.

It is also important to calm the parents.

Follow-up: Re-examine patient in 2 to 3 days to ensure that there are no signs of infection.

Sequelae: Rarely the disease progresses to the point where intubation or tracheostomy is necessary. For the most part, children recover completely, without any permanent respiratory system damage. Occasionally, bronchitis develops after an episode of croup. When this is suspected, appropriate antibiotic therapy should be instituted.

Prevention/prophylaxis: Children should avoid close contact with other children who exhibit signs and symptoms of croup or bronchitis. Prompt attention to and treatment of respiratory problems can improve outcomes for infants with croup.

Referral: If the disease does not respond to treatment within 1 to 2 days or if there is a worsening of symptoms, a pediatrician should be consulted.

Education: Parents should be taught how to treat a recurrence of a croup attack; they should go outside to expose the child to cold air or go into the bathroom, turn on the hot water, and mist the room. They should also be taught to inform the health care provider of the episode. If the child is in acute distress, they should bring the child immediately to the emergency department.

EPIGLOTTITIS

SIGNAL SYMPTOMS▶ croupy cough, drooling, sore throat, fever

Epiglottitis	ICD-9 CM: 464.3

Description: Epiglottitis is an acute and potentially fatal respiratory infection. Inflammation of supraglottic structures can rapidly cause acute airway obstruction. Epiglottitis is a pediatric emergency, and a physician should be present at all times during the patient's treatment.

Etiology: *H. influenzae* type B (almost always).

Occurrence: Generally in late fall or early winter.

Age: Primarily ages 3 to 7 years; however, *H. influenzae* epiglottitis may occur at any age, including infancy and older childhood.

Ethnicity: Not significant.

Gender: Male-to-female ratio is 3: 2.

Contributing factors: Sore throat is a possible factor.

Signs and symptoms: The parent usually reports a quick onset of fever, sore throat, and difficulty swallowing and breathing. For the most part, no other family members are ill. Auscultation reveals inspiratory and expiratory stridor. The pediatric nurse practitioner can observe nasal flaring and retractions. The pharynx is inflamed, and there is an increased amount of saliva, sometimes resulting in drooling. Some rhonchi may be heard on auscultation. If the disease progresses, increasing cyanosis, air hunger, and progression to coma may occur. A cherry-red, enlarged swollen epiglottis may be visualized, but the nurse practitioner should take care not to induce a laryngospasm when examining the throat.

 Clinical Pearl: Do not use a tongue depressor to visualize throat.

The child may be observed to sit leaning forward, with a hyperextended neck ("sniffing-dog" position).

Diagnostic Tests:

Test	Results Indicating Disorder	CPT Code
Complete blood count	Highly elevated WBC	85007
Blood culture	Usually positive for *H. influenzae* type B	87040
Radiographs of lateral neck	Reveal "thumbprint sign"	70360

Differential diagnosis:

Croup syndrome is generally diagnosed by a barking cough and is usually a nonprogressive disease.

Bacterial tracheitis has symptoms that develop more slowly and nearly always follows a viral infection. There is an accompanying brassy cough.

Pertussis is accompanied by a characteristic spasmodic, whooping cough.

Foreign bodies are differentiated by radiograph or direct inspection of the trachea and larynx.

Retropharyngeal abscess progresses more slowly, and palpation of the posterior wall reveals a fluctuant mass.

Treatment: Swift and careful management should be instituted in consultation with a physician.

 Clinical Pearl: The primary goal is to maintain an adequate airway.

It is imperative to plan treatment in advance. A patent airway should be maintained, and supplies to accommodate immediate intubation should be present with the patient at all times. Skilled personnel prepared to perform airway stabilization and ventilation support (anesthesiologist and otolaryngologist) should be present. The child should be kept calm, preferably in parent's arms. Staff must accompany the child to the radiology department.

Nasotracheal intubation or elective tracheotomy is the procedure of choice after diagnosis. Generally, children are intubated for 2 to 3 days.

Antibiotic therapy includes ampicillin (100–200 mg/kg IV divided into four doses) and chloramphenicol (25 mg/kg IV once daily for neonates; 50–100 mg/kg IV divided every 6 hours in children) until results of sensitivities are available.

Follow-up: One week after discharge from the hospital, the child should return to the primary care office.

Sequelae: Laryngeal obstruction, pneumonia, or cervical lymphadenitis may result from epiglottitis. If the disease progresses untreated, asphyxia and death occur.

Prevention/prophylaxis: Conjugated *H. influenzae* type B vaccine can be given.

Referral: Refer if epiglottitis is suspected. Hospitalize child immediately, and refer to anesthesiologist and otolaryngologist.

Education: Parents should be kept informed of the condition of the child. They should be educated regarding the possible treatment modalities, including intubation and tracheostomy.

EPISTAXIS

SIGNAL SYMPTOMS▶   nosebleed

Epistaxis	ICD-9 CM: 784.7

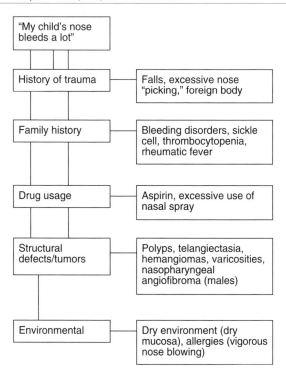

Figure 5–6. Evaluation of epistaxis.

Description: Epistaxis is blood loss from the nose arising from the Kiesselbach area.

Etiology: Commonly occurs as a result of trauma (picking nose) and excessive dryness of the mucous membrane. Less common causes are vascular malformation, hypertension, nasopharyngeal angiofibroma (adolescent boys), and allergic rhinitis (Fig. 5–6).

Occurrence: Common.

Age: Occurs in any age group.

Ethnicity: Not significant.

Gender: Occurs equally in males and females.

Contributing factors: Vigorous nose blowing, allergies, chronic bleeding disorder (von Willebrand's disease, thrombocytopenia), family history of bleeding disorder, other spontaneous blood loss, and aspirin usage.

Signs and symptoms: The child presents with a history of spontaneous nosebleed. The frequency may range from daily to monthly. Obtain a detailed history of the present nosebleed (e.g., trauma, extended use of nasal sprays containing phenylephrine, type of home heating system, nasal insertion of a foreign body, duration of nosebleed). Obtain a family history of bleeding disorders or illnesses such as rheumatic fever and sickle cell disease. Ask about color of stools (tarry stools indicate that the bleeding did not occur recently). On examination, the anterior portion of the nasal septum has a red, raw surface with crusts. Observe for the presence of a foreign body or polyps. Evaluate the Kiesselbach area for telangiectasia, hemangiomas, or varicosities (structural defects). Observe the color and character of the nasal mucosa to determine allergic rhinitis.

Diagnostic tests:

Test	Results Indicating Disorder	CPT Code
Hematocrit (as baseline and 5–12 hours after nosebleed)	Assess for anemia	85104

If there is a family history of bleeding disorder, easy bleeding, other spontaneous loss of blood, a nosebleed lasting more than 30 minutes, onset of nosebleed before age 2 years, or a drop in hematocrit after a nosebleed, obtain a hematologic workup.

Differential diagnosis:

In allergic rhinitis, rubbing, picking, and itching of the nose because of boggy, inflamed mucosa predispose patients to nosebleeds.

If the patient has a history of easy bleeding after lacerations or surgical procedures, together with family history of bleeding tendencies, an in-depth evaluation for a chronic bleeding disorder is indicated.

Treatment: If the child is having an active nosebleed, he or she should sit with head down, pinch nose at site for 10 minutes, then reapply pressure if bleeding is not stopped.

 Clinical Pearl: Use of cautery is contraindicated because of possible destruction of the septal tissue.

Remove any foreign bodies if identified. If simple anemia is present, treat with an iron supplement, 3 mg/kg per day, before breakfast for 2 months.

Follow-up: The patient should return in 6 to 12 hours for a follow-up hematocrit. If the patient is anemic and placed on iron therapy, re-evaluate hematocrit level in 2 months.

Sequelae: Mild anemia; less than 5% of children have a bleeding disorder.

Prevention/prophylaxis: Parent or patient should apply petroleum jelly daily until 5 days elapse without a nosebleed occurring, then weekly for 1 month; avoid giving aspirin; discourage vigorous blowing or picking of the nose; and increase humidity in patient's room in dry climates.

Referral: In cases of recalcitrant nosebleeds or a suspected bleeding disorder, refer to a primary care physician or otolaryngologist. To induce vasoconstriction, apply a pledget soaked with 0.25% phenylephrine nose drops; 1% lidocaine with 1:1000 epinephrine inserted into the nose is usually effective. The most potent vasoconstricting agent is 1% cocaine, but this is rarely used.

Education: Instruct parents in home techniques to stop bleeding. Caution parents about the causes of nosebleeds, such as insertion of foreign bodies and rubbing or picking the nose. Instruct parents as to measures to increase humidity in the home (e.g., using a vaporizer, simmering water on the stove). Parents should avoid giving the child aspirin. Reassure parents that the amount of blood loss always appears to be greater than what is actually lost; a normal hematocrit is comforting to parents.

FOREIGN BODIES IN THE NOSE

SIGNAL SYMPTOMS▶   odor emanating from nostrils

Foreign body in the nose	ICD-9 CM: 932

Description: A foreign body inserted into the nose can obstruct the nasal passage.

Etiology: The most common objects inserted are buttons, beans, nuts, and marbles.

Occurrence: Common.

Age: Usually children age 3 to 6 years.

Ethnicity: Not significant.

Gender: Occurs equally in males and females.

Contributing factors: The natural curiosity of the 3- to 6-year-old child and improper storage of objects most likely to be inserted.

Signs and symptoms: The child presents to the clinic with a history of known insertion of a foreign object (parent or caregiver saw the activity), the "nose smells," or abnormal sounds are heard on respiration. Often the first indication is a unilateral, purulent, foul-smelling rhinitis, with occlusion of the nasal passage. Inspection reveals the presence of a foreign body.

Diagnostic tests: None.

Differential diagnosis: None.

Treatment: Removal of the object. If child is cooperative, the pediatric nurse practitioner may attempt to remove the object by having the child vigorously blow nose while leaning over a basin to reduce risk of aspiration and irrigating the contralateral nasal passage with normal saline solution. The overflow of the solution into the closed passage often brings the object out. If any space around the object can be seen, insert a no. 8 balloon catheter past the object, inflate the catheter balloon, and gently remove the catheter, extracting the object. Treat inflammation or infection with amoxicillin, 40 mg/kg per day in three divided doses for 10 days.

Follow-up: None for simple removal with no evidence of infection. If infection is present, the patient should return in 10 days for evaluation of therapeutic response.

Sequelae: None.

Prevention/prophylaxis: Instruct the child not to insert anything into bodily orifices.

Referral: Refer to primary care physician or otolaryngologist if object is not easily removed or child is unable to cooperate.

Education: Instruct parents as to the proper storage of offending objects.

HEARING LOSS

SIGNAL SYMPTOMS▶ diminished hearing

Hearing loss	ICD-9 CM: 389
Conductive	ICD-9 CM: 389
Sensorineural	ICD-9 CM: 389.10

Description: Normal hearing ranges from 0 (threshold of hearing) to a 120-dB hearing loss, which is the threshold for pain. The following are hearing loss values for children:

Amount of Hearing Loss	Hearing Loss Value
Normal threshold for hearing	0–5 dB Hz
Minimal loss	≤25 dB Hz
Mild loss	25–40 dB Hz
Moderate loss	40–55 dB Hz
Moderately severe loss	55–70 dB Hz
Severe loss	70–90 dB Hz
Profound loss	>90 dB Hz

The two mechanisms are:

- Conductive—caused by a problem in the external or middle ear
- Sensorineural—caused by a problem medial to the stapes, inner ear, auditory nerve, or brain

Any hearing loss lasting up to 72 hours is classified as acute; any hearing loss lasting more than 72 hours is classified as chronic.

Etiology: Conduction abnormality resulting from middle ear disease, congenital infections such as rubella, perinatal complications such as kernicterus, or genetic deafness (mutations in the connexin 26 gene transmitted as an autosomal ressive).

Occurrence: Hearing loss is common: 1 to 2:1000 full-term infants at birth and 1% to 3% of all premature infants. Of cases, 33% to 50% have a genetic basis. Sensorineural loss is more common if hearing loss becomes more severe.

Age: All age groups.

Ethnicity: Not significant.

Gender: Occurs equally in males and females.

Contributing factors: Recurrent otitis media, chronic exposure to excessive noise either job related or through recreational activities (e.g., listening to music, recreational shooting of firearms).

Signs and symptoms: The parent may bring the child to the clinic at age 12 to 18 months with the complaint, "He is not talking like my other children"; alternatively the hearing loss may be discovered at a regular well-baby visit or as a result of testing because of otitis media. The child may complain that the ear is painful or feels full. History should include questions regarding family history of hearing loss; noise exposure associated with work or recreation; and past medical history, including medications, head trauma, history of flying or diving, and recurrent otitis media. If the hearing loss is acute, a prior viral infection or episodes of otitis media may be the cause.

Typical auditory symptoms found in conductive hearing loss include otalgia and otorrhea, which are compatible with the findings of either otitis externa or otitis media. The sensation of aural fullness is associated with otitis media and eustachian tube dysfunction. Fluctuation in hearing intensity is noted with otitis media, eustachian tube dysfunction, and genetic forms of hearing loss. Tinnitus and vertigo are noted less frequently; hyperacusis is not noted in conductive loss.

In sensorineural hearing loss, otalgia and otorrhea are absent; sensation of aural fullness and hearing fluctuation are present in mild forms. Sound sensations are overly loud and uncomfortable; the sensation of different pitches of the same tone (hypercusis and dipacusis) is strongly evident in sensorineural hearing loss.

Examination of the ear, external canal, and tympanic membrane (TM) may reveal cerumen in the canal, otitis externa, or otitis media. Pneumatic otoscopy may be helpful in establishing the diagnosis of tympanic immobility. Perforation of the TM may be noted.

Diagnostic Tests: Diagnostic testing should begin in the newborn nursery and at each well-baby visit. Most of these tests require a licensed audiologist.

Behavioral observational audiometry should be done at all visits during the regular physical examinations from birth to age 3 years. The bell is rung, and the observer watches for the reaction from the infant. By age 4 months, the child should turn the head toward the sound.

Office tympanograms can assist in determining the presence of effusion and eustachian tube dysfunction. Office audiometry can provide basic screening, identify a need for referral, and enhance effective treatment.

The Rinne test and the Weber test, using a 512-cycle tuning fork, can be performed on older children; these tests are not reliable in young children. The Rinne test, which evaluates air and bone conduction, is positive when air conduction of sound elicited from a 512-Hz tuning fork is twice as long as bone conduction. The Weber test for unilateral hearing loss is sensitive because sound localizes to the ear with the conductive hearing loss.

Differential Diagnosis: Examine the ear for underlying cause, such as otitis media with effusion or otitis externa with swelling that occludes the ear canal.

Treatment:

Nonpharmacologic
Remove the impacted cerumen, if indicated.

Pharmacologic
Treat the otitis media.

Follow-up: Return to clinic in 10 days for evaluation of otitis and for hearing reassessment.

Sequelae: Acute hearing loss resulting from head trauma or ototoxic drugs is irreversible. Progressive hearing loss occurs if hearing loss is not detected and treated early (e.g., if cause is recreational or work related, such as in situations with continuous exposure to loud sounds). Loss of communication occurs as a result of hearing loss.

Prevention and prophylaxis: Genetic counseling, improved prenatal care, prompt treatment of otitis media, and wearing ear plugs if hearing loss is work related.

Referral: Refer any suspicion of a sensorineural loss to an audiologist for definitive testing. Refer to primary care physician and otolaryngologist for definitive diagnosis, testing (audiologist), and treatment. Some children benefit from the use of hearing aids or cochlear implants. Refer parents to a parent-centered program for the hearing impaired and to a support group.

Education: Teach parents what behaviors to watch for to assess hearing loss, such as the child turning a radio or TV very loud or speaking in a loud voice or the child's failure to hear when being spoken to in a normal tone of voice.

OTITIS EXTERNA

SIGNAL SYMPTOMS▶   painful itchy ear canal

Otitis externa, acute	ICD-9 CM: 380.10
Otitis externa, chronic	ICD-9 CM: 380.23

Description: Otitis externa is an inflammation of the skin lining of the ear canals accompanied by swelling, pain, and itching; there is no hearing loss until the canal is occluded. There are four categories:

- Localized—an infected nodule is noted on the skin; it may be a furuncle or a boil
- Generalized—infection involves the entire ear canal
- Acute—tenderness is noted on traction of the pinna or pain on pressure over the tragus; patient may have regional lymphadenopathy
- Chronic—ear canal is dry, pruritic, not tender; cerumen is absent, and there may be some erythema of the skin.

Etiology: Conversion of the pH from acid to alkaline in the ear canal, trauma to the canal, contact dermatitis, or irritation from chronic drainage from a perforated TM. Localized, usual agent is *S. aureus*; generalized, usual agent is *Pseudomonas aeruginosa*; chronic, usually caused by a fungus.

Occurrence: Common, seen more often during the summer months.

Age: All age groups.

Ethnicity: Not significant.

Gender: Occurs equally in males and females.

Contributing factors: Contributing factors include use of hair sprays and dyes, accumulation of wax in the canal, and increased wetness or moisture in the canal.

Signs and symptoms: The child is brought to the clinic with the complaint of "pain in the ear." History should include the duration of the condition, location and quality of the pain, activities preceding the onset, and home treatment already given. Type of inflammation is categorized as follows:

- Localized—infection is localized, perhaps with purulent, bloody drainage
- Generalized—there may be a foul-smelling discharge and swelling of the canal
- Acute—canal is red and edematous; tenderness on traction of the pinna or pain on pressure over the tragus; regional lymphadenopathy present if disease has progressed
- Chronic—dry canal; skin may be slightly red and edematous, with no ear wax

Diagnostic tests:

Test	Results Indicating Disorder	CPT Code
Culture of ear drainage	Identification of organism	87070

Differential diagnosis:

Cellulitis usually involves the total auricle.

No foreign body is found on inspection of the canal in otitis externa.

TM rupture with drainage is not found on inspection of the canal
and TM with otitis externa.

Treatment:

Nonpharmacologic

Clean exudate from the canal, and insert an ear wick (1/4-inch sterile
gauze or a commercial product).

Pharmacologic

Give acetaminophen for pain.

Give hydrocortisone/acetic acid (V$\bar{o}$Sol) or
hydrocortisone/neomycin/polymyxin B (Cortisporin otic solution
sterile), 5 drops in the affected ear four times daily for 4 days, or
hydrocortisone/acetic acid or hydrocortisone/neomycin/colistin
ear drops (Coly-Mycin), 5 drops in the affected ear four times daily
for 4 days.

Perform ear cleaning and instill antifungal/steroid, 2 drops three
times daily, for 7 to 14 days for fungal infections.

When instilling ear drops, have the patient lie down with ear upward
for 5 minutes, or keep the head bent with the ear upward for 5
minutes.

 Clinical Pearl: Give systemic antibiotics only if there is fever or
lymphadenopathy.

Follow-up: The patient should return to the clinic in 2 days for removal
of the wick and evaluation of therapeutic response.

Sequelae: Allergic reaction to the neomycin in the ear drops.
Untreated, necrotizing otitis externa can result in damage to cranial
nerves and death from sepsis.

Prevention/prophylaxis: The parent or patient should be instructed
to (1) keep objects such as hairpins and swabs out of the ear canal, (2)
wear ear plugs when swimming to keep water out of the canal, and (3)
instill alcohol drops in the ears before and after swimming.

Referral: None except for recalcitrant cases.

Education: Teach children not to pick at their ears, especially with
sharp objects. Teach that the ear is self-cleaning and that poking the ear
with swabs just pushes the wax farther down the canal. Teach children to
wear ear plugs when swimming.

OTITIS MEDIA

SIGNAL SYMPTOMS▶ pain in ear, child may tug at ear, irritability, may
have nausea or diarrhea

Otitis media, acute	ICD-9 CM: 382.9
Otitis media with effusion	ICD-9 CM: 381.40

Description: Acute otitis media is an inflammation of the middle ear characterized by pain, a full or bulging eardrum, or a perforated eardrum with drainage of purulent material. Otitis media with effusion is fluid in the middle ear without signs and symptoms of infection. Otitis media is considered chronic or persistent if there are six episodes by the age of 6 years, five episodes in 1 year, or three episodes in 6 months.

Etiology: Bacterial infections (*S. pneumoniae, H. influenzae,* and *Moraxella catarrhalis* are the most common pathogens), viral infections (influenza A, RSV, coxsackievirus, adenovirus, and parainfluenza virus are the most common), immune reactivity, and allergic rhinitis.

Occurrence: Common. Occurs primarily in winter, but also fall and spring.

Age: Any pediatric age group, but most common from 6 to 36 months and from 4 to 6 years; incidence decreases after 6 years of age. Chronic otitis media is more common in children whose first episode occurred before 1 year of age.

Ethnicity: Otitis media is more prevalent among Native Americans and Alaskan and Canadian Eskimos; it occurs in African-Americans less than in whites. Effusion is more likely to occur in white children younger than age 2 and is more likely to be associated with allergy than infection. It has been suggested there may be a genetic predisposition.

Gender: Males are at greater risk than females.

Contributing factors: Risk is increased in premature infants, children with Down's syndrome, and infants fed in the supine position. Children who attend day care centers, have parents who smoke, and who have a family history of otitis media are also at greater risk. Continuous use of a pacifier has been implicated as a risk factor of increased incidence of otitis media.

Signs and symptoms: The child with acute or recurrent otitis media presents with a complaint of "tugging at ears," ear pain, fever, irritability, and sleep disturbances. Not all children have ear pain; nausea, vomiting, diarrhea, and upper left quadrant abdominal pain may also be evident.

In otitis media with effusion, the child is usually asymptomatic but may exhibit inattentiveness, or older children may complain of "ears being plugged."

Assess and describe the TM for position, mobility (response to positive and negative pressure), color, and degree of translucency.

 Clinical Pearl: When children cry, the TM becomes red.

Acute otitis media: The TM is usually bulging; mobility of the TM is diminished or absent. Abnormal color variations of the TM may be noted as red, yellow, white, or opaque, or the TM may have a cobblestone appearance.

Otitis media with effusion: The TM may be noted to be translucent, with the presence of an air-fluid level or the presence of air bubbles with an amber or bluish fluid, or retracted or convex, opaque with mobility diminished and blurred landmarks.

Diagnostic tests:

Test	Results Indicating Disorder	CPT Code
Tympanometry	Low static admittance (low peak height) indicates effusion Normal peak height but tympanogram that is too wide indicates oncoming or resolving effusion	92567 (impedance testing) 92568 (with acoustic reflex)
Audiometry	Threshold >20 dB in the better ear (threshold may vary by equipment manufacturer)	92551 (screening examination, pure tone only)

Persistent middle ear dysfunction is prognostic for the increased risk of recurrence. Children who have had otitis media with effusion for 3 months should undergo hearing tests.

Differential diagnosis:

- Toothache (examine mouth and tap each tooth to elicit tenderness)
- Foreign body in the ear (found on examination)
- Furuncle in the canal (found on examination)
- Temporomandibular joint dysfunction (pain radiates from jaw to ear)

Treatment:

Otitis Media

Children older than age 2, children without fever, and children with few clinical signs may be managed without antibiotics, with a follow-up examination in 24 to 72 hours.

Antibiotics

Acute otitis media (10–14 days of treatment): Amoxicillin (Amoxil), 40 to 50 mg/kg in three divided doses every 8 hours. Effective against non-β-lactamase, *H. influenzae,* penicillin-susceptible *Streptococcus*. A dosage of 70 to 90 mg/kg/day is recommended for cases of suspected *S. pneumoniae* or resistant *S. pneumoniae.*

Amoxicillin/clavulanate potassium (Augmentin), 45 mg/kg per day based on amoxicillin component in two divided doses for 10 days, has been found to be effective against *H. influenzae, M. catarrhalis, S. pneumoniae, Streptococcus pyogenes, S. aureus, Escherichia coli, Proteus mirabilis,* and *Bacteroides fragilis* and gives β-lactamase coverage.

Higher dosages (Augmentin ES), 90 mg/kg of amoxicillin, 6.4 mg/kg per day of clavulanate in two divided doses for 10 days, seem to be effective against penicillin-resistant strains.

Cefaclor (Ceclor), 40 mg/kg per day in three divided doses, every 8 hours. Effective against *M. catarrhalis, S. pneumoniae, S. pyogenes, E. coli,* and *P. mirabilis* and gives β-lactamase coverage and partial coverage for *H. influenzae* and *S. aureus.*

Cefixime (Suprax), 8 mg/kg per day single dose for children weighing less than 50 kg and younger than 12 years old. For children weighing more than 50 kg and older than age 12, give adult dosage, 400 mg. Effective against *H. influenzae, M. catarrhalis, S. pneumoniae, S. pyogenes, E. coli,* and *P. mirabilis* and gives β-lactamase coverage.

Cefpodoxime proxetil (Vantin), 10 mg/kg per day in two divided doses in children age 2 months to 12 years. Effective against *H. influenzae, M. catarrhalis, S. pneumoniae, S. pyogenes,* and *P. mirabilis* and gives β-lactamase coverage.

Cefprozil (Cefzil), 15 mg/kg every 12 hours in children age 6 months to 12 years. Effective against *H. influenzae, M. catarrhalis, S. pneumoniae, S. pyogenes, P. mirabilis,* and *E. coli* and gives β-lactamase coverage.

Cefuroxime axetil (Ceftin), 30 mg/kg divided twice daily for children younger than age 13; 250 to 500 mg twice a day if older than age 13. Effective against *H. influenzae, M. catarrhalis, S. pneumoniae, S. pyogenes, P. mirabilis, S. aureus,* and *E. coli* and gives β-lactamase coverage.

Erythromycin ethylsuccinate/sulfisoxazole acetyl (Pediazole), 50 mg/kg per day in four divided doses based on the erythromycin component every 6 hours. Effective against *H. influenzae, M. catarrhalis, S. pneumoniae, S. pyogenes,* and *S. aureus* and gives β-lactamase coverage.

Loracarbef (Lorabid), 30 mg/kg per day in two divided doses every 12 hours. Effective against *H. influenzae, M. catarrhalis, S. pneumoniae, S. pyogenes, S. aureus, E. coli,* and *P. mirabilis* and gives β-lactamase coverage.

Omnicef 125/5 cc, 1 tsp every 12 hours for 10 days.

Trimethoprim (TMP)/fulfamethoxozole (SMX) (Bactrim, Septra), 8 mg TMP/40 mg SMX daily in two divided doses. Effective against *H. influenzae, M. catarrhalis, S. pneumoniae,* most strains of *S. pyogenes, E. coli, S. aureus,* and *P. mirabilis* and gives β-lactamase coverage.

Trimethroprim hydrochloride oral solution (Primsol Solution), 10 mg/kg/day, maximum dose 400 mg, in two doses for 10 days.

For children in whom there is suspected noncompliance, vomiting, high fever, or concurrent bacterial infections: ceftriaxone, 50 mg/kg intramuscularly, single dose.

Azithromycin (Zithromax): 30 mg/kg × one dose only or 10 mg/kg on day 1, 5 mg/kg per day on days 2 through 5.

Shortened treatment regimens are not recommended for children younger than age 2 years, children with severe or complicated acute otitis media, children with chronic or recurrent acute otitis media, or children who attend day care centers.

Prophylactic treatment is recommended for recurrent acute otitis media if the child has three episodes in 6 months or four episodes in 1 year. Consider antibiotic prophylaxis during high-risk seasons (winter and spring): amoxicillin (Amoxil), 20 mg/kg per day, or sulfisoxazole (Gantrisin), 75 mg/kg per day twice a day.

Analgesics

Acetaminophen may be given for discomfort. Relief for ear pain may be obtained through the use of ear drops containing antipyrine and benzocaine (Auralgan).

Otitis Media with Effusion

Consider a trial of antibiotics (discussed previously).

Otitis media with effusion usually resolves spontaneously in 3 to 4 months. Amoxicillin/clavulanate, 40 mg/kg/day based on the amoxicillin component in three divided doses every 8 hours for 2 to 3 weeks, or clarithromycin (Biaxin), 15 mg/kg per day in two divided doses for 2 to 3 weeks, may be given.

The Clinical Practice Guidelines do not recommend corticosteroids, antihistamines, or decongestants for the treatment of otitis media with effusion.

Follow-up: Have the child return in 48 to 72 hours if there is no improvement. The child should return to the clinic in 10 days to evaluate therapeutic response. (*Note:* Fluid may remain behind the eardrum for 3–4 months before fully absorbed.) Re-evaluate children on prophylaxis at 2- to 3-month intervals for asymptomatic effusion.

Sequelae: Mastoiditis, labyrinthitis, petrositis, facial paralysis, and intracranial complications are all possible sequelae of otitis media and otitis media with effusion. Delayed language skill development may be associated with recurrent or chronic otitis media.

Prevention/prophylaxis: Parents should be taught to prevent otitis media by taking steps to avoid contributing factors: feeding infant in an upright position, keeping child away from day care and sick playmates (or using small day care facilities), and avoiding passive smoke. Mothers should breast-feed children during infancy. Prescribe prophylaxis as noted under Treatment.

Referral: If hearing loss occurs, prophylaxis fails to prevent recurrence, or the child is allergic to penicillins or sulfa drugs, refer to an otolaryngologist for tympanostomy tube evaluation and insertion. Children who fail to respond to medical treatment for otitis media with effusion in 3 to 4 months should be referred to an otolaryngologist for evaluation for tympanostomy tube insertion and evaluation of adenoids. Tonsillectomy is not recommended as a treatment option for otitis media with effusion.

Education: Instruct parents in ways to prevent ear infections: avoiding exposure of the child to passive smoke, not propping bottle, stopping use of pacifiers, keeping child away from sick children, and watching child's swimming habits (child should not dive and should not submerge his or her head in water >2 feet deep). The child may be more comfortable with chest and head elevated at bedtime. Parents should ensure the child takes all the medication, even if there seems to be improvement.

PHARYNGITIS/TONSILLITIS

SIGNAL SYMPTOMS▶ painful throat with postnasal secretions

Pharyngitis/Tonsillitis	ICD-9 CM 465.8

Description: Pharyngitis is an inflammation of the pharynx; the term *tonsillitis* is used when the tonsils are involved.

Etiology: In children younger than age 2, the agent is a virus (e.g., adenovirus, enteroviruses, Epstein-Barr virus, coxsackievirus A); in children older than age 5, the agent is group A streptococcus with an incubation period of 2 to 5 days; and in adolescents, the agents are *Clostridium haemolyticum, Mycoplasma* (10% of adolescents), and gonococcus.

Occurrence: Common; peak incidence is in late fall, winter, and spring.

Age: All age groups.

Ethnicity: Not significant.

Gender: Occurs equally in males and females.

Signs and symptoms: When observing the tonsils, grade enlargement on a scale of +1 to +4. With acute infections, an enlargement of +2 or greater may be expected. Normal enlargement of the lymphoid tissue may be rated +1 or +2.

Bacterial

Infants usually present with a low-grade fever with serous or serous-mucoid rhinitis; toddlers present with a low-grade fever, irritability, anorexia, and cervical adenitis; and adolescents present with a low-grade fever and sore throat. (*Note:* In group A β-hemolytic streptococcus, look for acute onset of sore throat, dysphagia, fever, malaise, vomiting, headache, abdominal pain, cough, and rhinorrhea.)

Findings in bacterial infections include erythematous pharynx, edematous uvula, enlarged tonsils with discrete yellow exudate, petechial stippling with moderate redness of the soft palate, and tender submandibular nodes. If the agent is a strain of streptococcus, there may be a red, finely punctate rash (sandpapery with Pastia's sign) starting on the trunk and spreading peripherally to cover the entire body, characteristic of scarlet fever.

Viral

Viral pharyngitis produces vesicular or ulcerative lesions and rash. There are six types of viral presentations:

- Infectious mononucleosis—exudative tonsillitis, cervical adenopathy, fever, palpable spleen, and presence of 20% atypical lymphocytes or positive mononucleosis test
- Herpangina—herpangina ulcer found on anterior tonsillar pillars and sometimes on the palate and uvula
- Lymphonodular pharyngitis—small, yellow-white nodules in the same distribution as in herpangina
- Hand, foot, and mouth disease—ulcers on tongue and oral mucosa; vesicles on palms, soles, and interdigital areas
- Pharyngoconjunctival fever—exudative tonsillitis, fever, and conjunctivitis
- Rubeola—small white specks (Koplik spots) on examination of the buccal mucosa

Diagnostic tests:

Test	Results Indicating Disorder	CPT Code
Complete blood count with differential	Assess infectious process	85014
Throat swab for rapid strep test Throat swab for culture and sensitivity	Identification of organism	86308 86403– 86406
Mono spot test	Differentiate infectious mononucleosis	86308
Throat culture for gonococcus if child abuse suspected or sexual history indicates participation in orogenital sex	Identify organism	87070
Throat cultures for children on prophylactic penicillin (e.g., children with sickle cell anemia) because of negative throat swabs	Identify organism	87070

Differential diagnosis:

Retropharyngeal abscess has asymmetrical swelling of tonsils, tonsillar fossae, and soft palate; uvula is shifted to opposite side.

Peritonsillar abscess has difficulty swallowing, hyperextension of the head, and possibly a forward bulge in the posterior pharyngeal wall.

Treatment:

Nonpharmacologic

Viral

Give supportive care; force fluids and gargles, soft foods, ices (e.g., Popsicles).

Bacterial

Force fluids.

Pharmacologic

Give analgesics for fever and discomfort.

Viral

Antibiotics are not recommended.

Bacterial

Antibiotics are recommended as follows.

Penicillin V (phenoxymethylpenicillin): Acid-resistant penicillin (Penicillin VK), supplied as tablets, oral suspension, and drops, 15 to 56 mg/kg per day every 8 hours. If patient is allergic to penicillin, erythromycin (macrolide antimicrobial), 30 to 50 mg/kg per day divided every 8 hours.

Azithromycin (Zithromax), 30 mg/kg $\times$ one dose or 10 mg/kg on day 1, 5 mg/kg per day on days 2 through 5.

First-generation cephalosporins:

Cephalexin (Keflex), 25 to 50 mg/kg per day

Cefadroxil (Duricef), 30 mg/kg per day

Second-generation cephalosporins:

Cefaclor (Ceclor), 40 mg/kg per day divided every 12 hours (*Note:* may cross-react with penicillin)

Cefuroxime axetil (Ceftin), 125 to 250 mg twice a day for children younger than 13; 250 to 500 mg twice a day for children older than age 13

Amoxicillin/clavulanate (Augmentin; β-lactam antibiotic with a β-lactamase inhibitor): Amoxicillin 20 to 40 mg/kg per day plus clavulanate 5 to 10 mg/kg per day divided every 8 hours.

Oral suspension: Amoxicillin 125 mg plus clavulanate 31.25 mg/5 mL, or amoxicillin 250 mg plus clavulanate 62.5 mg/5 mL

Tablets: Amoxicillin 250 mg/clavulanate 125 mg, or amoxicillin 500 mg/clavulanate 125 mg (*note:* may cause diarrhea, urticaria).

Child can return to school after 24 hours on antibiotics.

Follow-up: Patient should return in 1 week for assessment of therapeutic response. If caused by streptococcus, repeat throat screen at that time.

Sequelae: Complications include otitis media and peritonsillar abscess; if causative agent is streptococcus, acute rheumatic fever and acute glomerulonephritis (1–4 weeks postinfection) may ensue.

Prevention/prophylaxis: Prompt and complete treatment of infection. If streptococcus is the offending organism, screen and treat other symptomatic family members. Although there is a carrier stage, which is noncontagious and self-limiting, there is no specific test or treatment during this period.

Referral: Consult or refer for suspected peritonsillar abscess. Patients in whom infections continue to develop despite the use of prophylactic penicillin should be referred to an otolaryngologist for possible tonsillectomy.

Education: Stress the importance of increasing fluid intake and of prohibiting the sharing of drinking glasses and eating utensils.

RHINITIS

SIGNAL SYMPTOMS▶ erythematous nasal mucosa with discharge

Rhinitis	ICD-9 CM 472

Description: Rhinitis is an inflammation of the nasal mucosa characterized by congestion and increased nasal secretions. There are two groups of patients: those without associated nasal eosinophilia, who often experience increased symptoms related to changes in temperature and environmental pollutants, and those with associated nasal eosinophilia, who have no history of atopy and have negative skin tests. The latter is less common in children. Symptoms of allergic rhinitis are more severe in the morning.

Etiology: Alterations in nasal mucosa related to immune-mediated conditions, infection, overuse of topical decongestants, irritants, nasal polyps, and ciliary defects have all been suggested as probable causes. Two years of exposure to the allergens are required before child develops clinical symptoms.

Occurrence: Occurs in 40% of children younger than age 6 years.

Age: After ages 4 to 5.

Ethnicity: Not significant.

Gender: Occurs equally in males and females.

Contributing factors: Pollens, dust, and molds contribute to the allergic response, as well as smoke and chemical irritants.

Signs and symptoms: The child is brought to the clinic with the complaint of a "runny" nose. History should include onset, severity, type of nasal secretion, and the identification, if possible, of precipitating factors. Past and current medical history, including medications, should be obtained. Note the pattern of onset, season of the year, and time of day. Ask about family history of allergies and other allergic manifestations. Past history may include a history of recurrent epistaxis.

Inspection reveals a boggy, edematous nasal mucosa with a large amount of clear drainage. Pale mucous membranes with swollen turbinates are observed obstructing the nasal passage. Eyes may be watery, and the sclera and conjunctiva may be red. Purulent secretions indicate secondary infection. There are usually dark shadows under the eyes ("allergic shiners") and a transverse crease over the bridge of the nose (from the "allergic salute"). Other findings on physical examination include a high, arched palate; a geographic tongue; and mouth breathing.

Diagnostic tests:

Test	Results Indicating Disorder	CPT Code
Nasal smear for eosinophils	Elevated in allergic responses	89109
Allergy testing, radioallergosorbent testing (RAST)	Identify specific allergan	95010–95199

Differential diagnosis:

Purulent rhinorrhea suggests sinusitis; can be confirmed by changes on radiographic films.

Congenital abnormalities are usually observed during the neonatal period.

Foreign bodies are usually unilateral, with a bloody, purulent discharge.

Nasal polyps are uncommon in childhood.

Nonallergic rhinitis with eosinophilic syndrome has a negative family history of atopy, negative skin tests, and adult onset.

Vasomotor rhinitis is similar to nonallergic rhinitis, having autonomic nervous system imbalance as a suggested cause.

Treatment:

Nonpharmacologic

Environmental control should be exercised, avoiding or limiting contact with irritants.

Pharmacologic

Natural remedies: Many herbs and vitamin products have been suggested for use in allergic rhinitis. Ask caregiver what over-the-counter products they have been treating the child with before coming to the clinic.

Antihistamines: Use of sustained-release antihistamines is not recommended for children younger than age 7. Use the smallest dose that relieves symptoms. If the first drug used is not effective, switch drug classes.

Alkylamines: (1) chlorpheniramine maleate (Chlor-Trimeton), 0.35 mg/kg per day in four divided doses; (2) brompheniramine maleate (Dimetane), 0.5 mg/kg per day in three to four divided doses for children younger than age 6; for children older than age 6, 4 mg every 4 to 6 hours

Ethanolamines: (1) clemastine fumarate (Tavist-D Tablets), 1.34 to 2.68 mg (1–2 tablets) every 12 hours; (2) diphenhydramine hydrochloride (Benadryl), 4 to 6 mg/kg per day every 6 to 8 hours; (3) loratadine (Claritin), 10 mg/10 mL (>6 years old, 2/3 tsp per day; >12 years old, 10-mg chewable tablet daily); (4) cetirizine (Zyrtec), 10 mg once daily for children older than age 12; (6) fexofenadine hydrochloride (Allegra), 30 mg twice daily in children 6 to 11 years old

Nasal sprays: (1) cromolyn nasal sprays, in a metered nasal spray, 1 to 2 sprays twice daily; (2) topical nasal steroids, for use in resistant cases of allergic rhinitis or rhinitis medicamentosa (prescribe for 1–3 weeks); (3) Nasacort AQ 1 spray each nostril once a day; (4) flunisolide (Nasalide or Nasarel); mometasone (Nasonex), 1 spray two times a day for children 12 years old and older; budesonide (Rhinocort or Rhinocort Aqua), 2 sprays in each nostril two times per day or 4 sprays in each nostril 1 time per day for children older than 6.

Decongestants: Administer when antihistamine therapy is inadequate. Pseudoephedrine hydrochloride, 4 mg/kg per day in four divided doses.

Immunotherapy if positive testing has shown that the disease is an IgE-mediated allergy and environmental control measures have been taken. Immunotherapy is contraindicated if child has severe asthma, is immunosuppressed, has a malignancy, is younger than 5, or is being treated with topical β-blockers.

Follow-up: Patient should return in 1 week for assessment of therapeutic response.

Sequelae: Overuse of nasal decongestants can cause rhinitis medicamentosa, characterized by dry, sore nasal mucosa. Children often develop asthma.

Prevention and prophylaxis: To identify precipitating factors, have the family perform an environmental survey of heating system, presence of pets, carpeting, and exposures to noxious substances. Have the family avoid or limit the child's exposure to these factors.

Referral: Refer to primary care physician or an allergist for allergy testing.

Education: Instruct the family in methods of reducing allergens in the home: changing pillows, covering mattress and pillows with plastic, eliminating rugs in the bedroom, daily damp mopping of floors, and avoiding contact with pets and other precipitating factors. Instruct patient in the proper method of using nasal sprays.

SINUSITIS

SIGNAL SYMPTOMS pain over sinuses

Sinusitis	ICD-9 CM 473.9

Description: Sinusitis is an acute inflammation of the paranasal sinuses, most commonly the ethmoid and maxillary sinus.

Etiology: The infective agents most commonly identified include *S. pneumoniae, H. influenzae, M. catarrhalis,* and β-hemolytic streptococcus; viruses have been isolated in 10% of cases.

Occurrence: Common.

Age: Occurs in the ethmoid sinus after age 6 months, the maxillary sinus after age 1, and the frontal sinuses after age 10.

Ethnicity: Not significant.

Gender: Occurs equally in males and females.

Contributing factors: Edematous obstruction of the nasal ostia, decreased ciliary action in the paranasal sinuses, and increased mucus production promote the development of retention of secretions leading to sinusitis. Local factors that contribute are allergic rhinitis, upper respiratory infection, overuse of topical decongestants, nasal polyps, tumors, foreign bodies, swimming and diving, dental extractions, and cigarette smoke.

Signs and symptoms: The parent and child present with a complaint such as, "The cold won't go away, and the nasal drainage is green." The detailed history of the present illness should include time of onset, duration of symptoms, and change in symptoms. Usually the pediatric nurse practitioner discovers that the present illness has existed for 7 to 10 days as a "cold," with nasal discharge, postnasal drip, and a daytime cough. Often there has been a low-grade fever. Older children may complain of a headache or a sense of fullness in the head.

Findings may include halitosis (if a morning visit), painless periorbital swelling, and tenderness when the facial areas are palpated or percussed (older children). Location of the pain indicates specific sinus: ethmoid, retro-orbital, maxillary, upper malar or zygomatic, frontal, or over the eyebrows. In children older than 10, transillumination of the maxillary and frontal sinuses reveals clouding. Examination of the nares reveals injected mucosa with purulent drainage. Nasal patency is tested by compressing one side of the nostril and having the child blow through the nose. Examination of the throat reveals an exudate in the area of the tonsillar pillars. An examination of the chest may reveal wheezing in children with reactive airway disease.

Diagnostic tests:

Test	Results Indicating Disorder	CPT Code
Radiographic studies are not done routinely but are indicated if there is facial swelling with an unknown cause, acute sinusitis not responsive within 48 hours, or chronic or recurrent sinusitis of at least 3 months' duration. A Waters view (occipitomental) for the maxillary sinus is usually sufficient. Other views are the Caldwell view (anteroposterior) for the frontal and ethmoid maxillary and the submental-vertex and lateral views for the sphenoidal	Positive findings in children >1 year old show opacities of the involved sinus, air/fluid levels, or a mucosal thickening of >5 mm. These findings may also be present in children with colds or nasal allergies	71210–70220

Transillumination of the sinuses is not a reliable diagnostic tool.
If there are complications or the patient is immunocompromised, consider a sinus aspiration for diagnostic purposes.
In chronic sinusitis, evaluate for allergies, immune defects, and cystic fibrosis.

Differential diagnosis:

Viral upper respiratory infection resolves spontaneously.
Group A streptococcal infection is differentiated by a positive streptococcus test.
Cystic fibrosis may be ruled out by a negative sweat test.
Foreign body in the nose may be ruled out by tests of nasal patency and radiographic studies.
Dental infections may be ruled out by an inspection of the mouth and by tapping each tooth to evaluate tenderness.

Treatment:

Nonpharmacologic

Parents may restore moisture to the air by running a vaporizer; they may also place warm washcloths on the child's face. Always ask what the parent has been "doing" because they often are using herbal or complementary therapy and these have not been found to be efficacious, although some agents are undergoing study. Saltwater nose drops (1/4 tsp salt to 8 ounces boiled water) can be used.

Pharmacologic

Analgesics are given for pain.
Antibiotics are recommended as follows.

If the child is younger than 2, does not attend day care, and has not recently been treated with an antibiotic:

Amoxicillin (Amoxil), 45 mg/kg per day in two divided doses or 90 mg/kg per day in two divided doses for 10 days

If the child is allergic to amoxicillin:

Cefdinir, 14 mg/kg per day in one dose or

Cefuroxime, 30 mg/kg per day in two divided doses or

Cefpodoxime, 5 mg/kg twice daily (if allergic reaction was not a type I hypersensitivity reaction)

Clarithromycin, 15 mg/kg per day in two divided doses or

Azithromycin, 10 mg/kg per day on day 1, 5 mg/kg per day for days 2 through 5 (subject to Food and Drug Administration approval for treatment of sinusitis)

In children known to have a penicillin-resistant *S pneumoniae,* give clindamycin, 30 to 40 mg/kg per day divided into three doses.

If the child does not improve within 48 to 72 hours, attends day care, or has recently been treated with an antibiotic:

Amoxicillin/clavulanate, 80 to 90 mg/kg per day of amoxicillin and 6.4 mg/kg per day of clavulanate in two doses

Other antibiotics include cefdinir, cefuroxime, and cefpodoxime

The efficacy of decongestants has not been established.

 Clinical Pearl: Do not use antihistamines unless the child has allergies because antihistamines slow the movement of secretions.

Follow-up: The patient should return to the clinic in 48 hours if there is no improvement with therapy; otherwise, the patient should return in 2 weeks for evaluation of therapeutic response.

Sequelae: Chronic or recurrent sinusitis may develop in some patients. The most frequent cause is allergic rhinitis, but this sequela may also be caused by structural defects, such as a deviated septum, a nasal polyp, or a foreign body, or by diving into water feet first. Orbital cellulitis may occur if infection spreads into the orbit through the sinus wall.

Prevention/prophylaxis: Prevention of spread of upper respiratory infection by proper hand washing. The use of steam or saline reduces secretions and improves mucociliary clearance, producing a mild decongestant effect. The patient should avoid swimming and diving during the treatment period, avoid exposure to smoke-filled rooms, and stop smoking.

Referral: Patients with chronic or recurrent sinusitis not caused by diving or allergies should be referred to an otolaryngologist. Refer patient to a primary physician or otolaryngologist if an orbital cellulitis is suspected.

Education: Instruct the parents to run a vaporizer to add moisture to the air. Application of a warm, wet washcloth over the face may relieve some of the discomfort. The child is not to swim or dive during the duration of treatment. If the child smokes, emphasize the importance of stopping smoking.

REFERENCES

Concussion

American Academy of Pediatrics, Committee on Injury and Poison Prevention and Committee on Sports Fitness: In-line skating injuries in children and adolescents (RE9739). Pediatrics 101:720, 1998.

American Academy of Pediatrics, Committee on Quality Improvement: The management of minor closed head injury in children. Pediatrics 104:1407, 1999.

American Academy of Pediatrics, Committee on Sports Medicine and Fitness: Injuries in youth soccer: A subject review. Pediatrics 105:659, 2000.

Kushner, D: Concussion in sports: Minimizing the risk for complications. Am Fam Physician 64:1007, 2001.

Perriello, V, and Barth, J: Sports concussions: Coming to the right conclusions. Contemp Pediatr 2:132, 2000.

Sotier, C: Complications of mild traumatic brain injury. ADVANCE for NP 9:42, 2001.

Craniosynostosis

Rohan, A, et al: Infants with misshapen skulls: When to worry. Contemp Pediatr 2:47, 1999.

Head Trauma

American Academy of Pediatrics, Committee on Injury and Poison Prevention: Bicycle helmets. Pediatrics 108:1030, 2001.

American Academy of Pediatrics, Committee on Injury and Poison Prevention and Committee on Sports Medicine and Fitness: Trampolines at home, school, and recreational centers (RE9844). Pediatrics 103:1053, 1999.

American Academy of Pediatrics, Committee on Injury and Poison Prevention: All-terrain vehicle injury prevention: Two-, three-, and four-wheeled unlicensed motor vehicles (RE9855). Pediatrics 105:1352, 2000.

American Academy of Pediatrics, Committee on Quality Improvement: The management of minor closed head injury in children. Pediatrics 104:1407, 1999.

Feldman, K, et al: The cause of infant and toddler subdural hemorrhage: A prospective study. Pediatrics 108:636, 2001.

Schutzman, S, et al: Evaluation and management of children younger than two years old with apparently minor head trauma: Proposed guidelines. Pediatrics 107:983, 2001.

Macrocephaly

United States National Library of Medicine: Multiple congenital anomaly/mental retardation (MCA/MR) syndromes. Updated 1999.

Microcephaly

Bostwick, H, et al: Celiac disease presenting with microcephaly. J Pediatr 138:138, 2001.

Vargas, J, et al: Congenital microcephaly: Phenotypic featues in a consecutive sample of newborn infants. J Pediatr 139:210, 2001.

Cervical Lymphadenitis

Ferrer, R: Lymphadenopathy: Differential diagnosis and evaluation. Am Fam Physician 58:1313, 1998.

Habermann, T, and Steensma, D: Lymphadenopathy. Mayo Clin Proc 75:723, 2000.

Torticollis

Cheng, J, et al: Clinical determinants of the outcome of manual stretching in the treatment of congenital muscular torticollis in infants: A prospective study of eight hundred and twenty-one cases. J Bone Joint Surg Am 83:679, 2001.

Cheng, J, et al: Sternocleidomastoid pseudotumor and congenital muscular torticollis in infants: A prospective study of 510 cases. J Pediatr 134:712, 1999.

Aphthous Stomatitis

Barrons, R: Treatment strategies for recurrent oral aphthous ulcers. Am J Health-Syst Pharm 58:41, 2001.

CFM (44-10): Taking care of canker sores. Clinical Advisor 5:75, 2002.

Hartmann, R: Ludwig's angina in children. Am Fam Physician 60:109, 1999.

McBride, D: Management of aphthous ulcers. Am Fam Physician 62:149, 2000.

Shashy, R, and Ridley, M: Aphthous ulcers: A difficult clinical entity. Am J Otolaryngol 21:389, 2000.

Glossitis

Kelsch, R: Geographic tongue. Emed, Feb 27, 2002.

Herpes Simplex Stomatitis

Nadelman, C, and Newcomer, V: Herpes simplex virus infections: New treatment approaches make early diagnosis even more important. Postgrad Med 107:189, 2000.

Thrush

Brent, N: Thrush in the breasfeeding dyad: Results of a survey on diagnosis and treatment. Clin Pediatr (Phila) 40:503, 2001.

Nadelman, C, and Newcomer, V: Herpes simplex virus infections: New treatment approaches make early diagnosis even more important. Postgrad Med 107:189, 2000.

Chalazion

Carter, S: Eyelid disorders: Diagnosis and management. Am Fam Physician 60, 1998.

Conjunctivitis

Alessandrini, E: The case of the red eye. Pediatr Ann 29:112, 2000.

Altemeier, W: The importance of adenoviral infections in pediatrics. Pediatr Ann 30:439, 2001.

Medical Letter consultants: New drugs for allergic conjunctivitis. Med Lett Drugs Ther 42:39, 2000.

Morden, N, and Berke, E: Topical fluoroquinolones for eye and ear. Am Fam Physician 62:1870, 2000.

Wagner, R (Program Chairperson): Management of conjunctivitis: Mimics and nonbacterial disease. Contemp Pediatr (Suppl):1, 2000.

Eye Injuries

American Academy of Pediatrics, Committee on Injury and Poison Prevention: Fireworks-related injuries to children (RE020004). Pediatrics 108:109, 2001.

American Academy of Pediatrics, Committee on Sports Medicine and Fitness and American Academy of Ophthalmology Committee on Eye Safety and Sports Ophthalmology: Protective eyewear for young athletes (RE930). Pediatrics 98:311, 1996.

Forbes, B: Management of corneal abrasions and ocular trauma in children. Pediatr Ann 30:465, 2001.

Hordeolum
Carter, S: Eyelid disorders: Diagnosis and management. Am Fam Physician 60, 1998.

Nasolacrimal Duct Obstruction
Ballard, E: Excessive tearing in infancy and early childhood: The role and treatment of congenital nasolacrimal duct obstruction. Postgrad Med 107:149, 2000.

Wagner, R: Management of congenital nasolacrimal duct obstruction. Pediatr Ann 30:481, 2001.

Nystagmus
Mills, M: The eye in childhood. Am Fam Physician 60:907, 1999.

Strabismus
Broderick, P: Pediatric vision screening for the family physician. Am Fam Physician 60, 1998.

Clarke, M: The assessment and management of strabismus in childhood. Curr Paediatr 12:269, 2002.

Rubin, S: Management of strabismus in the first year of life. Pediatr Ann 30:474, 2001.

Common Cold
Pappas, D, et al: Treating colds: Keep it simple. Contemp Pediatr 12:108, 1999.

Croup
Bjornson, C, and Johnson, D: That characteristic cough: When to treat croup and what to use. Contemp Pediatr 10:74, 2001.

Consuelos, M, et al: Infantile stridor: An important factor to consider. Pediatr Ann 30:633, 2001.

Ewig, J: Croup. Pediatr Ann 31:125, 2002.

Kaditis, A, and Wald, E: Viral croup: Current diagnosis and treatment. Contemp Pediatr 60:139, 1999.

Rittichier, K, and Ledwith, C: Outpatient treatment of moderate croup with dexamethasone: Intramuscular versus oral dosing. Pediatrics 106:134, 2000.

Epiglottitis
Felter, R: Pediatrics, epiglottitis. Emed, June 5, 2001.

Epistaxis
Weaver, E, et al: Acute epistaxis: A step-by-step guide to controlling hemorrhage. Consultant March:901, 1999.

Foreign Bodies in the Nose
Cox, R: Foreign bodies, nose. eMedicine Journal 2, May 17, 2001.

Hearing Loss
American Academy of Pediatrics, Committee on Preventive and Ambulatory Medicine, and the Section on Otolaryngology and Bronchoesophagology: Hearing assessment in infants and children: Recommendations beyond neonatal screening. Pediatrics 111:436, 2003.

American Academy of Pediatrics, Task Force on Newborn and Infant Hearing: Newborn and infant hearing loss: Detection and intervention (RE 9846). Pediatrics 103, 1999.

Clemens, C, et al: The false-positive in universal newborn hearing screening. Pediatrics 106:e7, 2000.

Cohn, E, et al: Clinical studies of families with hearing loss attributable to mutations in the connexin 26 gene (GJB2/DFNB1). Pediatrics 103:546, 1999.

Feldman, K, et al: The cause of infant and toddler subdural hemorrhage: A prospective study. Pediatrics 108:636, 2001.

Garganta, C, and Seashore, M: Universal screening for congenital hearing loss. Pediatr Ann 29:302, 2000.

Kenna, M: Connexin 26 mutations tied to hearing loss in children. Arch Otolaryngol Head Neck Surg 127:1037, 2001.

Meyer, C, et al: Neonatal screening for hearing disorders in infants at risk: Incidence, risk factors, and follow-up. Pediatrics 104:900, 1999.

Rabinowitz, P: Noise-induced hearing loss. Am Fam Physician 61:2749, 2000.

Otitis Externa

Holten, K: Management of the patient with otitis externa. J Fam Pract 50:353, 2001.

Pray, W: Swimmer's ear: An ear canal infection. US Pharmacist 26, 2001.

Otitis Media

American Academy of Pediatrics, Section on Otolaryngology and Bronchoesophagology: Follow-up management of children with tympanostomy tubes. Pediatrics 109:328, 2002.

American Academy of Pediatrics, the Otitis Media Guideline Panel: Managing otitis media with effusion in young children. Pediatrics 94, 1994.

Bell, E: Antibiotic concentrations at the infection site: Implications for AOM. Infect Dis Child January, 2002.

Cohen, R, et al: One dose ceftriaxone vs ten days of amoxicillin-clavulanate therapy for acute otitis media; clinical efficacy and change in nasopharyngeal flora. Pediatr Infect Dis 18:403, 1999.

Dean, W, and Davison, M: Pediatric hearing loss. Clin Rev 12:60, 2002.

Hoberman, A, and Paradise, J: Acute otitis media: Diagnosis and management in the year 2000. Pediatr Ann 29:609, 2000.

Kenna, M: Otitis media: The otolaryngologist's perspective. Pediatr Ann 29:630, 2000.

Leibovitz, E, and Dagan, R: Pediatric infection: Otitis media therapy and drug resistance: Part 2. Current concepts and new directions. Infect Med 18:263, 2001.

Little, P, et al: Pragmatic randomized controlled trial of two prescribing strategies for childhood acute otitis media. BMJ 322:336, 2001.

Niemelä, M, et al: Pacifier as a risk factor for acute otitis media: A randomized, controlled trial of parental counseling. Pediatrics 106:483, 2000.

Pichichero, M: Acute otitis media: Part I. Improving diagnostic accuracy. Am Fam Physician 61:2051, 2000.

Roddey, O, and Hoover, H: Otitis media with effusion in children: A pediatric office perspective. Pediatr Ann 29:623, 2000.

Wetmore, R: Complications of otitis media. Pediatr Ann 29:637, 2000.

Pharyngitis/Tonsillitis

Hayes, C, and Williamson, H: Management of group A beta-hemolytic streptococcal pharyngitis. Am Fam Physician 63:1557, 2001.

Rhinitis

Buck, M: Intranasal steroids for children with allergic rhinitis. Pediatr Pharmacother 7:5, 2001.

Corren, J: The association between allergic rhinitis and asthma in children and adolescents: Epidemiologic considerations. Pediatr Ann 29:400, 2000.

Guilbert, T, and Taussig, L: Chronic cough in children: When is it serious? Patient Care April 30, 1998.

Hurwitz, M: Treatment of allergic rhinitis with antihistamines and decongestants and their effects on the lower airway. Pediatr Ann 29:411, 2000.

Kulig, M, et al: Development of seasonal allergic rhinitis during the first 7 years of life. J Allergy Clin Immunol 106:832, 2000.

LoBuono, C: Eliminating allergy triggers. Patient Care for the NP April:45, 2000.

Schenkel, E, and Berger, W: Treatment of allergic rhinitis with intranasal steroids and their effects on the lower airway. Pediatr Ann 29:422, 2000.

Thornhill, S: Natural treatment of perennial allergic rhinitis. Altern Med Rev 5:448, 2000.

Vinuya, R: Specific immunotherapy for allergic rhinitis and asthma. Pediatr Ann 29:425, 2000.

Sinusitis

American Academy of Pediatrics, Subcommittee on Management of Sinusitis and Committee on Quality Improvement: Clinical practice guideline: Management of sinusitis. Pediatrics 108:798, 2001.

Hayes, R: Pediatric sinusitis: When it's not just a cold. Clin Rev 11:53, 2001.

Ioannidis, J, and Lau, J: Technical report: Evidence for the diagnosis and treatment of acute uncomplicated sinusitis in children: A systemic overview. Pediatrics 108:e57, 2001.

Chapter 6

CHEST
DISORDERS

APPARENT LIFE-THREATENING EVENT

SIGNAL SYMPTOMS ▶ pathologic apnea in infants greater than 37 weeks' gestation; parent reports infant is found still, lifeless, and cold, sometimes cyanotic, and with stimulation rouses

Apparent life-threatening event   ICD-9 CM: 798

Description: An apparent life-threatening event (ALTE) is a respiratory pause that lasts a minimum of 20 seconds or is associated with bradycardia (heart rate <100 beats/min). Formerly called *near-miss sudden infant death syndrome* (SIDS), ALTE now refers to pathologic apnea that occurs in infants greater than 37 weeks' gestation.

Etiology: The etiology of ALTE is unclear. The condition seems to be related primarily to an unstable or depressed respiratory control system. Also implicated are depressed respiratory chemoreceptors, altered rapid eye movement (REM) sleep, and spontaneous airway obstruction. Of SIDS cases, 2% may be related to sodium channel gene mutations. Increased degranulation of mast cells in an allergic reaction has been suggested. Vertebral artery compression caused by head movement is under investigation.

Occurrence: The incidence of ALTE is not documented, but the incidence of SIDS-related deaths is 1.5 to 2 in 1000 live births per year. Approximately 80% of infants who die of SIDS have no identifiable risk and no history of ALTE. Siblings of infants who had SIDS are at increased risk for SIDS. Also at risk are infants born addicted to cocaine. Premature infants are especially prone to apnea.

Age: SIDS is rare during the first month of life, peaks between 2 and 4 months, then the rate declines.

Ethnicity: Blacks and Native Americans have higher rates of SIDS.

Gender: Occurs equally in males and females.

Contributing factors: Prematurity, congenital heart disease, hypoglycemia, hypocalcemia, electrolyte disorders, anemia, hypovolemia, intracranial hemorrhage, or seizures may be associated with apneic spells. No clear indicators for SIDS have been documented. Prone sleeping, sleeping on soft surfaces, maternal smoking, and overheating have been implicated.

Signs and symptoms: The parent reports that the infant was fine when it was put to bed but was found either not to be breathing at all or "breathing funny," having cool, bluish skin and not reacting to any stimulus. The following are the signs and symptoms seen in the infant with apnea: cessation of breathing, marked pallor or cyanosis, hypotonia, and bradycardia.

Diagnostic tests: There is no test to diagnose ALTE. Tests done to rule out an underlying cause include the following:

Test	Results Indicating Disorder	CPT Code
Pneumogram	Diagnostic for apneic spells	94772
Electroencephalogram	Rule out seizures	95816
Complete blood count with differential	Rule out infection	85007
Electrolyte panel	Rule out disorders of electrolytes	80051
Blood glucose	Rule out hypoglycemia	82947
Calcium	Low level indicates depression of respiratory centers	82310
Radiographic studies of neck	Rule out obstruction	70360
Radiographic studies of chest	Rule out pneumonia	71020
Arterial blood gases (if apnea is severe)	Hypoxia	82803
Pneumogram for premature infants or infants with a sibling known to have SIDS or ALTE	Documentation of apneic spells	94772

The definitive diagnosis of SIDS requires an autopsy, a death scene investigation, and a careful history. Only through postmortem findings can a case of SIDS be distinguished from a death attributable to severe child abuse, infection, inborn errors of metabolism, or accidental suffocation.

Differential diagnosis:

Sepsis is differentiated by fever, elevated white blood cells (WBCs), and progressive illness.

Seizures are differentiated by electroencephalography.

Gastrointestinal reflux resulting in gagging or choking is differentiated by upper gastrointestinal studies.

Metabolic disorders such as hypoglycemia and hypocalcemia are differentiated by serum-specific and urine-specific tests.

Munchausen syndrome by proxy is differentiated by the presence of pinch marks on the nares.

Infanticide is differentiated through investigation of the case and the scene.

Treatment: If a cause is found, treat the underlying cause. Infants with repeated episodes, siblings of two or more infants who died of apnea, symptomatic preterm infants, and infants with severe forms of central hypoventilation may wear an electronic monitor to reassure the parents. The monitor is left in place usually until the infant has been alarm-free for 2 months, but the period may be 9 months. Vigorous stimulation that consists of rubbing the trunk and thumping the feet is indicated during an episode.

 Clinical Pearl: Never shake the infant during an apneic episode.

Follow-up: The infant should be seen at regular (e.g., monthly) intervals, depending on the needs of the family. If no ALTE occurs for 9 months, the monitor can be discontinued.

Sequelae: Infants who have experienced an ALTE requiring vigorous stimulation are at risk of dying. It is estimated that 25% to 30% will die of SIDS.

Prevention/prophylaxis: For sleeping, place the infant on back, rather than on the stomach.

Referral: Refer to the primary care physician for consultation and perhaps admission to the hospital for observation and complete diagnostic evaluation.

Education: Parents should be instructed in cardiopulmonary resuscitation, and they should know the signs and symptoms of apnea.

ASTHMA

SIGNAL SYMPTOMS ▶ difficulty breathing, evidenced by audible wheezing, rapid breathing, or visible distress and restlessness caused by decreased oxygenation of blood

Asthma	ICD-9 CM: 493.9

Description: Asthma, a reversible obstructive airway disease, is characterized by hyperresponsiveness of the trachea and bronchi. Asthma has multiple triggers, but specific causes are often difficult to pinpoint. Although few children outgrow the disease during puberty, they usually experience a remission of symptoms.

Etiology: The specific etiology is unknown; however, there is a strong genetic predisposition.

Occurrence: 12% in the United States.

Age: Of affected children, 30% are symptomatic by age 1 year. Most (70%) have symptoms by 4 to 5 years of age.

Ethnicity: Slightly higher incidence of asthma in African-American children.

Gender: Occurs in 10% to 15% of boys and 7% to 10% of girls. Before puberty, twice as many boys are affected; after puberty, the incidence equalizes.

Contributing factors: Factors that may precipitate asthma include viral infection; allergens, either environmental or ingested; gastroesophageal reflux; emotional stress; and certain medications, specifically aspirin and β-adrenergic blockers.

Signs and symptoms: Obtain a history including when the symptoms began, any factors that preceded the attacks, and the first signs noted. Determine whether there is a familial history of asthma or allergies. Complaints include wheezing, coughing, and dyspnea.

Signs and symptoms depend on whether the attack is acute or insidious. Signs that are generally progressive are cough, dyspnea, shortness of breath, wheezing, restlessness, and irritability. The child has noisy respirations and may have retractions, nasal flaring, and cyanosis. Other more general signs include atopic signs; chronic or serous otitis media; pale, blue-gray, and boggy nasal turbinates; and clear drainage from the nose. Additional signs include atopic dermatitis, tachycardia, and, in chronic and recurrent asthma, barrel chest. High-pitched rhonchi and wheezing are noted on auscultation. Hyperinflation of the lungs is also noted (Fig. 6–1).

Diagnostic tests:

Test	Results Indicating Disorder	CPT Code
Peak flowmeter	<70% of expected baseline	94010–94070
Pulmonary function tests (for children >6 years old)	Decreased lung capacity	78596
Nasal cytology from nasal smear	>10% eosinophil count	89109
Allergy testing	Not to diagnose asthma but to help differentiate allergens that may trigger asthma attack	95010–95099
Chest radiograph	Helps to diagnose chest infiltrates in prolonged or severe attacks	71010

Differential diagnosis:

Bronchiolitis is manifested by predisposition to wheeze; however, children having this problem also have a positive respiratory syncytial virus (RSV) test.

Pneumonia is differentiated from asthma by the presence of fever, elevated WBCs, and a more acutely ill child.

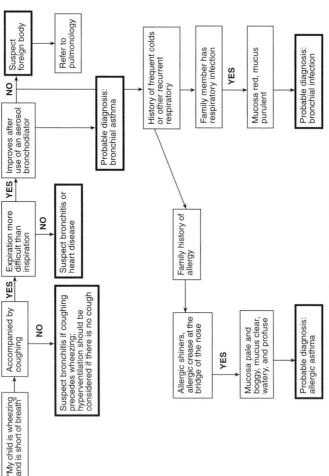

Figure 6–1. Evaluation of wheezing.

Croup is associated with a barking cough and stridor.

Tuberculosis (TB) is differentiated by a positive TB test and lymphadenopathy.

Bronchitis is difficult to differentiate because many symptoms are similar.

Bronchopulmonary dysplasia is generally seen in premature infants and may progress to asthma.

Congenital heart disease may be accompanied by a heart murmur, feeding problems, poor weight gain, and progressive symptoms including digital clubbing.

Treatment:

Nonpharmacologic

Nonpharmacologic treatment includes comfort measures.

Pharmacologic

Inhaled β_2-agonists are commonly used for symptomatic asthma. Theophylline (3–8 mg/kg each night for nocturnal asthma) is also used for most asthma patients. For moderate asthma, cromolyn sodium (2 puffs two to four times daily) is recommended along with an inhaled β-agonist taken three to four times daily. Sustained-release theophylline is recommended to achieve a serum concentration of 5 to 15 mg/mL. Sometimes a short course of oral corticosteroids is also given (2 mg/kg four times a day for 1 week).

A metered-dose inhaler (MDI) or home nebulization machine may be used to deliver β-agonist and cromolyn sodium (Table 6–1). For children younger than 2 years old, a nebulizer or an MDI with a spacer and mask is the most effective method of medication delivery. For children 2 to 4 years old, an MDI with a spacer is the most useful; for children older than 5, MDIs and powdered inhaler preparations are the most effective.

The pediatric nurse practitioner should treat asthmatics in close collaboration with a team of physicians, including a pulmonologist or allergist. For a complete therapy summary, see Table 6–1.

Follow-up: Parents should be instructed to return immediately to the clinic or emergency department if symptoms worsen. Routine follow-up should be scheduled in 1 to 2 weeks initially, then every month for 2 months. After that, a regular schedule should resume for health maintenance.

Sequelae: Possible complications include pulmonary atelectasis, pneumothorax, decreased growth, thoracic deformity, respiratory failure, psychological problems, and death. Children often have poor school performance, difficult relationships with peers, and a low self-esteem. In severe cases, depression and suicidal ideation are seen.

Prevention/prophylaxis: Avoidance of specific triggers, when known, is crucial for all asthmatic patients. Adequate treatment of infections, which can trigger asthmatic attacks, is also important. Getting adequate

Table 6–1 Asthma Medication Therapy Summary: Dosages for Therapy in Childhood Asthma

Medication	Dosage
β₂-Agonists	
Inhaled (*Examples:* albuterol, metaproterenol, bitolterol, terbutaline, pirbuterol)	
Mode of administration	
Metered-dose inhaler	2 puffs q 4–6 hr
Dry powder inhaler	1 capsule q 4–5 hr
Nebulizer solution*	Albuterol 5 mg/mL; 0.1–0.15 mg/kg in 2 mL saline q 4–6 hr; maximum 5 mg
	Metaproterenol, 50 mg/mL; 0.25–0.50 mg/kg in 2 mL saline q 4–6 hr; maximum 15 mg
Oral	
Liquids	
Albuterol	0.1–0.15 mg/kg q 4–6 hr
Metaproterenol	0.3–0.5 mg/kg q 4–6 hr
Tablets	
Albuterol	2- or 4-mg tablet q 4–6 hr
	4-mg sustained-release tablet q 12 hr
Metaproterenol	10- or 20-mg tablet q 4–6 hr
	2.5- or 5-mg tablet q 4–6 hr
Discus	
Advair 100/50	1 inhalation bid
Cromolyn Sodium	
Mode of administration	
Metered-dose inhaler	1 mg/puff; 2 puffs bid–qid
Dry powder inhaler	20 mg/capsule; 1 capsule bid–qid
Nebulizer solution	20 mg/2 mL ample; 1 ampule bid–qid
Theophylline	
Liquid	
Tablets, capsules	
Sustained-release tablets, capsules	Dosage to achieve serum concentration of 5–15 µg/mL
Leukotriene Receptor Agonist	
Accolate	10 mg bid
Singular	4 or 5 mg chewable tablet, once a day
Corticosteroids	
Inhaled†	
Beclomethasone	42 µg/puff, 2–4 puffs bid–qid
Triamcinolone	100 µg/puff, 2–4 puffs bid–qid
Flunisolide	250 µ/puff, 2–4 puffs bid
Pulmicort Torbihaler	200 µg/puff 1 puff bid
Oral‡	
Liquids	
Prednisone	5 mg/5 mL
Prednisolone	5 mg/5 mL
	15 mg/5 mL
Tablets	
Prednisone	1, 2.5, 5, 10, 20, 25, 50 mg
Prednisolone	5 mg
Methylprednisolone	2, 4, 8, 16, 24, 32 mg

* Premixed solutions are available. It is suggested that the "per kilogram" dosage recommendations be followed until symptoms are controlled.

† Use spacer devices to minimize local adverse effects and systemic effects.

‡ For acute exacerbations, doses of 1–2 mg/kg in single or divided doses are used initially and are modified. Reassess in 3 days because only a short burst may be needed. There is no need to taper a short (3- to 5-day) course of therapy. If therapy extends beyond this period, it may be appropriate to taper the dosage. For long terms dosage of oral steroids, the lowest possible alternate-day AM dosage should be established.

rest, eating a balanced diet, avoiding stress, and promptly identifying symptoms can decrease the severity of the disease. A yearly TB test and influenza vaccine are recommended for all patients with asthma.

Referral: Children who have a relapse within 10 days of an asthmatic attack or children who do not respond to initial treatment should be referred to an allergist or pulmonologist.

Education: Educate parents in the use of peak flowmeters and in the early signs of asthma, including breathing difficulty, coughing, wheezing, retractions, and dyspnea. Teach patients and families about potential complications and the signs and symptoms of problems such as severe hypoxia, dehydration, atelectasis, and pneumonia.

Teach parents the importance of giving extra fluids to maintain hydration and liquefy secretions (3000 mL per day unless contraindicated).

Educate parents regarding the purpose, dosage, side effects, and adverse and toxic effects of all medications. Teach families that they must continue medications and never abruptly stop any therapy. If steroid inhalers are used, the mouth should be rinsed to avoid candidiasis.

Teach patients relaxation techniques to improve breathing. Advise patients and families that regular exercise is needed, but that rest periods are also needed.

BRONCHITIS

SIGNAL SYMPTOMS most likely presentation is a persistent cough and cold symptoms that are usually preceded by rhinitis; child usually has a low-grade fever accompanied by substernal pain

Bronchitis	ICD-9 CM: 490.0

Description: Bronchitis is an inflammatory disease of the bronchi characterized by one or more of the following: hyperemia of the bronchial mucosa, increased production of mucus, and inflammatory exudate of mucus and WBCs.

Etiology: Viruses are the most common cause of acute bronchitis. Other common agents are the bacteria *Streptococcus pneumoniae, Haemophilus influenzae,* and *Mycoplasma pneumoniae.*

Occurrence: Seasonable occurrence has been noted, most frequently in the spring and winter.

Age: Not significant.

Ethnicity: Not significant.

Gender: Occurs equally in males and females.

Contributing factors: Exposure to persons with upper respiratory infections (URIs).

Signs and symptoms: There is a report of a dry, unproductive cough beginning a few days after rhinitis (Fig. 6–2). There may also be com-

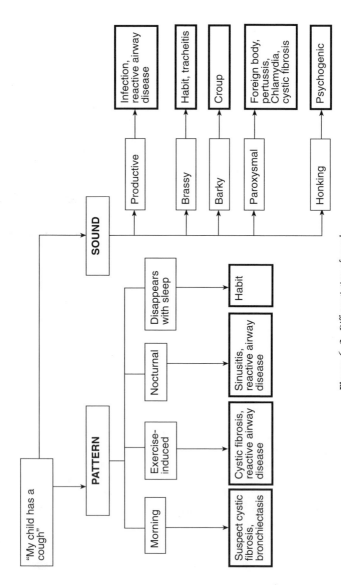

Figure 6–2. Differentiation of cough.

plaints of low substernal discomfort or a burning sensation in the chest. The parent may state that the cough became productive after a few days. Substernal pain aggravated by coughing is also reported. Signs of nasopharyngeal infection, conjunctivitis, and rhinitis are common. There may be fever of less than 101°F. Some shortness of breath can be observed. Chest is clear on percussion. Coarse breath sounds and moist rales are heard in the upper part of chest. Rhonchi may be high-pitched and may be similar to the sounds of wheezing. Bacterial bronchitis is frequently characterized by copious sputum (>2 tbsp a day). Viral bronchitis rarely causes more than 2 tbsp of mucopurulent sputum.

Diagnostic tests:

Test	Results Indicating Disorder	CPT Code
Chest radiograph	Indication of infiltrates	70101
Sputum culture	Only positive in bacterial infections	87999

Differential diagnosis:

Bronchopneumonia is differentiated by radiograph.

TB and other chronic pulmonary diseases are differentiated by skin tests (purified protein derivative [PPD], tine, histoplasmosis tests) and radiograph.

Bronchial asthma is differentiated by symptoms, including marked inspiratory wheezing.

Treatment:

Bronchitis with Production of Less than 2 tbsp Mucoid or Mucopurulent Sputum per Day

Nonpharmacologic

Nonpharmacologic treatment measures include rest and a vaporizer or humidifier for increasing the humidity in the air, making it easier to breathe.

Pharmacologic

Acetaminophen (Children's Tylenol), or ibuprofen (Children's Advil) is indicated for discomfort (see Tables 3–5 and 3–6).

Cough suppressants, such as dextromethorphan hydrobromide, may be used sparingly (30 mg every 6–8 hours orally as needed; 240 mL is enough for 6 days).

Expectorants may be used, although there is debate as to their efficacy. Guaifenesin (Tussi-Organidin NR) is available alone or in combination with cough suppressants; dosage is 200 to 400 mg (100 mg/tsp) orally every 4 hours as needed (comes in 4- and 8-ounce bottles).

Bronchitis with Production of More than 2 tbsp Purulent Sputum per Day (Usually Associated with Systemic Symptoms)

Nonpharmacologic

Nonpharmacologic treatment measures include rest and a vaporizer or humidifier for moisture (this is of most value in winter).

Pharmacologic

Children's Tylenol (325 mg orally, 2 tablets every 4–6 hours) or Children's Advil (200–400 mg orally every 6 hours) is given for discomfort. An expectorant and antibiotic therapy are also indicated. Some suggestions for antibiotics are as follows:

Cephalexin (Keflex) is indicated for treatment of *Escherichia coli,* group A β-hemolytic streptococcus, *H. influenzae, S. pneumoniae,* and staphylococcus. Children's dosage is 6 to 12 mg/kg orally every 6 hours with a maximum dose of 25 to 50 mg/kg every 6 hours.

Amoxicillin is indicated for gram-negative and gram-positive organisms. Children's dosage is 20 to 40 mg/kg orally daily in divided doses every 8 hours.

Ampicillin is used for gram-negative and gram-positive organisms. Dosages are 50 to 100 mg/kg orally daily in divided doses every 6 hours.

Omnicef 125/5, 1 tsp q12 h for 10 days.

Tetracycline is effective against gram-positive and gram-negative organisms. Children older than 8 should be given 25 to 50 mg/kg per day orally every 6 hours.

Trimethoprim (TMP)/sulfamethoxazole (SMX) (Bactrim) is effective for children with penicillin allergy. Dosage is 8 mg/kg TMP and 50 mg/kg SMX orally every 24 hours.

Clarithromycin (Biaxin) is effective against streptococcus and *S. pneumoniae.* Doses are 15 mg/kg per day in two divided doses.

Azithromycin (Zithromax) is effective against *H. influenzae, Moraxella,* staphylococcus, and streptococcus. Dose is 10 mg/kg day 1, then 5 mg/kg daily days 2 through 5.

If chest tightness and wheezing are present, metaproterenol or albuterol inhaler, 2 puffs every 4 hours, should be used. To decrease respiratory problems, avoid bronchial irritants, such as smoke.

Follow-up: Return visit if no improvement occurs in 72 hours, fever increases, or pleuritic pain develops.

Sequelae: Bronchitis can progress to more serious infections, such as pneumonia, but most cases resolve with no future problems.

Prevention/prophylaxis: Avoid contact with persons with URIs.

Referral: Referral should be made if there is significant respiratory distress or failure to improve within 72 hours.

Education: To avoid progression of the disease, parents should be encouraged to report respiratory problems to health care providers. Most of the time treatment is symptomatic; response needs to be monitored. Because bronchitis is usually caused by a viral infection, parents need to understand that antibiotics are not always needed.

CHEST WALL TRAUMA

SIGNAL SYMPTOMS a sudden alteration in oxygenation, which occurs as a result of an accident or injury, that is evidenced by difficulty breathing, intense pain, or death

Chest wall trauma   ICD-9 CM: 959.1

Description: Chest wall trauma, which results in a variety of chest injuries, accounts for 25% of all traumatic deaths. Injuries associated with chest trauma include fractured ribs, pulmonary contusions, pneumothorax, hemothorax, sternal fractures, and widened mediastinum. Aortic rupture, which often accompanies widened mediastinum, is fatal in 80% to 90% of all cases. If three or more adjacent ribs are fractured, "flail chest" may develop. Flail chest impairs the bellows action of the chest, causes intense pain, and affects the child's ability to cough and clear secretions. If a pulmonary contusion occurs, there is a greater risk of impaired oxygenation, and the pulmonary system is compromised. Pneumothorax can result from a blunt or penetrating chest trauma. Occasionally a pneumothorax can develop spontaneously. Pneumothorax can be closed or open; open pneumothorax results from a penetrating chest injury.

Hemothorax, another injury resulting from chest trauma, is defined as a collection of blood in the pleural space, which results from laceration of the chest wall, heart, great vessels, or lung tissues. A hemothorax results in impaired ventilation, but the greatest danger associated with this problem is hypovolemic shock. A sternal fracture, characterized by pain, can result in additional problems, including cardiac arrhythmias, right ventricular impairment, cardiac tamponade, and ventricular aneurysms. A widened mediastinum may result in an aortic tear, which is potentially fatal.

Etiology: Chest wall trauma results from blunt or penetrating injuries. These injuries can be the result of a motor vehicle accident, seat belt injury, stabbing, shooting, crushing injuries, or other forms of trauma.

Occurrence: Although the incidence of chest wall trauma is not available, 25% of all deaths result from traumatic chest injuries.

Age: Any age.

Ethnicity: Not significant.

Gender: Slightly higher in males than females.

Contributing factors: Risk-taking behaviors may contribute to the incidence of chest wall injuries. Abuse should be considered when there is no evidence of accidental injury.

Signs and symptoms: Generally a traumatic incident is reported in which the chest has suffered a penetrating or blunt injury. There may be a report of respiratory difficulty, chest pain, or hemoptysis. The time and type of injury should be elicited, if possible, from either the patient or the person accompanying the patient.

Inspection commonly reveals shallow breathing and splinting of chest. Poor color (cyanotic or pale) and uneven chest expansion are noted. In the case of an open pneumothorax, the pediatric nurse practitioner may feel or hear air escaping from the chest. Bruising, swelling, and bleeding also may be observed.

Touching the patient often elicits a pain response. Swelling at each site of the injury is also noted. Diminished or unequal expansion of the chest, crepitus, or deformity over fracture sites is felt with rib fractures. Right jugular distention and peripheral edema occur with right-sided heart failure. Absent or rapid pulses may be felt.

When a pneumothorax is present, auscultation with the stethoscope often reveals decreased air exchange. Various cardiac and pulse arrhythmias may be noted. Hypotension is present in a tension pneumothorax, whereas tachycardia is present in a hemothorax. Pulmonary rales are often heard; when cardiac tamponade has occurred, muffled sounds are auscultated.

Diagnostic tests:

Test	Results Indicating Disorder	CPT Code
Radiographic studies of chest	Identification of fractures Identification of a pneumothorax	71010
ECG	Irregular cardiac functioning	93000
Arterial blood gases	Indication of need for supplemental oxygen	82803
Hemoglobin and hematocrit	Indication of bleeding	83036

ECG, electrocardiogram

Differential diagnosis: None.

Treatment: Refer patient immediately to a tertiary care setting. The goals of treatment are to maintain satisfactory respiration; stabilize cardiac problems; and treat shock, bruises, contusions, and fractures as promptly as possible. Cover open chest wounds quickly, but allow one side of the dressing to remain slightly open. If the patient shows signs of deterioration, open the dressing completely to allow air to escape, then close dressing with only one side open. A thoracotomy is the required treatment for pneumothorax. Treatment for a hemothorax includes oxygenation, volume replacement, surgical intervention, and chest tube insertion. Providing supplementary oxygen is also a priority. Because this treatment regimen is complicated and requires specialized care, the nurse practitioner should refer the child to a physician in a tertiary care or trauma setting.

Follow-up: All follow-up examinations should be appropriate for the particular injury. Generally an appointment should be made for 2 weeks after hospitalization. Patients should be told to call the health care provider if any changes occur before their appointment date.

Sequelae: Respiratory failure and death can be the result of a simple blunt trauma injury. Pay careful attention to all aspects of the patient's condition. Lingering pain from a rib fracture may persist for several months.

Prevention/prophylaxis: Safety measures can prevent these types of injuries. Seat belt injuries do account for a measurable portion of blunt chest injuries in a motor vehicle accident, however.

Referral: All cases of chest wall trauma should be immediately referred to a tertiary care setting for supervision by a physician.

Education: The importance of safety measures, such as seat belts and child restraints, should be taught to all parents. The dangers of traumatic injuries should be stressed.

CONGENITAL CARDIAC DEFECTS

SIGNAL SYMPTOMS the complexities of these defects make one signal symptom difficult to predict, but cardiac irregularities, either with or without cyanosis, can usually be evidenced by poor growth and feeding patterns of children

Congenital Lesions

Tetralogy of Fallot (TOF)	ICD-9 CM: 745.2
Tricuspid atresia (TA)	ICD-9 CM: 746.1
Pulmonary atresia	ICD-9 CM: 747.3
Truncus arteriosus	ICD-9 CM: 745.0
Transposition of great arteries (TGA)	ICD-9 CM: 745.10

Acyanotic Lesions

Patent ductus arteriosus (PDA)	ICD-9 CM: 747.0
Atrial septal defect (ASD)	ICD-9 CM: 745.5
Ventricular septal defect (VSD)	ICD-9 CM: 745.4
Truncus arteriosus	ICD-9 CM: 745.0
Atrioventricular (AV) canal defect	ICD-9 CM: 745.69

Cyanotic lesions

Pulmonary stenosis (PS)	ICD-9 CM: 745.3
Atrial stenosis (AS)	ICD-9 CM: 747.22
Coarctation of the aorta (COA)	ICD-9 CM: 747.10

Description: Congenital cardiac defects, the most common group of congenital anomalies encountered in infants, are structural abnormalities of the heart. Although all congenital anomalies are present at birth, congenital cardiac defects are recognized any time from the early neonatal period up until later in childhood and in some cases not until adulthood. The severity and type of anomaly usually directly relate to how early it is discovered, with the most severe anomalies being identified at birth or within 48 hours of birth. This coincides with the time necessary for the change from fetal to neonatal circulation.

Congenital anomalies are classified into three categories:

- Cyanotic lesions—TOF, TA, pulmonary atresia, truncus arteriosus, and TGA
- Acyanotic lesions—PDA, ASD, VSD, truncus arteriosus, and AV canal defect
- Obstructive lesions—PS, AS, and COA

Etiology: Chromosomal abnormalities, familial association, a combination of genetic and environmental catalysts, and teratogens. Deficiency of fetal growth or failure of component parts to align or fuse in utero can also cause cardiac defects.

Occurrence: Congenital cardiac defects affect approximately 1% of the North American population. Of that 1%, the specific incidence of defects is as follows. VSD, the most common defect, occurs 25% of the time. Because of the frequency of this disorder, VSD is treated as a separate protocol in this chapter. Other acyanotic defects occur in the following frequency:

- PDA, 12%
- Truncus arteriosus, 2%
- AV canal defect, 2%
- ASD, 10%

Obstructive defects occur in the following frequency:

- COA, 6%
- AS, 5%
- PS, 10%;
- Endocardial cushion defect (ECD), 4%

Cyanotic defects occur in the following frequency:

- TGA, 4%
- TOF, 5% to 9%
- TA, 2%

Age: These are congenital abnormalities present at birth.
Ethnicity: Not significant.
Gender: For the most part, gender is not a factor, but COA and PDA occur in a male-to-female ratio of 2:1. In ASD, the female-to-male ratio is 2:1.

Contributing factors: Prematurity and increased altitude may increase the incidence of PDA. There is an increased incidence of ASD among children with Down's syndrome and Ellis-van Creveld syndrome. Other factors include maternal exposure to certain teratogens, use of addictive drugs including cigarettes, and exposure to certain viruses or illnesses during the prenatal period.

Signs and symptoms: If congenital cardiac defects are evident at birth, there is usually tachycardia and tachypnea or apnea. These signs may be accompanied by hypothermia and feeding or swallowing difficulties with poor intake of fluids. The prenatal history may reveal exposure to rubella or other teratogens, use of medications, illness history, and bleeding during the prenatal period. There may be a positive family history of congenital heart disease. The parents may report repeated gastroesophageal reflux in younger children. Older children may have a history of exercise intolerance, fatigue, and episodes of squatting. Parents may also report that the child frequently sighs. The following is a list of the specific symptoms for individual congenital cardiac defects (Fig. 6–3 and Table 6–2):

TGA:

> Cyanosis from birth
> Dyspnea
> Slow weight gain
> Feeding difficulties

TOF:

> Cyanosis from birth
> Dyspnea with exercise
> Squatting, hypoxia
> Irritability
> Tachycardia followed by weakness and syncope
> Exercise intolerance
> TET spells
> Increased fatigability
> Hypercyanotic spells worsened by crying, defecation, or feeding (age 2–3 months)

AS:

> Mild exercise intolerance
> Chest pain or syncope or both with exertion

Table 6–2   Gradation of Heart Murmurs

Grade 1: Barely audible in quiet room by experienced examiner
Grade 2: Soft, but easily audible; limited radiation
Grade 3: Moderately loud; moderate to wide radiation
Grade 4: Loud; associated with palpable thrill
Grade 5: Audible with stethoscope chest piece in incomplete contact with skin
Grade 6: Audible with stethoscope chest piece 1 cm away from skin

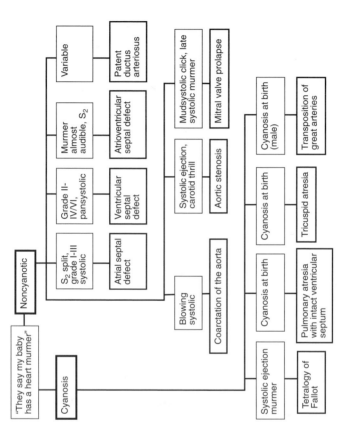

Figure 6–3. Noncyanotic versus cyanotic heart disease.

ASD:

Increased incidence of respiratory infections

Slight physical underdevelopment

Increased fatigue and exertional dyspnea

PDA:

Asymptomatic in newborns

Diaphoresis during feeding

Poor feeding

Falling asleep during feedings

Truncus arteriosus:

Cyanosis

Dyspnea on exertion

Increased fatigability

Occasional hypoxic spells

AS:

Fatigability

Dyspnea

Occasional angina

Syncope

A cardiac thrill or heave is detected in ASD, VSD, PS, and ECD. In COA, pulse rate is decreased in the dorsalis pedis and in the femoral and popliteal areas; the brachial, radial, and carotid arteries have bounding pulses; and increased blood pressure is noted in the arms, with corresponding decreased blood pressure in the legs. In AS, there is a difference between the peripheral pulses (right arm greater than left arm); the skin and mucous membranes may appear cyanotic or pale; and there is a narrow pulse pressure. In TOF, hepatomegaly is present, with an observable sternal lift owing to right ventricular hypertrophy. Also, there is clubbing of the fingers and toes; these digits feel cooler to touch. In TGA, hepatomegaly is noted.

In AS, a systolic ejection click murmur transmits to the neck. In ASD, there is a wide, fixed split S_2, ejection systolic murmur, and a diastolic flow murmur that is best heard at the left lower sternal border. In ECD, there is an abnormally split S_2 and either a diastolic flow murmur at the apex of the heart or a pansystolic murmur. In PS, an abnormally split S_2, a systolic ejection click, and an ejection systolic murmur may be heard over the pulmonic area. In VSD, there is an accentuated S_2, with either a diastolic flow murmur at the apex or a pansystolic murmur heard. In COA, there may be an audible ejection systolic murmur heard over the intrascapular area of the back. In TGA, there is a sharp S_1 and a loud single or narrowing split S_2. In TOF, there is a loud or harsh systolic ejection murmur or a holosystolic murmur at the mid lower sternal border. In truncus arteriosus, there is a grade III–IV/VI harsh, pansystolic ejection murmur in the upper right sternal border. When AS is present and the problem is located at or in the valve itself, an opening snap is heard.

When the lesion is severe, there is a pronounced S_2 split. In PS, there is a grade III–IV/VI harsh murmur in the mid to late ejection phase murmur at the upper left sternal border in the pulmonic region. In severe or pronounced cases, cardiomegaly or hepatomegaly may be revealed when percussion is performed on the abdomen.

Diagnostic tests:

Test	Results Indicating Disorder	CPT Code
ECG	Abnormal results	93000
Chest radiograph	Enlarged heart or portion of the heart	71010
Arterial blood gases	Poor oxygenation or indications of respiratory or metabolic acidosis or alkalosis	82803
Hemoglobin and hematocrit	<10 abnormal	85007
Echocardiogram	Abnormal results	93303

Specific results indicating particular disorders are as follows:

ASD: Chest radiograph reveals cardiomegaly. Abnormal ECG shows a right axis deviation and paradoxical motion of the ventricular septal wall.

VSD: In a small shunt, radiograph reveals few findings. In larger defects, cardiomegaly is noted, the aorta is small to normal, and the pulmonary markings are increased. The ECG is normal in small defects; in larger ones, there is pronounced left ventricular hypertrophy. An echocardiogram reveals defects of 4 mm or greater, generally pinpointing their location.

PDA: If shunt is large, radiograph reveals an enlarged heart; ECG shows left ventricular hypertrophy. Cardiac catheterization shows an increased oxygen saturation near the pulmonary artery.

For any cyanotic defect, the following tests along with an echocardiogram may be useful in diagnosing a problem. A radiograph shows a boot-shaped contour of the heart and increased vascular markings. The ECG is normal at first and later reveals prominent P waves, right axis deviation, or right ventricular hypertrophy. Cardiac catheterization reveals the right-to-left shunt and the size of the defect.

Differential diagnosis:

- For cyanotic heart defects, acyanotic defects
- For acyanotic defects, cyanotic defects
- Functional murmur
- For VSD, peripheral pulmonic stenosis
- Metabolic abnormalities, which can be differentiated by tests to exclude cardiac problems
- Polycythemia, not related to a congenital cardiac defect
- Heart failure during the first few days of life, which is related to

metabolic disorders, thyroid diseases, hypomagnesemia, or hypocalcemia

Treatment: When a congenital cardiac defect is suspected, referral to a pediatric cardiologist is required and should be done as quickly as possible. The following are specific treatment regimens:

ASD: Elective surgery may be performed between ages 2 and 4.

VSD: Small defects generally close on their own; if large, the defect should be closed during the first year of life.

PDA: The ductus arteriosus usually closes spontaneously during the first 2 years of life. In the preterm infant in whom closure is needed, indomethacin (0.1–0.3 mg/kg) is given by mouth every 8 to 24 hours or parenterally every 12 hours with a maximum of three doses. Surgery is done only if the shunt is severe.

TGA: Prostaglandin E_1 (0.05–0.2 mg/kg per minute) is given to delay closure of PDA. Morphine sulfate (0.1–0.2 mg/kg) is given to relax the right ventricle; supplemental oxygen is used. Surgery is necessary, but still considered risky. Closure is sometimes delayed when certain defects (e.g., TGA and COA) require surgery, but the surgery needs to be postponed.

TOF: Instruct the parents to hold the child in the knee-chest position during hypoxic episodes. Surgery (Blalock-Taussig procedure) is done in infants aged newborn to 4 months; this procedure increases the oxygen saturation and the pulmonary outflow, but complete repair is done when the child is 10 kg, or by 9 to 12 months.

AS: Surgery, if performed during the neonatal period, has a high mortality rate. The parents and child need to be cautioned to avoid sports because of the high rate of sudden death associated with these activities.

COA: Surgery, either as an emergency during the neonatal period or electively between ages 2 and 4 years, should be performed. The stenotic area is excised, and the ends of the artery are reanastomosed.

PS: Valvuloplasty is done in a catheterization facility.

Follow-up: When a defect is suspected during the neonatal period, the infant should be referred to a cardiologist for follow-up. Referral is usually done during the first weeks of life or, when the defect is thought to be life-threatening, immediately. Follow-up continues for life; although some problems necessitate monthly visits, others are followed on a yearly basis. If surgery is done, the same follow-up schedule holds true in that rarely does the surgery have to be repeated, although some procedures are done in stages. Routine checkups should be maintained; immunizations should be given as scheduled, including vaccines for pneumonia and influenza.

Sequelae: With early identification, appropriate intervention can be achieved, allowing these children to lead normal lives. Some (e.g., children with severe defects or AS) may not be able to participate in certain sports activities. Occasionally, parents become overly protective, refusing to allow the child to partake fully in activities; an emotional tug of war between the child and parent can result in conflict. For some of the more severe anomalies, death can occur when a child is not treated early or as a result of the intervention (surgery).

Referral: All children with suspected congenital cardiac defects must be referred to a pediatric cardiologist immediately.

Education: Parents need to know what treatments (medication or surgery) are needed and the prognosis of the specific defect. The rationale for various treatment regimens should also be carefully explained to the parents. When necessary, psychological counseling may be recommended for parents and children who are not coping with the diagnosis. Long-term outcomes of the disease should be reviewed at each visit to assess children's and parents' level of understanding.

COSTOCHONDRITIS

SIGNAL SYMPTOMS dull respiratory chest pain, occurs in center of chest, radiating to back and abdomen

Costochondritis	ICD-9 CM: 733.6

Description: Costochondritis is the unilateral inflammation of the costochondral junctures, usually the left side, involving the fourth to sixth ribs. The pain radiates to the back and abdomen. There is either minimal or no swelling. Tietze's syndrome involves the second sternochondral junction at the right sternoclavicular junction, is accompanied by painful swelling at the junctions, and is aggravated by respiratory movement.

Etiology: Unknown.

Occurrence: Common.

Age: School-age children, usually adolescents.

Ethnicity: Not significant.

Gender: Occurs equally in males and females.

Contributing factors: Unknown.

Signs and symptoms: The child presents with a history of chest pain that radiates to the back or abdomen or both. The pain, which varies in intensity, is accentuated by palpation or movement. There is marked tenderness on palpation over the costochondral junctions with minimal or no swelling. The pain is not increased by coughing or swallowing (Fig. 6–4).

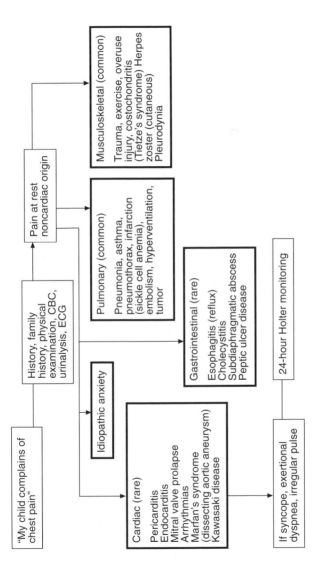

Figure 6–4. Differential diagnosis of chest pain in children and adolescents.

Diagnostic tests:

Test	Results Indicating Disorder	CPT Code
Chest radiograph	Rule out pulmonary or diaphragmatic causes of chest pain	71010
ECG	Rule out cardiac causes of chest pain	93000

Differential diagnosis:

Pericarditis presents with sharp, stabbing chest pain that increases with deep breathing, coughing, swallowing, or twisting of the thorax.

Pleurisy produces sharp pain that increases with deep breathing, coughing, and arm movements.

Slipped rib syndrome is characterized by sudden onset of pain. The eighth, ninth, or tenth rib is usually involved.

Precordial catch (Texidor twinge) causes sharp, shooting pain at the left sternal border or cardiac apex.

Muscle strain or spasm involves the muscles. There is a history of participation in strenuous sports.

Treatment: Analgesics for the discomfort.

Follow-up: None.

Sequelae: None.

Prevention/prophylaxis: None.

Referral: None.

Education: Instruct parents that costochondritis is a self-limiting illness. Reassure the parents and child that the child is not having a heart attack.

HYPERTENSION

SIGNAL SYMPTOMS complaints of headaches, epistaxis, visual disturbances, and shortness of breath; a sense that the heart is beating too fast may also be reported

Hypertension	ICD-9 CM: 401.9

Description: Hypertension occurs when blood pressure is above the 95th percentile for age. Because hypertension is a potentially serious problem, all children should have their blood pressure taken routinely, starting at age 3 years (See Table 1–4).

Systolic blood pressure, which gradually increases with age, should be correlated with weight and height throughout adolescence. Hypertension may be either primary or secondary.

Etiology: Of all cases of hypertension, 60% can be genetically linked. In primary hypertension, heredity, salt intake, diet, stress, and obesity all may contribute to primary hypertension. Secondary hypertension is found most frequently in children with renal disorders. Certain foods or substances (e.g., sodium, nicotine, caffeine, licorice), medications (e.g., oral contraceptives, sympathomimetics, monoamine oxidase inhibitors, corticosteroids), or toxic exposure to certain elements (e.g., lead) or drugs (e.g., amphetamines, cocaine) can also lead to hypertension.

Occurrence: In infants and young children, secondary hypertension is more common than primary. Hypertension (primary and secondary) occurs in about 5% to 7% of all children and 10% to 15% of the adult population.

Age: All age groups.

Ethnicity: Hypertension occurs more often in African-Americans than in any other group.

Gender: The prevalence of hypertension is slightly increased among males, but females are found to have hypertension with increasing frequency.

Contributing factors: Heredity, obesity, and smoking are the leading contributors to the incidence of primary hypertension. Physical problems, particularly renal problems and congenital cardiac defects, and certain medications can also contribute.

Signs and symptoms: Because hypertension is generally a silent disease, there are often no signs. Of greater importance is a known familial history of hypertension. Occasionally the child has frequent headaches, nosebleeds, visual difficulties, or shortness of breath. Also, there may be a history of renal problems or unexplained febrile episodes throughout childhood.

Inspection may reveal short stature; otherwise, there are not any visible signs. Obesity may be obvious.

Palpation may reveal a significant difference in upper and lower extremity pulses, especially with COA. Edema may be present, and kidney abnormalities may be evident. The abdomen should be carefully assessed for masses and costovertebral angle tenderness. In neonates, respiratory distress, irritability or lethargy, vomiting, apnea, or seizures may be observed.

The presence of café-au-lait spots or depigmented areas of skin may signify hypertension secondary to neurofibromatosis. Fundus examination may reveal arterial changes, exudate, or hemorrhages. Auscultation may reveal a murmur with hypertension secondary to COA. If renal artery stenosis is present, a bruit may be heard over the costovertebral angle.

Diagnostic tests: The most useful tool is to take the child's blood pressure with the appropriate size cuff in two positions (sitting, standing, or lying) and on both arms and at least one leg. If elevated on two or more occasions, other tests should be initiated.

Test	Results Indicating Disorder	CPT Code
Urinalysis	Hematuria, proteinuria, leukocyturia	81000
Blood urea nitrogen	Elevated—indicating renal disease	82540
Serum creatinine	Elevated—indicating renal disease	82565
Metabolic panel	Hypokalemia, hypochloremia, or metabolic alkalosis may reveal a kidney problem causing hypertension	80048
ECG	Usually normal until much later in the disease but part of the standard of care	93000
Chest radiograph	Usually normal until later in the disease, but should be done as part of standard of care	71010

Differential diagnosis:

White coat hypertension is a rise in blood pressure that occurs only when the patient is in the health care provider's office.

Renal diseases, cardiac abnormalities, or renovascular hypertension may present with hypertension.

Lead toxicity may be indicated by a serum lead level greater than 10 but more likely greater than 50.

Drug toxicity, especially illicit drugs, can be detected by urine or blood screening.

Obesity is associated with hypertension.

Treatment: In children, the first step is to discover the underlying cause. If mild hypertension exists, treatment initially should be a non-pharmacologic regimen including weight reduction, moderate sodium reduction (80–100 mEq per day), increased calcium and potassium intake, aerobic exercise, and behavior modification.

If intervention is ineffective after a minimum of 3 months or a maximum of 6 months, drug treatment should be initiated. Single-agent therapy is preferred. For young children, the drugs of choice are hydralazine (1–2 mg/kg per day twice daily) and propranolol (2.0–3.0 mg/kg per day two times daily). Other drugs used, in the order given, are clonidine (0.002–0.06 mg/kg per day twice daily), prazosin (0.05–0.1 mg/kg per day twice daily), captopril (0.3–2.0 mg/kg per day three times daily), nifedipine (0.25–1.0 mg/kg per day two or four times daily).

Follow-up: Initially, weekly monitoring for 4 to 6 weeks, then every 2 months for 2 to 6 months, and finally every 6 months or when symptoms warrant a visit.

Sequelae: Headaches and epistaxis are common if the blood pressure is elevated. These should be reported immediately to the health care provider. Stroke, although rare in children, is a possibility.

Prevention/prophylaxis: Risk assessment, including hereditary factors, should be done on each child. Children should be taught to avoid cigarettes and drugs. The importance of aerobic exercise, decreasing salt, and decreasing fat should be stressed.

Early identification is essential; at each visit, children aged 3 years and older should have their blood pressure taken.

Referral: Refer to a physician if secondary hypertension is suspected. Consult with a pediatrician and refer to a cardiologist if primary hypertension is suspected.

Education: Children and parents should be taught the dangers of obesity, drug use, smoking, and lack of exercise. Parents should be reassured that with adequate control, morbidity is significantly decreased. Adequate control also improves the growth and overall well-being of the child. Although heredity cannot be controlled, certain factors can be avoided. The importance of maintaining the assigned regimen should be stressed. Environmental and teratogenic agents can be avoided. The importance of maintaining the assigned regimen should be stressed.

INFLUENZA

SIGNAL SYMPTOMS usually seen as a cold accompanied by a sense of weakness, myalgia, and fever

Influenza	ICD-9 CM: 487.1

Description: Influenza—an acute, contagious, viral illness—often occurs in epidemics. This disease is characterized by fever, malaise, myalgia, and respiratory symptoms.

Etiology: Caused by one of three myxoviruses having similar properties and categorized as influenza virus types A, B, and C. Influenza A viruses have shown an unusual ability to mutate, resulting in new antigenic strains that frequently produce worldwide epidemics.

Occurrence: Every 4 to 7 years.

Age: All ages.

Ethnicity: Not significant.

Gender: Occurs equally in males and females.

Contributing factors: Epidemics occur usually in cooler weather and during the rainy season in the tropics.

Signs and symptoms: Parents report that the child complains of a headache, malaise, lassitude, and occasional prostration. Some vomiting and diarrhea may be reported in young children. There is a complaint of generalized myalgia. Clear nasal drainage is noted. A nonproductive cough is heard. Photophobia is often noted. Fever, often 102°F to 103°F, is present. Rhonchi and occasionally scattered rales are auscultated. A rapid, weak pulse may be seen if myocarditis is present.

Diagnostic tests: None.

Differential diagnosis:

Other viral respiratory infections, including RSV, are differentiated by a positive RSV test.

The symptoms of the common cold are much less severe, with fever less than 102°F.

Croup is differentiated by the classic barking cough, normal or only slightly elevated temperatures, and absence of generalized aching in joints.

Bacterial URIs cause elevated WBCs, with an increased band count and granulocytes; this does not occur in influenza.

Treatment:

Nonpharmacologic

Fluid intake should be increased to help liquefy secretions.

Pharmacologic

Amantadine (Symmetrel) (given to children aged 1–9 in a dose of 4.4 to 8.8 mg/kg per day and to children aged 9–12 twice daily; maximum dose 200 mg per day) may decrease the severity of symptoms.

Acetaminophen (given to children >10 years old; children weighing <40 kg receive 5 mg/kg per day; children weighing >40 kg receive 200 mg per day) may be given for fever.

Rimantadine (Flumadine) (100 mg twice a day for 5 days) is indicated for prophylaxis against influenza A in children older than 12. For children 1 to 9 years old, the dosage is 5 mg/kg per day for 5 days.

A mild cough suppressant, such as guaifenesin plus dextromethorphan hydrobromide (Robitussin-DM) may be given to help the child rest and decrease the frequency of coughing spells.

Follow-up: As indicated. Generally the child should be seen within 2 weeks for follow-up to check for resolution of symptoms; the child should be seen sooner if his or her condition worsens.

Sequelae: Influenza pneumonia or secondary bacterial pneumonia may be seen if disease progresses. Encephalitis and myocarditis rarely occur, unless there is an underlying pathology or influenza is unresponsive to treatment.

Prevention and prophylaxis: Children should avoid close contact with other children exhibiting flu-like symptoms. Parents should consider keeping children home from day care centers during epidemics. When appropriate, give influenza virus vaccine.

Referral: Refer to a pediatrician if the patient is severely ill, experiences respiratory distress, or has widespread rales or rhonchi on physical examination. Pregnant patients should be referred to their obstetrician.

Education: Parents should be taught that the disease is generally self-limiting. Symptoms should be treated as needed; worsening of symptoms may indicate progression of disease, requiring referral to a physician.

KAWASAKI SYNDROME

SIGNAL SYMPTOMS ► fever that continues for 5 days or more, accompanied by sore throat; conjunctivitis; polymorphic rash; chapped or cracked lips; and desquamation of skin, particularly hands, feet, and genital areas

Kawasaki syndrome ICD-9 CM: 446.1

Description: Kawasaki syndrome, also called *mucocutaneous lymph node syndrome,* is an acute illness affecting multiple systems in infants and young children.

Etiology: Unknown. Possible causes include Epstein-Barr virus, retrovirus, *Rickettsia,* group A streptococci, *Staphylococcus aureus, Propionibacterium,* and *Candida.*

Occurrence: Most likely to occur in December through May.

Age: Most common in children younger than 2, with 85% of all cases occurring by age 5.

Ethnicity: The incidence is highest in Asians and lowest in African-Americans.

Gender: More males than females contract the disease (1.5:1).

Contributing factors: Ancestry and predisposing factors. Avoid contact with others known to have the disease.

Signs and symptoms: There is a history of a rash and fever greater than 103°F lasting for 5 or more days. Inspection reveals at least four or more of the following features: polymorphic rash, bilateral conjunctivitis, cracked or dry lips, swollen lips, strawberry tongue, edema, erythema, desquamation of extremities or groin area.

Palpation reveals cervical lymphadenopathy and guarding in the right upper quadrant during assessment of the gallbladder. Auscultation may reveal a cardiac murmur.

Diagnostic tests:

Test	Results Indicating Disorder	CPT Code
Complete blood count	Marked leukocytosis with shift to left	85032
Erythrocyte sedimentation rate	Elevated	85651
Platelet count	By week 3, >800,000/mm^3	85585
IgE	Moderately elevated	82657
ECG	Normal unless coronary aneurysm present	93000
Echocardiogram	Presence of coronary aneurysm	93303

Differential diagnosis:

Measles, rubella, and scarlet fever are differentiated by
characteristics of disease not present (e.g., platelet elevation,
prolonged fever).

Rocky Mountain spotted fever is differentiated by laboratory tests.

Juvenile rheumatoid arthritis (JRA) usually has pain as the primary
symptom.

Mercury poisoning is differentiated by laboratory test.

Treatment: The child diagnosed with or strongly suspected to have
Kawasaki syndrome should be hospitalized. Consultation with pediatrician should be initiated.

In the acute phase, aspirin is given in high doses (80–100 mg/kg per
day) in four divided doses for 14 days. Intravenous gamma globulin,
2000 mg/kg in one dose, is given over a 12-hour period.

After 14 days, if the patient is afebrile, aspirin (3–5 mg/kg per day) is
given once daily for 6 to 8 weeks from the onset of disease. This should
be done after an echocardiogram reveals no abnormalities.

Follow-up: An echocardiogram should be repeated 2 to 3 weeks after
disease onset. Periodic physical examinations should be done until normal platelet, erythrocyte sedimentation rate, and liver function tests are
obtained.

Sequelae: Cardiovascular findings, specifically myocarditis, pericardial
effusion, mitral regurgitation, and—most important—coronary
aneurysms, are the most serious complications.

Prevention/prophylaxis: Prompt treatment and referral can prevent
an aneurysm. Long-term cardiac follow-up should be offered to all children diagnosed with Kawasaki syndrome.

Referral: Immediate referral to a pediatrician when findings suggest the
disease, with follow-up by a pediatric cardiologist.

Education: Parents should be taught the importance of maintaining the
treatment regimens. This disease lasts for 3 to 8 weeks, but that follow-up may be for life.

PNEUMONIA

SIGNAL SYMPTOMS▶   cold-like symptoms accompanied by fever to
104°F, cough, chills, decreased appetite, and restlessness; in infants,
grunting, nasal flaring, and retractions may also be noted

Pneumonia	ICD-9 CM: 486

Description: Pneumonia, an infectious disease of the lower respiratory
tract, can be classified in two ways—by the area it affects or by its cause.

Classified by area, it can be subclassified as lobar, interstitial, and bronchopulmonary. Classified by cause, it can be subclassified as viral, bacterial, or aspiration. Pneumonia affects the lungs by altering normal lung secretions, inhibiting phagocytosis, changing the normal bacterial flora of the lungs, and disrupting the epithelial layer of the lungs. Children who are immunocompromised or have chronic lung problems are often more susceptible to these infections.

Etiology: *S. pneumoniae* is estimated to cause approximately 90% of all bacterial pneumonia. Other bacterial agents that cause pneumonia include *Pneumococcus, Staphylococcus, H. influenzae, Klebsiella, Pseudomonas aeruginosa,* and *Mycobacterium tuberculosis*. Viral agents include cytomegalovirus and influenza virus. *Pneumocystis carinii, Coxiella burnetii, M. pneumoniae, Treponema pallidum, Chlamydia,* and *Chlamydia psittaci* are other causes. Finally, mycotic agents include *Aspergillus, Histoplasma, Candida,* and *Blastomyces*. Aspiration (e.g., amniotic fluids, food, foreign bodies, lipids, or hydrocarbons) is another cause of pneumonia.

Occurrence:

- Bacterial: commonly acquired, 1200/100,000; nosocomial, 800/100,000
- Mycoplasmal: commonly acquired,130/100,000; viral nosocomial,60/100,000

Age: Can occur at any time, but children younger than 4 are more likely to acquire bacterial pneumonia. Mycoplasmal pneumonia is more likely to occur in children older than 5.

Ethnicity: Not significant.

Gender: Occurs equally in males and females.

Contributing factors: Chronic lung diseases, human immunodeficiency virus (HIV) infection (in infants), any other problem related to defects in swallowing or airway clearance, or altered secretions of the lung may increase the risk of pneumonia. Neonates born to mothers infected with *Chlamydia trachomatis* are at increased risk for this type of pneumonia. Bacterial pneumonia is more prevalent among persons living in overcrowded conditions.

Signs and symptoms: In infants and young children with pneumonia, there is usually a report of rhinitis or a stuffy nose, fever (104°F), decreased appetite, cough, and restlessness accompanied by chills or shaking. For older children and adolescents, there is a brief period of symptoms including a mild URI followed by the sudden onset of chills and a high fever. There is a report of alternating periods of restlessness and sleepiness; a dry, hacking cough; and decreased appetite.

In chlamydial pneumonia in infants, there is no fever, but there may be a report of previous conjunctivitis. In viral pneumonia, there is a slower, less dramatic progression of symptoms. Other facts may be given, such as a history of chronic lung or respiratory tract illnesses, exposure to another person with similar symptoms, HIV-positive history, or aspiration of a foreign body.

The infant with bacterial pneumonia appears ill, having nasal flaring, retractions, and grunting. Tachypnea and cyanosis may also be observed. There may be abdominal distention. Some nuchal rigidity is noted, indicating right upper lobe involvement but not meningitis. For the older child, retractions may be noted with a splinting effect on the affected side. There may be circumoral cyanosis if the disease is severe. In bacterial pneumonia, there are fine crackling rales and diminished breath sounds over the area of the pneumonia.

In viral pneumonia, there is marked tachypnea, cough, and retractions. There are also rales, wheezing, and diminished breath sounds. If the causative agent is mycoplasmal pneumonia, the patient has general symptoms of a URI—dry, hacking cough; sometimes a sore throat; and a fever. Infants with chlamydial pneumonia have a repetitive cough, tachypnea, and air hunger, and, in some cases, conjunctivitis. In chlamydial pneumonia, rales are heard, but wheezing is a rare finding.

In mycoplasmal pneumonia, there are harsh breath sounds and rhonchi.

Diagnostic tests:

Test	Results Indicating Disorder	CPT Code
Complete blood count	Leukocytosis with a shift to the left	85031
Chest radiograph	Presence of lobar consolidation. In mycoplasmal pneumonia, increased bronchovascular markings are noted. In chlamydial pneumonia, hyperinflation of lungs with diffuse infiltrates is present. In viral pneumonia, patchy infiltrates are noted	71010
Blood culture	Positive for specific agent	87040
Arterial blood gases	Hypoxia	82803
Eosinophil count	300–400/mm^3	85651
IgM and IgG	Elevated	82657

 Clinical Pearl: In staphylococcal pneumonia, the right lobes are affected about 65% of the time.

Differential diagnosis:

RSV in infants is differentiated by an RSV-positive nasopharyngeal swab.

TB is differentiated by positive sputum cultures or chest radiograph.

Acute bronchiectasis resulting from aspiration of a foreign body may be detected on radiograph, but in small children this often necessitates consultation so that a bronchoscopy can be performed.

Because of the pain in the right lower quadrant of the abdomen, right lobar pneumonia may be confused with appendicitis; radiographs help differentiate this diagnosis.

Viral, fungal, and bacterial pneumonia can be differentiated with the appropriate cultures of nasopharyngeal secretions, sputum, or blood.

Treatment: Treatment depends on determination of the causative agent.

For viral pneumonia, supportive treatment of symptoms is all that is required.

For bacterial pneumonia, penicillin, methicillin, cefuroxime, and gentamicin are the drugs of choice. Erythromycin and TMP-SMX can be used for children who are allergic to penicillin. Erythromycin is used for mycoplasmal and chlamydial pneumonia. Often humidified oxygen is used for infants; when necessary, supplemental oxygen is used for children with severe hypoxemia. Intravenous fluids are used for any child who requires hospitalization and is not receiving the required amount of fluids by mouth (Table 6–3).

Follow-up: A follow-up radiograph probably would not show significant improvement for about 6 weeks; the radiograph should be done at that time. Repeat cultures are not necessary unless the child's symptoms worsen, then the cultures are done to see whether a new, previously unidentified bacterial infection is present. If the patient is treated on an

Table 6–3 Common Antibiotic Therapy for Pneumonia

Medication	Dose	Causative Agent
Penicillin G	100,000 units/kg/day	Streptococcus pneumoniae or β-hemolytic streptococcus
	600,000 units IM followed by oral penicillin	
Erythromycin	30-50 mg/kg/day PO in divided doses qid 15-20 mg/kg/day IV in divided doses q 4 or 6 hr	Penicillin-resistant patients
Methicillin	200 mg/kg/day IV	Staphylococcus aureus
Cefuroxime	100 mg/kg/day	Haemophilus influenzae
Gentamicin	2-2.5 mg/kg IM or IV q 8 hr (if <1 week, q 12 hr)	Pseudomonas, Escherichia coli Klebsiella, Enterobacter, Staphylococcus
Trimethoprim/ sulfamethoxazole	15 mg/kg/day in 3 divided doses	Pneumocystis carinii
Erythromycin	500 mg q 6 hr × 10-14 days if >9 years; 30-50 mg/kg/day for 10-14 days, if <9 years of age	Mycoplasma Chlamydia

outpatient basis, there should be close contact (every day or every other day) with the health care provider.

Sequelae: Overall mortality rate is about 5%. In the otherwise healthy child or adult, improvement is noted within 1 to 3 days. Patients with the poorest outcomes are the very young or the immunocompromised.

Possible complications include empyema, pulmonary abscess, pericarditis, pleurisy, and superinfections. A protracted course can occur when positive cultures are obtained or if the sensitivity and effectiveness of the medications are not adequate.

Prevention/prophylaxis: Children considered at high risk for pneumonia (e.g., children with chronic lung disease, immunocompromised children) should be given a yearly influenza immunization. A pneumococcal vaccine (Pneumovax) should be given to all children who are older than 2 and included in a high-risk group.

Referral: Refer when aspiration of a foreign object is suspected so that the child can undergo bronchoscopy to rule this out. Also, all children in a high-risk group should be referred to a pediatrician. Children requiring hospitalization should be treated collaboratively with a pediatrician.

Education: All parents of children who are at increased risk for serious complications should be taught the importance of immunizations to decrease or eliminate the possibility of pneumonia. Also, if a child is seen with a mild URI, parents should be taught when to bring the child back and what specific signs and symptoms may indicate that the disease is progressing. The importance of giving all medications on schedule and completing the course of therapy should be stressed.

RESPIRATORY SYNCYTIAL VIRUS

SIGNAL SYMPTOMS ▶ rhinitis and persistent coughing accompanied by decreased appetite, irritability, and lethargy; as disease progresses, signs of severe respiratory distress often seen

Respiratory syncytial virus	ICD-9 CM: 079.6

Description: RSV infection, an acute respiratory illness, is the most serious cause of bronchiolitis and pneumonia in infants and young children. Adults with RSV have minor symptoms of an upper respiratory tract illness. In infants and children, the symptoms may be minimal initially but can progress to major signs requiring hospitalization and highly specialized treatment.

Etiology: This disease is caused by RSV, a large RNA virus seen in two major strains, A and B, usually occurring together. It is spread by human contact through exposure to infected droplets that are aerosolized. Incubation is 2 to 8 days.

Occurrence: Annual epidemics are seen generally in the winter and early spring.

Age: Initial infection generally occurs in the first year of life.

Ethnicity: Not significant.

Gender: More prevalent in boys, by a ratio of 1.5:1.

Contributing factors: Exposure to symptomatic or nonsymptomatic infected persons causes the disease. Nosocomial infection in hospitals often occurs during epidemics.

Signs and symptoms: Mild-to-severe respiratory symptoms are reported. Other symptoms seen are lethargy, irritability, poor feeding, and apneic spells. Auscultation reveals diffuse rhonchi, fine rales, and wheezing. Chest radiographs are usually normal. Signs that the disease is severe include compromised cardiac, pulmonary, or immune function. Children with RSV exhibiting significant or severe symptoms should be hospitalized.

Diagnostic tests:

Test	Results Indicating Disorder	CPT Code
Nasopharyngeal culture	Presence of RSV virus	86756
Complete blood count	WBCs sometimes elevated with a shift to the right or left	85031
Chest radiograph	Presence of RSV pneumonia seen with evidence of infiltrates or consolidation	70101

Differential diagnosis:

Bronchitis has a more insidious onset, with no wheezing or fever, and occurs in slightly older children.

Asthma is differentiated by increased wheezing and past history.

Pneumonia is a febrile illness with little or no wheezing.

Croup is characterized by a barking cough.

Treatment: Treatment should be given for symptoms. Patients who exhibit respiratory distress should be hospitalized. Humidified oxygen with nebulization treatments should be considered. Respiratory isolation should be instituted. Ribavirin, which is used only in severe cases for hospitalized patients, is administered by small-particle aerosol for 12 to 20 hours each day for 3 to 5 days.

Follow-up: For the hospitalized child, follow-up should occur 10 to 14 days after discharge.

Sequelae: Bronchitis, pneumonia, and death have been reported.

Prevention/prophylaxis: Control of nosocomial RSV is complicated because there is a continued chance of introduction of the virus by others not exhibiting any symptoms. Avoidance of contact with persons who may have the virus is perhaps the only control. For infants considered high risk, palivizumab (Synagis) should be given up to the age of 24 months. Dosage is calculated on mg/kg, and the package insert should be consulted.

Referral: A child who continues to worsen after 24 hours of treatment should be referred to a pediatrician or pediatric pulmonologist.

Education: Parents should be taught the early signs of respiratory problems so they can seek early treatment and the appropriate diagnoses. Also, avoidance of contact with children who are known to be RSV-positive should be stressed.

RHEUMATIC FEVER

SIGNAL SYMPTOMS▶ a cold or sore throat that is not improving despite treatment often the first sign; a rash accompanied by joint pain also is often seen

| Chronic, old | ICD-9 CM: 398.90 |
| Acute | ICD-9 CM: 391.9 |

Description: Rheumatic fever (RF), an inflammatory disease process, occurs after a group A β-hemolytic streptococcal infection. There has been a resurgence of RF. In the 1950s and 1960s, RF and its major complications were significant worldwide health problems. The incidence declined until the late 1980s, when the increase was first noted; however, the reasons for this increase are not yet known. RF causes cardiac tissue damage and is a leading cause of acquired heart disease.

Etiology: The main agent is group A β-hemolytic streptococcus.

Incidence: There are an increased number of RF cases in the fall, winter, and early spring. RF develops in approximately 3% to 5% of patients with untreated or undertreated group A β-hemolytic streptococcal infection.

Age: Occurs most often in children between age 5 and 15.

Ethnicity: Not significant.

Gender: Occurs equally in males and females.

Contributing factors: Groups who experience overcrowding, poverty, and social disadvantages are at increased risk for contracting RF. Patients who have had a URI in which streptococcus was the causative agent and who have had inadequate or no treatment at all are predisposed to the development of RF.

Signs and symptoms: The parent or child reports that the child has had a URI or sore throat for which there was either no treatment or ineffective treatment. They may report fever, joint pain, rash on the trunk and extremities, easily changeable moods, and a racing heart. They may also report that the child has a history of RF.

The child appears ill, and the skin is warm or hot to the touch. A macular ecthymatous rash is present, mainly on the trunk and extremities. Palpation of the scalp, joints, and spine reveals pea-sized nodules that are nontender and firm, called *subcutaneous nodules,* and two or more joints with severe pain, tenderness, warmth, swelling, and redness.

When percussing the chest, the nurse practitioner may note (1) cardiomegaly, or a heart size greater than expected; (2) a heart murmur that is new and fairly significant; and (3) an increased heart rate.

Diagnostic tests:

Test	Results Indicating Disorder	CPT Code
Throat culture	Positive for Group A β-hemolytic streptococcus	87070
Erythrocyte sedimentation rate	Elevated	86561
ECG	Look for prolonged PR interval	93000

There are no specific tests that address RF, and the diagnosis is determined based on the Jones criteria (Table 6–4).

Differential diagnosis:

JRA is differentiated from RF by the following: (1) antistreptococcal agents produce no significant improvement in JRA, and (2) antinuclear antibody (ANA) test is positive in JRA.

Infective endocarditis is differentiated by blood cultures and endocarditis (in RF, there is pancarditis).

Connective tissue disease, particularly systemic lupus erythematosus, is differentiated by a speckled ANA test result.

Lyme disease is differentiated by a positive Lyme titer.

Treatment: Treatment of RF involves three major components. First, the group A β-hemolytic streptococcal infection should be treated. Benzathine penicillin G, 1,200,000 units (600,000 if patient weighs <27 kg) should be given intramuscularly. Oral medicines may also be used, including penicillin V (250 mg/kg per day twice daily for 10 days) or erythromycin (40 mg/kg per day twice or three times daily, not to exceed 1 g in 24 hours). Second, anti-inflammatory agents should be used to reduce the arthralgia associated with the disease. These include steroids, given in a dosage of 2.5 mg/kg per day divided into two doses over 2 to 3 weeks. After treatment, the patient should be gradually weaned from

Table 6–4   Jones Criteria for Rheumatic Fever*

Major Criteria	Minor Criteria
Carditis	Fever
Migratory polyarthritis	Arthralgia
Erythema marginatum	Previous RF
Chorea	Elevated ESR
Subcutaneous nodules	Prolonged PR interval on the ECG

* Diagnosis of RF may be made if the patient meets two major criteria or one major and two minor criteria and has had preceding group A β-hemolytic streptococcal infection.

ECG, electrocardiogram; ESR, erythrocyte sedimentation rate; RF, rheumatic fever.

the steroids. Salicylates should be given so that blood levels of 20 to 25 mg/dL are achieved. This requires giving about 90 to 120 mg/kg per day in four divided doses.

The patient should be given supportive therapy to treat other problems associated with RF, particularly congestive heart failure and carditis. Often the use of salicylates alone is effective for carditis, but a physician should be consulted to institute treatment for congestive heart failure.

Follow-up: Children who have been diagnosed with RF should have regular follow-up examinations at 1- to 2-week intervals for the first month, then about once per month; during these visits, antibiotic prophylaxis is given to ensure that the disease does not recur. Injections with benzathine penicillin G should be given once per month for 5 years after the diagnosis, although this is still controversial.

Sequelae: The most frequent sequela is the development of rheumatic valvular heart disease. Untreated, RF may result in death.

Referral: When cardiac involvement is suspected, the pediatric cardiologist should be consulted for treatment and follow-up. The nurse practitioner should consult with a pediatrician for all children who have a presumptive diagnosis of RF.

Prevention/prophylaxis: The best way to prevent this disease is to initiate prompt treatment of all cases of streptococcal infection.

Education: Parents and children should be taught the importance of compliance with drug regimens, especially antibiotic prophylaxis to prevent a recurrence of the disease. Families should be taught that the child will need prophylaxis before dental work for the rest of his or her life.

Prompt identification and treatment of β-hemolytic streptococcal infections should be stressed to families.

SEVERE ACUTE RESPIRATORY SYNDROME (SARS)

SIGNAL SYMPTOMS▶ acute and extremely rapid onset of respiratory symptoms that include cough, congestion, shortness of breath, fever, and in some cases accompanying diarrhea.

Severe acute respiratory syndrome (SARS)	ICD-9-CM 486

Description: SARS is an acute respiratory illness that is viral in origin and can be life-threatening. It is characterized by a rapid onset, and by symptoms similar to pneumonia; it is highly contagious.

Etiology: It is caused by a previously unrecognized coronavirus.

Occurrence: At the publishing of this book, the worldwide occurrence is nearly 5,000 cases, with more than 200 deaths being attributed to this disease. Currently, the mortality rate for this disease is 4%. The incubation time for this disease is 2–7, days with a maximum of 10 days.

Age: The population at greatest risk includes very young children (infants), the aged population, immunocompromised persons, or those with previously diagnosed respiratory problems.

Ethnicity: Asian and Canadian individuals currently have the highest rate of occurrence.

Gender: Occurs equally in males and females.

Contributing Factors: Exposure to other infected individual(s), international travel (particularly to areas of high incidence of the disease), immunocompromised state or influenza, preexisting respiratory conditions.

Signs and Symptoms: The major symptoms seen are fever > 38°C (100.4°F), dry cough, shortness of breath, and difficulty breathing that is rapidly progressive.

Diagnostic Tests: Initial diagnostic testing should include the following based on the information now available related to SARS:

Test	Results Indicating Disorder	CPT Code
Radiographic studies of chest	Rule out atypical pneumonia	71020
Pulse oxymetry	Readings below 92% indicate compromise	94760
Sputum culture and Gram stain	Positive for specific organism	87070
RSV Testing	Will be negative for SARS	87280

Differential diagnosis: Influenza A and B, RSV, *Legionella*, bacterial and viral pneumonia should all be considered in the differential diagnosis. These can be differentiated by specific viral and bacterial cultures.

Treatment: Currently, treatment is supportive and symptomatic. The use of supplemental oxygen to assist breathing, intravenous steroids, and airborne isolation measures should be used. If the nurse practitioner has a presumptive case of SARS the patient should be referred to the collaborating physician, and hospitalization should be considered.

An experimental treatment is currently being used in some areas and it involves the use of high dose steroids IV or PO, along with ribaviron, also PO or IV. These measures should not be instituted by the PNP. The patient who is not severely compromised may be treated at home, but isolation measures there, including quarantine, should be instituted.

Follow-up: The patient should be seen at regular intervals during the illness itself if at home, and after resolution of the symptoms follow-up should continue for about two weeks. Family contacts should also be screened and followed closely for about 10 days following exposure to a presumptive case of SARS.

Sequelae: Little is known at this time as to the long-term effects of this disease. It is presumed that, depending on the severity of the illness, long-term respiratory complications may result.

Prevention/prophylaxis: Avoidance of travel to Hong Kong, China, and Toronto has been advised at this time. The use of facemasks may be helpful in persons who feel that they have an increased risk of exposure, e.g., because of necessary business or military travel. Strict handwashing is recommended, and at this time avoidance of large crowds in high-incidence areas is recommended. It is thought, however, that, long-term exposure is required for an increased risk of the disease and that casual contact is not a cause of the illness.

Referral: Referral should be made for all possible or presumptive cases to both the collaborative physician as well as the health department in the area as soon as the diagnosis is made.

Education: Patients should be taught the risks of the illness and how to avoid contact or decrease the risk of infection.

SYNCOPE

SIGNAL SYMPTOMS ▸ lightheadedness or actual fainting in which the patient remembers nothing of the incident except waking on the floor

Syncope	ICD-9 CM: 480.2

Description: Commonly known as fainting, syncope is generally a benign event that may occur when a person experiences severe pain, anxiety, or high levels of emotion or stands erect for a long period. If syncope occurs more than once, however, more serious causes must be ruled out.

Etiology: Syncope secondary to vasovagal stimulation results in a partial or total loss of consciousness for a short period.

Occurrence: Common; about 50% of children have experienced at least one syncopal episode.

Age: Any age.

Ethnicity: Not significant.

Gender: Occurs equally in males and females.

Contributing factors: Severe anxiety, stress, or standing for a long period.

Signs and symptoms: The child or parent reports a period of partial or total unconsciousness that may be idiopathic in origin or can be related to stress, pain, or standing for a long period. Further evaluation is important if other family members have had the same problem (Fig. 6–5).

The syncopal event may be sudden or may have a prodromal period. The child may be diaphoretic and pale. The time the child is unconscious should be recorded; the time may vary from a few seconds to several minutes. There is a transient loss of muscle tone.

Skin is cool and diaphoretic. Pulse rate can vary from absent to rapid

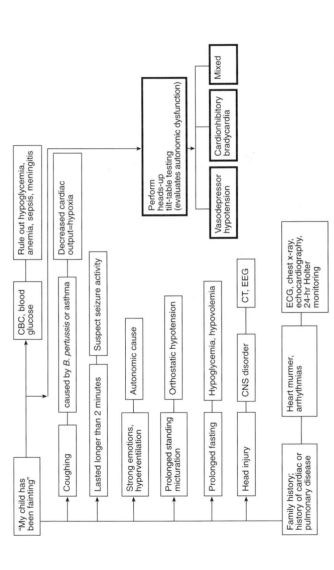

Figure 6–5. Evaluation of syncope. (CBC, complete blood count; CT, computed tomography; CNS, central nervous system; EEG, electroencephalogram; ECG, electrocardiogram.)

and should be evaluated and recorded. The child may experience palpitations or bradycardia.

Diagnostic tests: For the first episode, tests may be deferred. When syncope occurs in the absence of pain, anxiety, and standing for a long time, some tests should be performed.

Test	Results Indicating Disorder	CPT Code
ECG	May be normal or have a prolonged QT interval or show abnormal AV conduction indicating Wolff-Parkinson-White syndrome or show tachycardia or bradycardia, which may indicate a heart block	93000
Chest radiograph	Cardiomegaly	71010

Differential diagnosis:

Prolonged QT syndrome is differentiated by an ECG, which shows this phenomenon.

Congenital cardiomyopathies are differentiated by history, abnormal ECG, echocardiogram showing defect, or chest radiograph.

Severe autonomic disease is characterized by repeated episodes of syncope.

Wolff-Parkinson-White syndrome is differentiated by an ECG that shows abnormalities in AV conduction.

Heart block is differentiated by an ECG.

Treatment:

Nonpharmacologic

Protect the child from injury. Obtain a detailed history that includes questions related to the nature of the fainting spell, events that preceded the loss of consciousness, proximity to exercise, and any seizure activity during the event.

Pharmacologic

If syncope is due to heart block, a pacemaker is recommended. If the problem is related to a prolonged QT syndrome, a cardiologist may start β-blockers, steroids, or a combination of the two.

Follow-up: After initial episode, the child should be re-evaluated immediately if there is a repeat syncopal episode. If all tests are normal, follow-up should be done in accordance with the routine recommended schedule.

Sequelae: Occasionally injury may occur as a result of the fall that occurs during syncope. Untreated or unrecognized cardiac abnormalities can result in death.

Prevention/prophylaxis: Stress modification should be taught. If standing event was the problem, the child should be taught to alter pressure slightly in the legs and to move slightly during the period required to stand.

Referral: Unexplained or recurrent episodes of syncope should be referred to a pediatric cardiologist.

Education: Parents should be taught the importance of reporting the occurrence of syncopal events and of giving a detailed history of each episode.

SPONTANEOUS PNEUMOTHORAX

SIGNAL SYMPTOMS ▶ sudden severe pain in chest accompanied by difficulty breathing

Spontaneous pneumothorax	ICD-9 CM: 512.8

Description: Pneumothorax is the dissection of air from the alveolar spaces into the interstitial spaces of the lung.

Etiology: Unknown. It may occur as a complication of infection, a tracheostomy, ventilatory support, or chest trauma.

Occurrence: Pneumothorax occurs more commonly in children with asthma or cystic fibrosis.

Age: Spontaneous pneumothorax occurs in children older than age 10 and young adults.

Ethnicity: Not significant.

Gender: Occurs more often in males than females.

Contributing factors: Underlying obstructive or restrictive lung disease, smoking cigarettes.

Signs and symptoms: Child complains of respiratory distress. Observation reveals retraction and often a shift of the larynx, trachea, and heart toward the unaffected side. Auscultation reveals decreased chest wall movement and markedly decreased breath sounds on the affected side, percussion is tympanic, and tachycardia is usually present.

Diagnostic tests:

Test	Results Indicating Disorder	CPT Code
Radiograph of chest	Assess severity of the pneumothorax	71010
	Differentiate between pneumopericardium (air surrounding the heart) and pneumomediastinum (heart and mediastinum outlined with air)	

Differential diagnosis:

Diaphragmatic hernia, lung cysts, congenital lobar emphysema, and cystic adenomatoid malformations may be distinguished by chest radiographs.

Treatment:

Small pneumothorax: Observation. Administration of 100% oxygen increases the nitrogen pressure gradient between the lung air and the blood, hastening resolution.

Large or symptomatic pneumothorax: Needle aspiration and insertion of chest tube drainage.

Follow-up: None.

Sequelae: Pneumopericardium and pneumomediastinum are life-threatening.

Prevention/prophylaxis: None.

Referral: Refer to pediatrician or surgeon for immediate hospitalization and insertion of chest tube in symptomatic cases.

Education: None.

TUBERCULOSIS

SIGNAL SYMPTOMS persistent cough accompanied by night sweats and weight loss

Tuberculosis	ICD-9 CM: 011.9

Description: TB is an infectious, inflammatory disease primarily affecting the lungs and is chronic in nature. Because of the danger TB poses to the community, it is a reportable disease, and when it is diagnosed, the health care provider is mandated to report the case and all contacts to the local health department. Although the lung is the primary site, other sites are affected; the bacilli can lodge in any organ of the body. In the United States, the most common mode of transmission is inhalation of infected droplet nuclei. In other parts of the world, bovine spread is more common.

Etiology: The most common causative agent is *M. tuberculosis*. Other atypical causes are *M. bovis, M. avium, M. intracellulare, M. kansasii, M. simiae,* and *M. szulgai*.

Occurrence: Approximately 7.5 million cases of TB were reported in 1990; the incidence is growing. The World Health Organization has predicted that 4.5 million children will die of TB between 2000 and 2010.

Age: Any age, but more recent reports indicate that children younger than 15 are at greater risk.

Ethnicity: Incidence is greater in nonwhite racial and ethnic minorities.

Gender: Occurs equally in males and females.

Contributing factors: HIV, increasing world poverty, living in urban areas, and living in areas in Asia and Africa increase the likelihood of contracting TB. Other factors include chronic illness, diabetes, renal failure, advanced age, occupation (health care workers), and race.

Signs and symptoms: The primary caregiver may relate that the child has been in contact with someone who was diagnosed with TB. There may be reports of coughing, weight loss, and night sweats. Most children are asymptomatic, and the diagnosis is made by skin testing and chest radiograph. Infants have failure to thrive, coughing, fever, and rales. Children who have hypertension also exhibit significant pulmonary signs.

No obvious signs are seen except in infants, who look frail and exhibit signs of failure to thrive. Lymphadenopathy is the most common finding in children. Auscultation may reveal rhonchi, rales, or silence—indicating atelectasis. Because few overall symptoms or signs are seen, heard, or felt, a chest radiograph should be obtained to confirm the diagnosis.

Diagnostic tests:

Test	Results Indicating Disorder	CPT Code
Mantoux (PPD) test	Positive. It should be read after 48–72 hours and is positive if the induration is >15 mm. If immunocompromised, >10 mm is positive	86580
Chest radiograph	Positive findings	70101

 Clinical Pearl: Sputum cultures are often negative for acid-fast bacilli in children and are not indicated.

Differential diagnosis:

Fatigue is related to disrupted sleep patterns.

Pneumonia is determined by radiograph and serum blood cultures that are negative for TB indicators.

Failure to thrive has a negative chest radiograph or PPD.

HIV is differentiated by Western blot, enzyme-linked immunosorbent assay tests, and viral load counts.

Treatment: The routine regimen is isoniazid and rifampin for 4 months and pyrazinamide for 2 months (Table 6–5). If isoniazid resistance is known, ethambutol or streptomycin may be used. When isoniazid or rifampin cannot be used because of demonstrated resistance, therapy is extended from 6 months to 12 months.

Directly observed therapy, which means that the health care provider directly observes the patient taking the medicine, is the most effective therapy.

Follow-up: Children diagnosed with TB should have yearly chest radiographs taken.

Sequelae: In children younger than 6, tuberculous meningitis can occur 2 to 6 months after a diagnosis of TB. Tuberculomas (space-occupying lesions), bone and joint infections, and superficial lymphadenitis may also occur. Ultimately, TB can cause death.

Prevention/prophylaxis: TB skin testing should be performed yearly on all children beginning at age 12 months. In a person who has signs and symptoms of TB, has had recent contact with a person with TB, has

Table 6–5 Pediatric Tuberculosis Drugs

Drug	Daily Dosage	Adverse Reactions
Isoniazid*	10–20 mg/kg PO or IV (maximum dose 300 mg/day)	Elevated liver enzymes, hepatitis, peripheral neuropathy
Rifampin*	10–20 mg/kg PO or IV (maximum dose 300 mg/day)	Orange coloration of body fluids, emesis, hepatitis, flu-like symptoms, thrombocytopenia
Pyrazinamide*	20–30 mg/kg PO or IV (maximum dose 2 g/day	Hyperuricemia, rash, joint pain, hepatoxicity
Ethambutol*	15–25 mg/kg PO (maximum dose 2.5 g/day)	Visual disturbance including loss of vision and color blindness, body rash
Capreomycin†	15–30 mg/kg IM (maximum dose 1 g/day)	Ototoxicity, nephrotoxicity
Ciprofloxacin†	20–30 mg/kg bid (maximum dose 1.5 g; only for >16 yrs of age)	Headache, rash, photosensitivity, gastrointestinal disturbances
Ethionamide†	15–20 mg/kg PO bid	Hepatotoxicity, gastrointestinal upsets
Cycloserine†	15–20 mg/kg PO bid	Personality changes, psychosis, rash, seizures
Kanamycin†	25–30 mg/kg IM	Ototoxicity, nephrotoxicity

* First-line drugs.
† Second-line drugs.

HIV or other chronic debilitating illness, or has recently immigrated to the United States from Asia, Africa, Latin America, or Oceania, testing should be done at least every 6 months.

Referral: A physician should be consulted if there are signs of drug resistance or worsening of the condition.

Education: Communities and parents should be educated about the prevalence of TB. There has been a loss of vigilance regarding TB, but as poverty and HIV increase in children, there needs to be active participation of family and community in seeking out routine screening for all children and adults.

The importance of taking medicines according to the prescribed schedule should be stressed, as should the need for patients and families to reveal all contacts.

VENTRICULAR SEPTAL DEFECT

SIGNAL SYMPTOMS ▶ usually no signal symptom exhibited by the patient, but the nurse practitioner hears a murmur that is pansystolic or a flow murmur and there is an accentuated S_2; parents may report increased fatigue and poor growth, and the child may appear small for age

VSD	ICD-9 CM: 745.4

Description: VSD is a common anomaly defined as a hole or defect in the intraventricular septum of the heart, resulting in a right-to-left shunt. Blood crosses the defect during systole and flows out to the pulmonary artery, causing pulmonary overload. The hemodynamic effects depend on the size of the defect.

Etiology: In most cases, the cause of VSD is unknown; however, it may accompany a chromosomal abnormality.

Occurrence: VSD occurs in 1.5 to 2.5 in 1000 live births. There was a marked increase in the occurrence of VSD during 1980s and 1990s. It occurs more frequently in premature or low-birth-weight infants.

Age: Usually detected between 2 and 6 weeks of age, but may be detected on day 1 of life.

Ethnicity: Not significant.

Gender: Occurs equally in males and females.

Contributing factors: When any of the following are present, the risk of VSD increases: Down's syndrome, trisomy 13 and 18, maternal exposure to rubella, maternal alcohol problems resulting in fetal alcohol syndrome, and phenylketonuria.

Signs and symptoms: Parents report no symptoms if the defect is small. In the case of a large VSD with a significant shunt volume, there may be a report of tachypnea, fatigue, exercise intolerance, dyspnea on exertion or with feedings, a slow growth rate, or frequent URIs. No cyanosis is noted. The child may be smaller than expected or may experience difficulty feeding. Palpation with a small VSD may or may not reveal a thrill at the lower left sternal border. With a moderate VSD, there may be a louder left ventricular apical impulse with or without a thrill. In a large VSD, there is a right ventricular lift and thrill. If the patient is in heart failure, there is also hepatomegaly.

Percussion may reveal slight cardiomegaly, but in the early days this would not be detected. In small VSDs, a normal S_1 and S_2 are heard with a holosystolic or long systolic, harsh, blowing murmur at the left and right sides of the sternum.

In a moderate VSD, a frequently heard wide split between S_1 and S_2 may or may not be accentuated. There is a harsh, holosystolic blowing murmur.

In a large VSD, S_1 may be accentuated, whereas S_2 is narrowly split. There may also be a thudding sound at the apex. There is usually a holosystolic, blowing murmur at the left sternal border.

Diagnostic tests:

Test	Results Indicating Disorder	CPT Code
Chest radiograph	Normal with small VSD but some cardiomegaly with larger defects	71010
ECG	Moderate-to-large VSD results in left ventricular hypertrophy, left axis deviation, or left atrial enlargement. If right ventricular hypertrophy is present, suspect pulmonary hypertension	93000

Differential diagnosis:

ASD is differentiated by an echocardiogram and the position and quality of the murmur.

Congestive heart failure, which can accompany the VSD, is differentiated by an echocardiogram and the presence of elevated cardiac electrolytes; ECG usually is essentially normal.

Treatment: Spontaneous closure occurs in 50% of all cases with no intervention. If congestive heart failure secondary to VSD occurs, however, surgical intervention is warranted. Large defects require vigorous treatment of respiratory problems.

Follow-up: Every 6 months, close monitoring with a pediatric cardiologist is important.

Sequelae: Generally, small VSDs have no significant sequelae. A large untreated defect that does not close can lead to congestive heart failure.

Prevention/prophylaxis: None—VSD is a congenital defect.

Referral: The patient should be referred to a pediatric cardiologist when the murmur is first detected. The nurse practitioner along with the cardiologist can provide continued follow-up.

Education: Reassure parents that most VSDs close spontaneously. Parents must schedule health visits regularly with primary health care provider and the cardiologist. The parents should also be taught to identify signs that the condition is worsening, such as poor weight gain, feeding problems, and shortness of breath.

REFERENCES

Apparent Life-Threatening Event

American Academy of Pediatrics Committee on Child Abuse and Neglect: Distinguishing sudden infant death syndrome from child abuse fatalities (RE0036). Pediatrics107:437, 2001.

American Academy of Pediatrics Committee on Child Abuse and Neglect: Distinguishing sudden infant death syndrome from child abuse fatalities (addendum). Pediatrics108:812, 2001.

American Academy of Pediatrics Task Force on Infant Sleep Position and Sudden Death Syndrome: Changing concepts of sudden infant death syndrome:

Implications for infant sleeping environment and sleep position (RE9946). Pediatrics 105:650, 2000.

Carolan, P, et al: Potential to prevent carbon dioxide rebreathing of commercial products marketed to reduce sudden infant death syndrome risk. Pediatrics 105:774, 2000.

Gold, Y, et al: Hyper-releasability of mast cells in family members of infants with sudden infant death syndrome and apparent life-threatening events. J Pediatr 136:460, 2000.

Guntheroth, W, and Spiers, P. Thermal stress in sudden infant death: Is there an ambiguity with the rebreathing hypothesis? Pediatrics 107:693, 2001.

Kemp, J, et al: Unsafe sleep practices and an analysis of bedsharing among infants dying suddenly and unexpectedly: Results of a four-year, population-based, death-scene investigation study of sudden infant death syndrome and related deaths. Pediatrics 106:e41, 2000.

Nakamura, S, et al: Review of hazards associated with children placed in adult beds. Arch Pediatr Adolesc Med 153:1019, 1999.

Ottolini, M, et al: Prone infant sleeping despite the "Back to Sleep" campaign. Arch Pediatr Adolesc Med 153:512, 1999.

Pamphlett, R, et al: Vertebral artery compression resulting from head movement: A possible cause of the sudden infant death syndrome. Pediatrics 103:460, 1999.

Persson, S, et al: Parallel incidences of sudden infant death syndrome and infantile hypertropic pyloric stenosis: A common cause? Pediatrics 108:e70, 2001.

Scheers, N, et al: Sudden infant death with external airways covered: Case-comparison study of 206 deaths in the United States. Arch Pediatr Adolesc Med 152:540, 1998.

Asthma

Barnes, P: Current issues for establishing inhaled corticosteriods as the anti-inflammatory agents of choice in asthma. J Allergy Clin Immunol 101:S427, 1998.

Chan, D, et al: Multidisciplinary education and management program for children with asthma. Am J Health Syst Pharmacol 58:1413, 2001.

Cordina, M, et al: Assessment of a community pharmacy-based program for patients with asthma. Pharmacotherapy 21:1196, 2001.

Hanne-Herborg, B, et al: Improving drug therapy for patients with asthma: Part I. J Am Pharm Assoc 41:539, 2001.

Hanne-Herborg, B, et al: Improving drug therapy for patients with asthma: Part II. Use of antiasthma medicationsJ Am Pharm Assoc 41:551, 2001.

Stoloff, S, et al: Improved asthma control after changing from low-to-medium doses of other inhaled corticosteroids to low-dose fluticasone propionate. Medscape General Medicine 3, 2001.

Werk, L, et al: Beliefs about diagnosing asthma in young children. Pediatrics 105:585, 2000.

Bronchitis

Fried, V, et al: Ambulatory health care visits by children: Principal diagnosis and place of visit. National Center for Health Statistics. Vital Health Stat 13:1, 1998.

Shay, D, et al: Bronchiolitis-associated hospitalizations among US children, 1980–1996. JAMA 282:1440, 1999.

Chest Wall Trauma

Bratton, S, et al: Serious and fatal air gun injuries: More than meets the eye. Pediatrics 100:609, 1997.

Jackman, G, et al: Seeing is believing: What do boys do when they find a real gun? Pediatrics 107:1247, 2001.

Link, M, et al: Reduced risk of sudden death from chest wall blows (commotio cordis) with safety baseballs. Pediatrics 109:873, 2002.

Silen, M, et al: Rollover injuries in residential driveways: Age related patterns of injury. Pediatrics 104:7, 1999.

Winston, F, et al: Hidden spears: Handlebars as injury hazards to children. Pediatrics 102:596, 1998.

Congenital Cardiac Defects

Braunwald, E, et al: Heart Disease: A Textbook of Cardiovascular Medicine, ed 6. WB Saunders, Philadelphia, 2001.

Lam, J, Tobias, J. Follow up survey of children and adolescents with chest pain. South Med J 94:921, 2001.

Pelech, A. The cardiac murmur: When to refer. Pediatr Clin N Am 45:107, 1998.

Porter, V. Summer camp for children with heart diseases. Medscape Infectious Diseases 3, 2001.

Woods, S, and Ray, U: Maternal smoking and the risk for congenital birth defects: A cohort study. J Am Board Fam Pract 14:330, 2001.

Costochondritis

Flowers, L, and Wippermann, B: Costochondritis. EMed J 2, 2001.

Hypertension

Arafat, M, and Mattoo, T: Measurement of blood pressure in children: Recommendations and perceptions on cuff selection. Pediatrics 104:30, 1999.

Flynn, J: Differentiation between primary and secondary hypertension in children using ambulatory blood pressure monitoring. Pediatrics 110:89, 2002.

Influenza

Chiu, S, et al: Influenza A infection is an important cause of febrile seizures. Pediatrics 108:63, 2001.

Cohen, G, and Nettleman, M: Economic impact of vaccination in preschool children. Pediatrics 106:973, 2000.

Edwards, K, and Poehling, K: Influenza virus continues to pose a new challenge. Pediatrics 108:1004, 2001.

James, J: The burden of influenza illness in children with asthma and other chronic medical conditions. Pediatrics 110:453, 2002.

Poland, G, and Hall, C: Influenza immunization of schoolchildren: Can we interrupt community epidemics? Pediatrics 106:1280, 1999.

Winther, B, et al: Viral respiratory infection in schoolchildren: Effects on middle ear pressure. Pediatrics 109:826, 2002.

Kawasaki Syndrome

Gardner-Medwin, J, et al: The clinical features of Kawasaki disease and incomplete Kawasaki disease in an incidence cohort. San Francisco, American College of Rheumatology 65th Annual Scientific Meeting, November 11–15, 2001.

Shibata, M, et al: Isolation of a Kawasaki disease associated bacterial sequence from peripheral leukocytes. Pediatr Int 42:467, 1999.

Strigl, S, et al: Is there an association between Kawasaki disease and *Chlamydia* pneumonia? J Infect Dis 181:2103, 2000.

Pneumonia

Bergh, K: The patient's differential diagnosis: Unpredictable concerns in visits for acute cough. J Fam Pract 46:153, 1998.

Gleason, P: The emerging role of atypical pathogens in community acquired pneumonia. Pharmacotherapy 22:2s, 2002.

Gundrum, B, et al: What do we really know about antibiotic pharmacodynamics? Pharmacotherapy 21:302s, 2001.

Guthrie, R, et al: Treating Resistant Respiratory Infections: I. Primary Care Settings: The Role of the New Quinolones. University of Cincinnati College of Medicine, Cincinnati, OH, 2001.

Margolis, P, and Jadonski, A: Does this infant have pneumonia? JAMA 279:308, 2001.

Tile, T, et al: Management of community acquired pneumonia: An appropriate use tool. Infect Med 18:462, 2001.

Respiratory Syncytial Virus

Committee on Infectious Diseases, Committee on Fetus and Newborn, American Academy of Pediatrics: Prevention of respiratory syncytial virus infections: Indications for the use of palivizumab and update on the use of RSVIGIV. Pediatrics 102:1211, 1998.

Joffe, S, et al: Cost effectiveness of respiratory syncytial virus prophylaxis among preterm infants. Pediatrics 104:419, 1998.

Randolph, A, Wang, E: Ribavirin for respiratory syncytial virus infection of the lower respiratory tract. Cochrane Library 4, 2001.

Respiratory syncytial virus activity—United States, 2000–2001 Season. MMWR Morb Mortal Wkly Rep 51:26, 2002.

Scott, L, and Lamb, H: Paivizumab. Drugs 58:305, 1999.

Wang, E, and Tang, N: Immunoglobulin for preventing respiratory syncytial virus infection. Cochrane Library 4, 2001.

Weber, M, et al: An in home synagis program for RSV prevention in high risk infants. J Managed Care Pharmacol 7:476, 2001.

Rheumatic Fever

Berhman, R, Kleigman, R: Nelson's Essentials of Pediatrics. WB Saunders, Philadelphia, 1999

Severe Acute Respiratory Syndrome (SARS)

Pottininger, M: Treating a medical mystery. The Wall Street Journal, April 3, 2003, B1–B4.

Department of Health and Human Services, CDC: Severe acute respiratory syndrome: treatment and background, corona virus sequencing, 4/20/03, *www.cdc.gov/ncidod/sars*.

Department of Health and Human Services, CDC: Updated interim domestic guidelines for triage and disposition of patients who may have severe acute respiratory syndrome (SARS), 4/12/03, *www.cdc.gov/ncidod/sars/ic-closecontacts.htm*.

Syncope

Bowen, J: Dizziness: A diagnostic puzzle. Hosp Med 39, 1998.

Evans, R, and Nasii, N: Dr. Lecter's convulsive syncope. Medscape General Medicine 3, 2001.

Friedman, D: Syncopal episodes following vaccination. Medscape Pediatrics 4, 2002.

Spontaneous Pneumothorax

Sahn, S, and Hefner, JE: Spontaneous pneumothorax. N Engl J Med 342:868, 2000.

Tuberculosis

Ampofo, K, and Saiman, L: Pediatric tuberculosis. Pediatr Ann 31:98, 2002.

Dye, C, et al: Global burden of tuberculosis: Estimated incidence, prevalence and mortality by country. WHO Global Surveillance and Monitoring Project. JAMA 282:677, 1999.

Institute of Medicine: Ending Neglect: The Elimination of Tuberculosis in the United States. National Academy Press, Washington, DC, 2001.

Nierengarten, M, and Ma, E: Tuberculosis in the 21st century: Still not history. Medscape Infectious Diseases 3, 2001.

Wilkinson, D: Drugs for preventing tuberculosis in HIV infected persons. Cochrane Library 1, 2001.

Ventricular Septal Defect

Sinaiko, A, and Prineas, R: Reduction of cardiovascular disease: What is the role of the pediatrician? Pediatrics 102:61, 1998.

Chapter 7

ABDOMINAL DISORDERS

ASCARIASIS

SIGNAL SYMPTOMS ▶ passage of long white worm rectally or orally

Ascariasis	ICD-9-CM: 127.0

Description: Ascariasis is the infestation of the body by the parasite *Ascaris lumbricoides* resulting from accidental ingestion of the eggs.

Etiology: Ingestion of parasitic eggs through contaminated food, water, or dirt.

Occurrence: Common in endemic areas (Southern states).

Age: Usually seen in toddlers.

Ethnicity: Not significant.

Gender: Occurs equally in males and females.

Contributing factors: Associated with day care centers, infected pets, travel to endemic areas, and eating infected soil.

Signs and symptoms: The child presents with a cough, abdominal discomfort, or bloating depending on the stage of development of the parasite.

- Pulmonary—cough, blood-tinged sputum, and transient infiltrates on the lung (owing to larvae migrating through the lung in the developmental processes) (Löffler's syndrome)
- Intestinal—abdominal discomfort and distention

Sometimes the parent has observed the passage of the worms, either in the stool or in the sputum.

Diagnostic tests:

Test	Results Indicating Disorder	CPT Code
Stool for OCP	Shows and identifies infecting agent	87177
Complete blood count	Eosinophil count may be elevated	85022

OCP, ova, cysts, and parasites.

Differential diagnosis:

In appendicitis, white blood cell (WBC) count is elevated ($>15,000$ cells/mm^3), neutrophils are elevated, and the patient presents with vomiting.

Biliary colic pain is crampy and primarily in the right upper quadrant; there is also occasional jaundice.

Treatment: Give pyrantel pamoate, 11 mg/kg single dose (maximum 1 g), or mebendazole, 100 mg twice day for 3 days for children older than 2 years.

Follow-up: Re-evaluate in 2 weeks and perform a recheck stool examination.

Sequelae: Biliary obstruction resulting from migration of the worms to the biliary duct is rare, as is intestinal obstruction owing to tangled masses of adult worms.

Prevention/prophylaxis: Wearing shoes, not allowing children to play in possibly contaminated areas, and providing for adequate disposal of fecal material are preventive measures.

Referral: None.

Education: Instruct in proper hand-washing techniques and disposal of fecal material. Advise parents of the risk of children eating dirt from contaminated areas in play areas.

ENCOPRESIS

SIGNAL SYMPTOMS▶ persistent fecal soiling

Encopresis	ICD-9-CM: 787.6

Description: Encopresis is the daytime or nighttime incontinence of formed stools in children older than age 4 to 5. There are four types.

Retentive encopresis (psychogenic megacolon) comprises withholding of stool, development of constipation, fecal impaction, and seepage of stool. Examination reveals a large amount of feces in the rectal vault. The soiling usually distresses children.

Continuous encopresis occurs in children who have never gained primary bowel control and have never received consistent bowel training; parents are usually disadvantaged.

Discontinuous encopresis usually occurs in response to a stressful situation after children have gained primary control, often as an expression of anger. Children are usually indifferent to the soiling.

Encopresis caused by toilet phobia is an infrequent cause. The toilet is viewed as a place to be avoided, and the child fears being flushed away with the feces.

Etiology: Inefficient intestinal motility; overuse of laxatives, enemas, or suppositories; anal fissures or rashes that cause pain on defecation; and parental demands regarding bowel training.

Occurrence: Occurs in 1% of first and second graders.

Age: Occurs after age 4 to 5 years; rare in adolescence.

Ethnicity: Not significant.

Gender: Primarily occurs in males (80% of cases).

Contributing factors: Children often have no sense of the need to defecate; often associated with UTIs, psychosocial stresses or illness, and irrational fears of the toilet.

Signs and symptoms: The child presents with a history of mild-to-severe soiling of underwear by feces. Obtain history of bowel patterns since birth, attempts to control or manage the incontinence, presence of stressors, and impact on the child and family. A rectal examination reveals stool in the rectal vault. The child may or may not have abdominal pain.

Diagnostic tests:

Test	Results Indicating Disorder	CPT Code
Radiographs of the abdomen	Reveal feces in the colon and ampulla	7400–74022
Urinalysis	Normal	81000
Rectal examination	Positive for feces	45999

Differential diagnosis:

Hirschsprung's disease has a history of passing small, ribbon-like stools; disease is present from birth.

Chronic impaction may be related to dietary intake.

Anal fissures foster withholding of stool.

Childhood depression may be presenting symptom of encopresis.

Attention-deficit hyperactivity disorder is often concomitant with encopresis.

Treatment:

In Home (Immediate Catharsis)

MODERATE-TO-SEVERE RETENTION

Initiate three to four 3-day cycles as follows.

Day 1: Give hypophosphate enemas (Fleet Adult) twice daily.

Day 2: Give bisacodyl (Dulcolax) suppositories twice daily.

Day 3: Bisacodyl (Dulcolax) suppositories are given once.

MILD RETENTION

Prescribe senna, 1 tablet daily for 7 to 14 days.

Obtain a follow-up abdominal radiograph to confirm adequate catharsis.

If child experiences discomfort, alter dosage and frequency. Give no lubricating agent at this time. Consider hospitalization if there is a small yield.

In Home (Maintenance)

The child sits on a toilet 10 minutes twice daily at the same time each day. A kitchen timer is helpful.

Light mineral oil, 2 tbsp twice daily, may be put into juice, cola, or any other food or beverage. Duration of mineral oil regimen may be 4 to 6 months. Give multiple vitamins twice daily at times other than when mineral oil is administered. Give oral laxative (senna) for 2 to 3 weeks, then every other day for 1 month, then discontinue.

Polyethylene glycol 3350 (Miralax) powder: 1/2 cup every other day for 2 weeks, then 1 or 2 times per week as needed.

Diet should be high in roughage (e.g., bran, cereal, fruits, vegetables).

Follow-up: Visits every 4 to 10 weeks to evaluate therapeutic response.

Sequelae: Relapses are common. Signs of relapse are excessive oil leaks, large stools, abdominal pain, decreased frequency of stools, and soiling.

Prevention/prophylaxis: Teach parents developmental milestones related to bowel training.

Referral: In cases of relapse related to psychological stressors, referral to a mental health professional is advisable, as is a referral to a physician for further evaluation for organic disease syndromes. Consider referral for biofeedback training because improvement has been noted with this technique.

Education: Teach parents normal growth and development. Bowel training is usually achieved between ages 2 and 3 years. Reassure parents by teaching about the disorder. Explain the treatment plan.

ENTEROBIUS (PINWORMS)

SIGNAL SYMPTOMS▶ anal itching at night

Enterobius (Pinworms)	ICD-9-CM: 127.4

Description: *Enterobius* infestation is caused by accidental ingestion of the eggs of the intestinal nematode *Enterobius vermicularis.*

Etiology: Ingestion of the eggs of the causative parasite, *E. vermicularis.*

Age: Any age group, but usually seen in children younger than 10.

Ethnicity: Not significant.

Gender: Occurs equally in males and females.

Contributing factors: Crowding and sleeping in an infested bed.

Signs and symptoms: The child presents with a history of nocturnal anal pruritus and sleeplessness. Caregiver may have seen the parasites in the perianal area. May observe excoriations of the perianal area or vaginal discharge in girls.

Diagnostic tests:

Test	Results Indicating Disorder	CPT Code
Slide/tape test of anal area	Positive for eggs and worms	87172

Differential diagnosis: None.

Treatment:

Give pyrantel pamoate (now available over the counter as Pin-X), 11 mg/kg, single dose (maximum 1 g); repeat in 2 weeks.

Alternatively, give mebendazole (Vermox), 100 mg, single dose; repeat in 2 weeks.

Alternatively, give albendazole, 400 mg, single dose; repeat in 2 weeks.

Repeat therapy may be needed because of reinfection. Treatment of all family members is recommended.

Follow-up: Re-evaluate in 2 weeks and at 4 weeks for efficacy of treatment.

Sequelae: If appropriately treated, none; if untreated, vaginitis or salpingitis may develop as a result of worm migration.

Prevention/prophylaxis: Preventive measures include hand washing and keeping the house dusted and cleaned because eggs are laid in house dust and on bed clothes.

Referral: None.

Education: Teach parents that they must thoroughly clean the house on a regular basis.

GASTRITIS

SIGNAL SYMPTOMS epigastric burning and tenderness

Gastritis	ICD-9-CM: 535.5

Description: Gastritis is an irritation of the lining of the stomach; it may lead to ulcer formation.

Etiology: Illness may follow viral infections, ingestion of medications (aspirin, nonsteroidal anti-inflammatory drugs [NSAIDs]), chemotherapeutic agents, or corrosive agents.

Occurrence: Common.

Age: All age groups.

Ethnicity: Not significant.

Gender: Occurs equally in males and females.

Contributing factors: Trauma, hypersensitivity drug reactions, and "acting-out" behaviors are factors to be considered in younger children; in adolescents, chronic alcohol usage may be the cause.

Signs and symptoms: The child presents with a history of abdominal pain, nausea, vomiting, and possibly hematemesis. Palpation reveals epigastric or generalized abdominal tenderness. Hyperactive bowel sounds may be heard on auscultation (Figs. 7–1 and 7–2).

Diagnostic tests:

Test	Results Indicating Disorder	CPT Code
Complete blood count	May indicate a viral or bacterial infection	85022–85025

Endoscopy and barium studies are not helpful.

Differential diagnosis: Peptic ulcer disease (PUD), which is more common in males and whites, can cause pain after eating; in PUD, however, the complete blood count is normal.

Treatment:

Nonpharmacologic

　Avoid irritating substances, such as aspirin.

　Implement a liquid to soft diet for 24 to 48 hours.

　Avoid irritating foods.

Pharmacologic

　Antacids can be given. In infants younger than 2 years, give 0.5 to 2.5 mL/kg every 1 to 2 hours or 1 to 3 hours after meals and before bedtime. Alternate magnesium-based and aluminum-based antacids to control diarrhea.

　Antacids alone are used in children younger than 2 years. Antacids may be used in older children in conjunction with other therapies.

　H_2-receptor antagonists (not recommended for infants because they increase gastrin secretion) can be used as follows:

　　Ranitidine, 2 to 4 mg/kg per day in two divided doses

　　Cimetidine, 20 to 40 mg/kg per day in four divided doses (not recommended for children <16 years old)

　Proton-pump inhibitors (not recommended for infants because they increase gastrin levels) can be used as follows:

　　Omeprazole, in children weighing more than 20 kg, 20 mg daily (take before eating); in children weighing less than 20 kg, 10 mg/kg

Follow-up: Initially, patient should return in 1 week, then every 2 weeks as therapy is continued for 6 to 8 weeks.

Sequelae: Untreated may result in PUD, perforation, obstruction, or uncontrolled bleeding.

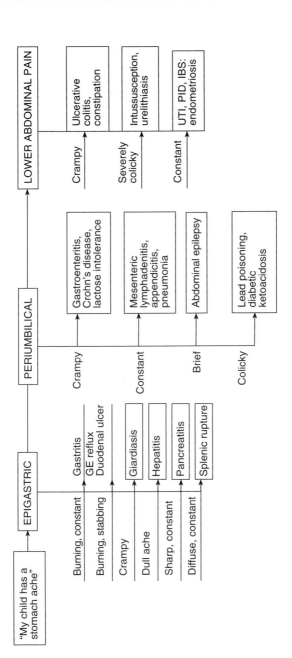

Figure 7–1. Defining characteristics of abdominal pain. (GE, gastroesophageal; UTI, urinary tract infection; PID, pelvic inflammatory disease; IBS, irritable bowel syndrome.)

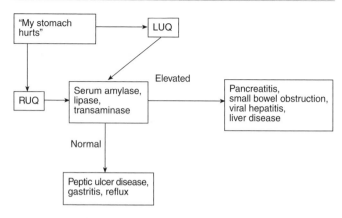

Figure 7–2. Evaluation of upper quadrant abdominal pain. (RUQ, right upper quadrant; LUQ, left upper quadrant.)

Prevention/prophylaxis: Observation for effects of drugs, proper storage of toxic agents, and avoidance of irritating substances.

Referral: Immediate referral for increased bleeding or for medical intervention for ingestion of toxic agents.

Education: Instruct parents in proper storage of medicines and toxic agents.

GASTROENTERITIS

SIGNAL SYMPTOMS ▶ explosive diarrhea

Gastroenteritis	ICD-9 CM: 009.0

Description: Gastroenteritis is an acute inflammatory process of the gastrointestinal tract manifested by severe diarrhea and occasional vomiting, which has a usual incubation period of 2 to 4 days. Several organisms are causative agents. *Salmonella, Shigella, Escherichia coli,* rotavirus, Norwalk virus, *Giardia lamblia,* and *Staphylococcus aureus* are among the most common.

 Clinical Pearl: Salmonellosis and shigellosis are reportable diseases.

Etiology: Causative agents are spread by fecal contamination through hand-to-mouth contact primarily with food. Heavy metals, such as antimony, cadmium, copper fluoride, lead, tin, and zinc, are sources of food poisoning when acidic foods are stored in such containers and the toxin is leached out.

Occurrence: Common. Occurs in outbreaks in day care centers, schools, and hospitals and during the winter.

Age: All age groups.

Ethnicity: Not significant.

Gender: Equally in males and females.

Contributing factors: Factors such as crowding, close contact, and improper hand washing have all been implicated. Undercooked meat products, especially chicken and hamburger, and improper storage of foods are additional factors.

Signs and symptoms: The child usually presents with nonbilious, nonbloody vomiting (first 24–48 hours). Degree of temperature elevation varies, and rash may be present in enteroviral infections. Stools are watery, frequent, and usually foul smelling. A thorough history related to onset; activities before onset; number and frequency of stools; consistency, color, and smell of stools; and presence of blood or mucus is essential. History of vomiting, fluid intake, and urinary output is important. There is usually a history of a similar illness among friends or family (Figs. 7–3 and 7–4).

Skin turgor may be poor, based on the degree of dehydration; oral mucosa is dry if the patient is dehydrated. The patient may have a fine, red, macular rash that is viral in origin. The abdomen may be distended, with increased bowel sounds. The child may appear listless.

Diagnostic tests:

Test	Results Indicating Disorder	CPT Code
Urinalysis and specific gravity	Evidence of dehydration	81000
Complete blood count	Differentiate between bacterial and viral infections	85007
Erythrocyte sedimentation rate	Elevated in bacterial enteritis	85651
Serum electrolytes	Assess degree of dehydration	80051
Stool for OCP, WBC Culture and sensitivity	Evidence of intestinal parasites, infectious processes, type of infectious agent	87177 87045/87046

Differential diagnosis:

Shigellosis is associated with high fever, febrile seizure, and change in mental status.

Severe abdominal pain indicates a more serious problem, such as appendicitis, intussusception, or volvulus.

Suspect obstruction, poisoning, or hepatitis when vomiting continues for 48 hours without diarrhea.

Treatment: The goal is to re-establish, correct, and maintain fluid and electrolyte status.

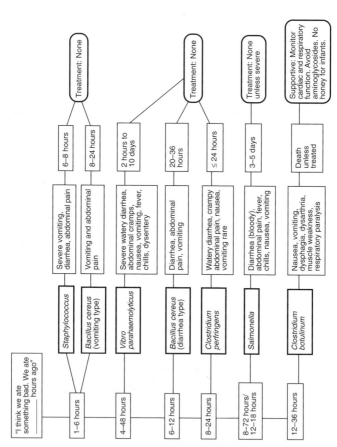

Figure 7–3. Evaluation of food poisoning.

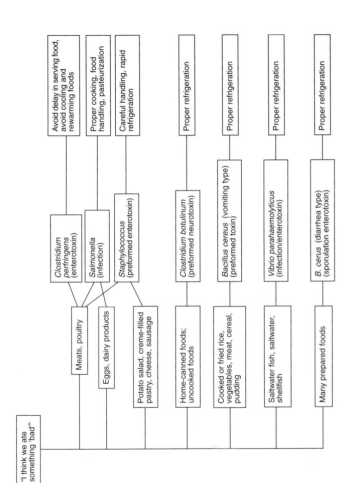

Figure 7–4. Sources and prevention of food poisoning.

Nonpharmacologic

First 12 hours: If infant is breast-feeding, mother should maintain infant at breast, but discontinue any supplemental feedings and give clear liquids instead.

For older infants, parents should discontinue diet and formula, and give small amounts of clear liquids (e.g., Gatorade, Pedialyte, Kool Aid, ginger ale). Parents should offer liquids every 3 to 4 hours if child is not vomiting; otherwise, give small amounts more frequently.

Second 12 hours: As diarrhea improves, parents should begin to offer formula at half strength; if well tolerated, it is safe to go to full strength. If unable to tolerate, child should resume drinking clear liquids, then start lactose-free formula at half strength.

Next 24 hours: If no further vomiting, offer normal diet as tolerated. The BRAT (bananas, rice, applesauce, and tea) diet is no longer considered appropriate because applesauce is high in sugar content, rice is not well tolerated by the intestine, and tea has no nutritional value.

Pharmacologic

Parents should increase fluid intake to rehydrate. If dehydration is severe (see Table 3–4), admit to the hospital for intravenous fluid replacement. Antidiarrheal agents, which are usually unnecessary, can be dangerous in cases of inflammatory enteritis (shigellosis).

If diarrhea has a bacterial cause, antibiotics specific for the organism may be given. Do not treat a *Salmonella* infection with antibiotics because they prolong the carrier state; however, treating shigellosis with antibiotics is usually indicated.

Follow-up: Patient should return in 24 and 48 hours for evaluation of progress, particularly hydration status.

Sequelae: Dehydration is the most important acute complication. Keeping the child on clear liquids may result in persistent loose stools and loss of weight. Occasionally, a milk protein allergy follows a bout of gastroenteritis; an elemental formula should be given in such cases.

Prevention/prophylaxis: Parents and children should use good hand-washing techniques after diaper changing and defecating. A rotavirus vaccine is being evaluated.

Referral: Refer patient to primary care physician for consultation regarding dehydration, severe abdominal pain, moderate amount of blood in the stool, failure to improve after 48 hours, and the need for hospital admission.

Education: Instruct parents and children in good hand-washing techniques and the importance of good hygienic practices. Instruct parents in the normal bowel patterns of children and in the effects of diet or medication on bowel functioning. Teach parents how to monitor and record fluid intake, vomiting, and bowel movements. Teach parents measures for safe handling of food, including storage, preparation, and preparation.

GASTROESOPHAGEAL REFLUX

SIGNAL SYMPTOMS nonviolent backward flow of ingested food

Gastroesophageal reflux	ICD-9-CM: 530.8

Description: Gastroesophageal reflux (GER) is the flow back or return of acidic gastric contents into the esophagus; 85% of cases are self-limiting by age 12 months (because of child's erect posture and the addition of solids to the diet).

Etiology: May be caused by delayed gastric emptying, a large hiatal hernia, or inappropriate relaxation of the lower esophageal sphincter.

Occurrence: Common during the first year of life; occurs in 3% of newborns.

Age: Peak age of onset is 1 to 4 months of age.

Ethnicity: Not significant.

Gender: Occurs three times more often in males than females.

Contributing factors: GER, which is common in neurologically impaired infants, may be associated with hiatal hernia, premature infants, infants with cystic fibrosis, asthma or other respiratory diseases, and cow's milk allergy.

Signs and symptoms: The child presents with a history of effortless spitting up, nonprojectile vomiting, difficulty feeding, and recurrent respiratory problems. The older child may complain of retrosternal burning or dysphagia or both and may awaken with abdominal pain or discomfort. May observe Sandifer's syndrome (lateral head tilt with arching of back); otherwise the physical examination is normal (see Fig. 7–4).

Diagnostic tests:

Test	Results Indicating Disorder	CPT Code
Barium swallow	May reveal anatomic causes such as pyloric stenosis	72420
24-hour monitoring of esophageal pH	Reveals prolonged periods when pH is <4 in the esophagus	91000

Differential diagnosis:

Colic occurs in 23% of 6-week-old infants, who show symptoms including crying 3 hours per day, 3 days per week, and 3 weeks in a row.

Pyloric stenosis is differentiated by the characteristic projectile vomiting and findings on radiographic studies.

Treatment:

Nonpharmacologic

> *Positioning:* To avoid aspiration, parents should elevate infant's head by 30° at all times. They should not involve infant in vigorous play after feeding.

> *Feeding:* Parents should feed infant frequently with small amounts of thickened formula (e.g., ratio of 1 tbsp rice cereal to 6 ounces of formula). Parents should burp infant frequently and avoid giving carbonated beverages. Older children should avoid foods that reduce esophageal sphincter pressure, such as chocolate, fatty foods, and onions. Drugs such as calcium channel blockers, diazepam, theophylline, and progesterone-containing contraceptives also reduce esophageal sphincter pressure. Parents should not allow child to lie down until 4 hours after eating (i.e., bedtime snacks should be prohibited) and should elevate the head of the child's bed 4 to 6 inches. Patients should avoid smoking and drinking coffee or alcoholic beverages. Tomato and citrus juices have also been implicated in GER.

Pharmacologic

> Give antacids, 0.5 mL/kg with meals. Antacids alone are used in children younger than 2 years.

> Give H_2-receptor antagonists (not recommended for infants because they increase excessive gastrin secretion).

>> Ranitidine, 2.5 mg/kg per day in divided doses

>> Cimetidine, 5 mg/kg per dose at mealtime and bedtime

> Give proton-pump inhibitors (not recommended for infants because they increase gastrin levels).

>> Omeprazole, 20 mg per day (in children weighing >20 kg) or 10 mg per day (in children weighing <20 kg)

> Prokinetic agents may be helpful.

>> Metoclopramide, 0.1 mg/kg before meals or

> Give acetaminophen, 0.1 mg/kg for pain every 4 to 6 hours as needed.

Surgical

Surgical intervention consists of a Nissen fundoplication, whereby the fundus of the stomach is wrapped around the distal esophagus. Gastric distention after eating increases the pressure around the wrap and prevents reflux.

Follow-up: Follow patient weekly to assess weight gain.

Sequelae: Aspiration pneumonia, chronic cough, apneic spells, failure to thrive, esophagitis with bleeding, and anemia are all possible complications.

Prevention/prophylaxis: None except lifestyle changes and avoidance of foods known to cause discomfort.

Referral: Refer patient to surgeon in the following cases: medical intervention fails after 2 to 3 months, there is persistent vomiting with failure to thrive, patient has apneic spells or chronic pulmonary disease, or patient is older than 18 months and has a hiatal hernia.

Education: Reassure parents that the condition is self-limiting. Instruct parents in appropriate feeding techniques.

GIARDIASIS

SIGNAL SYMPTOMS▶ periumbilical pain

Giardiasis	ICD-9 CM: 007.1

Description: Giardiasis is the infestation of the gastrointestinal tract by *G. lamblia,* caused by accidental ingestion of the cysts.

Etiology: Ingestion of cysts from a person with giardiasis or from contaminated food or water.

Occurrence: Common.

Age: All age groups.

Ethnicity: Not significant.

Gender: Occurs equally in males and females.

Contributing factors: Contaminated water or food and crowded conditions are associated factors.

Signs and symptoms: The child presents with a history of periumbilical pain, anorexia, nausea, abdominal distention, and diarrhea. On palpitation, there may be periumbilical tenderness. Auscultation may reveal distention.

Diagnostic tests:

Test	Results Indicating Disorder	CPT Code
Stool for OCP	Reveal causative organism	87177
Duodenal washings	Reveal causative organism	89100
Biopsy of small bowel	Reveal causative organism	44020

Microscopic examination of stools, duodenal washings, or biopsy specimen of the small bowel reveals the causative organism.

Differential diagnosis:

Gastroenteritis is an acute, self-limiting illness usually lasting 3 days. School phobic children often present with abdominal pain. Discuss feelings related to the school situation with the child and parent.

Treatment:

- Quinacrine, in children, 0.9 mg/lb three times daily after meals for 7 days; in teenagers, 100 mg three times daily for 5 to 7 days
- Furazolidone, 5 mg/kg per day in four doses for maximum of 7 days or

- Tinidazole, 50 mg/kg single dose (maximum 2 g) or
- Metronidazole, 15 mg/kg per day in three doses for 5 days or
- Paromomycin, 25 to 30 mg/kg per day in three doses for 7 days

Follow-up: Re-evaluate patient in 2 weeks to determine efficacy of treatment.

Sequelae: Usually none.

Prevention/prophylaxis: Proper hand washing, proper preparation of food, and clean drinking water are all prevention measures.

Referral: None.

Education: Instruct parents in techniques of proper hand washing, proper food preparation, and water sterilization.

HEPATITIS

SIGNAL SYMPTOMS persistent flu-like symptoms most common; jaundice is an indicator that this may be hepatitis

Hepatitis A	ICD-9 CM 070.1
Hepatitis B	ICD-9 CM 070.30
Hepatitis C	ICD-9 CM 070.51

Description: Hepatitis is an inflammation of the liver, which is the result of infection by a virus, most commonly hepatitis A, B, or C.

Etiology: Hepatitis is caused by one of three viruses: hepatitis A, hepatitis B, or hepatitis C (HCV) virus.

 Clinical Pearl: In children, hepatitis A is most common.

Occurrence: There are approximately 60,000 cases per year reported of hepatitis A, B, and C. It occurs in about 1.8% of the general population with about 0.2% occurring in infants younger than 2 years and 0.4% in children 12 to 19 years old.

Age: Hepatitis A affects primarily young children and infants, whereas hepatitis B and C occur in all ages. There are approximately 500 million carriers of hepatitis C; 5000 die annually from hepatitis B.

Ethnicity: Not significant.

Gender: Not significant.

Contributing factors: For the newborn, having a hepatitis B–positive or hepatitis C–positive mother increases the probability of contracting the disease. Intravenous drug use, sharing of needles, and obtaining a tattoo or body piercing can also contribute to the incidence of hepatitis.

Signs and symptoms: Usually this disease presents initially as flu-like symptoms. These include increased fatigue, decreased appetite, abdominal pain, nausea and vomiting, and fever. There may be dark colored urine, and most striking is jaundice.

Diagnostic tests:

Test	Results Indicating Disorder	CPT Codes
Liver function test	Elevated ALT, AST	80076
Hepatitis Panel	Positive for A, B, or C	86704–86708 86803–86804
Bilirubin	Elevated	82247
Serum transaminase	Elevated	84450/84460
IgG IgM	Positive for antibody	86001 82657

ALT, alanine aminotransferase; AST, aspartate aminotransferase.

Differential diagnosis:

- Liver cancer differentiated by biopsy
- Physiologic jaundice in the newborn
- Hemolytic disease
- Hemolytic-uremic syndrome
- Medication toxicity

 Clinical Pearl: The introduction of orange, yellow, or red fruits and vegetables into the child's diet can result in carotenemia, which can cause a discoloration or pseudojaundice of the skin.

Treatment: For all cases of uncomplicated hepatitis, the treatment is supportive. Bed rest is not indicated, but a decrease in strenuous activities is recommended. In some cases, a low-fat diet is helpful in decreasing gastrointestinal symptoms.

Follow-up: Regular visits over the first 2 weeks of the diagnosis of hepatitis are recommended with follow-up as needed beyond that time because this is usually a self-limiting disease when uncomplicated.

Sequelae: Hepatitis can progress to a chronic state, and hepatitis B and C can be precursors to liver cancer. In severe acute hepatitis, progressive liver failure and hepatic encephalopathy can result.

Prevention/Prophylaxis: Prophylaxis with the hepatitis B vaccine is now required of all school-age children. In areas of increased incidence of the disease, hepatitis A vaccine is also recommended. Using or sharing needles, taking intravenous drugs, and obtaining tattoos or body piercing can also increase the incidence of hepatitis. Hand washing after each bathroom use should be practiced by all. Household contacts of hepatitis A patients should receive 0.02 mL/kg of immune globulin as soon as the diagnosis is made. If a child younger than 1 year old is exposed to hepatitis B, 0.5 mL of hepatitis B immunoglobulin and the initial dose of the hepatitis B vaccine should be given.

Referral: Collaboration with a pediatrician or infectious disease specialist is recommended for the treatment of all infants and children with hepatitis.

Education: Instruct parents in techniques of proper hand washing.

INGUINAL HERNIA

SIGNAL SYMPTOMS▶   bulge close to pubic tubercle

Inguinal hernia   ICD-9 CM: 550.9

Description: Inguinal hernia is the protrusion of abdominal structures into the scrotum or inguinal canal; patients present with a painless inguinal swelling. Unilateral, right-sided hernias account for 85% to 90% of the total number of hernia cases.

Etiology: The persistence of the peritoneal sac, which normally becomes fibrotic late in gestation, or a weakness of the musculature. Congenitally acquired cases are due to the incomplete closure of the processus vaginalis.

Occurrence: Inguinal hernias occur in about 2% of males with a small percentage (<0.5%) occurring in females.

Age: Any pediatric age group; 50% of cases are diagnosed during the first year of life, but most cases are diagnosed by age 3 months.

Ethnicity: Not significant.

Gender: Males or females, but mostly males (5 to 6:1 to 9:1).

Contributing factors: Coughing, vomiting, or standing for long periods may be factors. Of premature infants, 5% to 30% are born with inguinal hernias.

Signs and symptoms: The child presents to the clinic because the caregiver finds a mass in the inguinal canal, scrotum, or labia. This mass is particularly noticeable when the child cries or strains. Usually the mass is reducible, and there is no pain. Complaints of vomiting, small stools, melena, irritability, and abdominal distention are suggestive of incarceration.

Findings include the palpation of a mass in the scrotum or labia; the size of the mass is enhanced by the increase in intra-abdominal pressure when the child cries or strains. If the neck of the sack closes over the herniated abdominal contents, the hernia may become incarcerated. If the area is tender and swollen, there is strangulation. Bilateral inguinal hernias with palpable contents in females should be investigated for an endocrine or genetic problem. Silk glove sign—a feeling of two surfaces sliding across each other during palpation along the inguinal canal—is evident.

Diagnostic tests:

Test	Results Indicating Disorder	CPT Code
Ultrasound of inguinal area	Assists in differentiating between hydrocele and hernia Assists in identifying contents of inguinal sac	76870

Differential diagnosis:

Inguinal lymph nodes present with multiple, discrete masses.

Transillumination is successful with a hydrocele.

Undescended testicle is movable along the canal and absent in the scrotum.

Lymphadenopathy may be accompanied by increased WBC and lymphocyte counts.

Neoplasms and other masses are differentiated by computed tomography or ultrasound.

Treatment: Surgical intervention to repair the intestinal obstruction.

Follow-up: Monitor patient at each well-child visit. Arrange a visit post-operatively.

Sequelae: Untreated, incarcerated hernia may develop into bowel gangrene. Incarceration or potential strangulation of hernia occurs in about two thirds of all hernias in children younger than 1 year old.

Referral: In suspected cases of inguinal hernia, referral to a surgeon or urologist to be seen in 1 to 3 weeks. Suspected cases of incarcerated or strangulated hernia should be referred to a surgeon immediately.

Prevention/prophylaxis: None; this is a congenitally acquired condition.

Education: Teach the caregiver the technique for reducing the hernia. Teach the caregiver the signs and symptoms of incarceration and strangulation, including increased pain, erythema, vomiting, and abdominal distention. The parents should be instructed, if these symptoms arise, to call a surgeon or urologist or to go to the emergency department.

IRRITABLE BOWEL SYNDROME

SIGNAL SYMPTOMS▶ intermittent diarrhea

Irritable bowel syndrome (IBS)	ICD-9 CM: 564.1
Ulcerative colitis	ICD-9 CM: 556.9
Crohn's disease	ICD-9 CM: 555.9

Description: IBS is a lifelong problem of continuous symptoms of abdominal pain and disordered defecation lasting at least 3 months. Crohn's disease and ulcerative colitis are severe manifestations of IBS. Crohn's disease affects any area of the intestine; the surface of the gut has a cobblestone appearance. Ulcerative colitis affects only the colon and occasionally the ileum.

Diagnostic criteria as adapted by the International Congress of Gastroenterology are as follows. Continuous or recurrent symptoms last at least 3 months and include:

- Abdominal pain relieved with defecation or associated with a change in frequency or consistency of stool
- An irregular (varying) pattern of defecation at least 25% of the time; altered stool frequency
- Altered stool from hard to loose or watery
- Altered stool passage (straining or urgency, feeling of incomplete evacuation)
- Passage of mucus
- Bloating or feeling of abdominal distention

Etiology: There is no universally accepted causative mechanism, but suggested multifactorial causes include genetics, individual immune systems, and the environment. Suggested causative factors include altered colonic motility, abnormal colonic muscle tone, abnormal small bowel motility, altered pain perception, and psychopathology.

Occurrence: Occurs in 5% to 15% of children.

Age: Occurs at any age, but typical onset is 5 to 15 years of age; has been seen between ages 6 and 20 months, clearing spontaneously at 36 months.

Ethnicity: Whites and descendants of Middle European Ashkenazic Jews are at higher risk.

Gender: Occurs more often in females than males.

Contributing factors: Cultures that allow females to report somatic complaints but inhibit males from doing so, stress (e.g., entering high school, going to college, getting married, sibling rivalry), sexual abuse, menstruation, and family history.

Signs and symptoms: The child presents to the clinic usually with a history of abdominal pain and bowel changes. Obtain a complete history, using the above-mentioned criteria for diagnosis of IBS as a guide. The history should include items related to diet, travel, laxative abuse, and psychological issues. The child may present with a history of nausea and vomiting, lethargy, and diarrhea. Nocturnal enuresis, fears, and sleep disturbances are noted in 30% of young children with IBS. There may be joint manifestations of IBD. These may occur in two patterns: the peripheral joints (knees, ankles, wrists, elbows, and hips) and the axial form (affects the spine and sacroiliac joints). Other extraintestinal signs and symptoms include growth failure and skin lesions.

Physical findings are usually negative except for abdominal tenderness, most often in the left lower quadrant.

Diagnostic tests:

Test	Results Indicating Disorder	CPT Code
Complete blood count	Rule out infection	85007
Erythrocyte sedimentation rate	Microcytic anemia	85651
Stools for OCP, fat, and blood	Negative in IBS, positive in infectious processes	87177, 82705–82715, 82270
Barium enema in older patients (diagnostic accuracy of 95% after 5 years)	Shows characteristic changes in the bowel wall	74270
Refer for flexible sigmoidoscopy	Evaluates sigmoid musculature	45331

Differential diagnosis:

Lactose intolerance is differentiated by history and breath test.

Parasitic infection is differentiated by stool examinations isolating the parasite.

Diverticular disease is differentiated by muscular hypertrophy of the sigmoid colon.

Food intolerance, manifested by the presence of mucus and undigested food in the feces, is differentiated in children younger than age 3 years; colic differentiated in the first 3 months of life; history of food intolerance, loose feces with abdominal pain, pain relieved by evacuation, and presence of undigested vegetables in the feces differentiated in children older than 3 years.

Acute appendicitis is differentiated by blood tests and computed tomography of abdomen.

Treatment:

Nonpharmacologic

Treatment comprises dietary management with elimination of foods not tolerated, fiber supplementation to increase stool volume, and smaller more frequent meals.

Pharmacologic

Give psyllium agents, 1 to 2 tsp twice daily.

Give loperamide (Imodium), 1 to 2 mg per day in one to three doses (dose is weight dependent), to decrease urgency, stool frequency, loose stools, and pain.

Give budesonide (Entocort EC), 9 mg daily up to 8 weeks.

Give sulfasalazine (Azulfidine EN-tabs) for ulcerative colitis, initially 1 to 2 g per day; increase gradually to 3 to 4 g per day in equally divided doses after meals until symptoms abate; maintenance dose is 2 g daily. Children older than age 2 years receive 40 to 60 mg/kg per day in three to six doses; maintenance dose is 30 mg/kg per day in four doses.

Give olsalazine (Dipentum) for ulcerative colitis, 500 mg twice a day with meals, to patients who are intolerant of sulfasalazine.

Follow-up: Monthly initially to develop rapport with the patient and evaluate progress.

Sequelae: Growth failure, malnutrition, delayed puberty.

Prevention/prophylaxis: None.

Referral: Refer to primary care physician or internist for flexible sigmoidoscopy and for diagnosis and treatment of depression, if indicated. Refer patient to a psychiatrist for short-term therapy to reduce stress and depression.

Education: Instruct patient in relaxation techniques to reduce pain. Instruct patient to increase intake of fruits, fiber, and fluids; to avoid caffeine, nicotine, and alcohol; and to avoid foods that seem to trigger episodes. Instruct patient to eliminate sources of stress and to increase exercise.

INTUSSUSCEPTION

SIGNAL SYMPTOMS intestinal obstruction; sausage-shaped mass

Intussusception	ICD-9-CM: 560.

Description: Intussusception occurs when one segment of bowel telescopes into the distal segment. It usually starts proximal to the ile cecal valve; invagination is ileocecal, resulting in impairment of venous return causing swelling, hemorrhage, and incarceration with necrosis of the invaginated bowel. Prognosis depends on the duration of the condition.

Etiology: Unknown; lymphoid hyperplasia (Peyer patches) may form a lead point at the proximal segment.

Occurrence: The most frequent cause of intestinal obstruction in the first 2 years of life; after age 6, lymphomas are the most common lesion.

Age: Occurs primarily in infants age 6 to 18 months; 10% of cases occur in children older than 3 years.

Ethnicity: Not significant.

Gender: More prevalent in males (3:1).

Contributing factors: Predisposing factors include cystic fibrosis, Schönlein-Henoch purpura, Meckel's diverticulum, lymphoma, and polyps.

Signs and symptoms: The child presents with acute-onset, intermittent, colicky lower abdominal pain. During episodes of pain, the child cries, draws up knees, and may vomit. Late findings may include lethargy, fever, and currant jelly–colored stools. A sausage-shaped mass may be palpated in the upper abdomen, which is tender and distended.

Diagnostic tests:

Test	Results Indicating Disorder	CPT Code
Barium enema (in 75% of cases, barium enema reduces the intussusception)	Confirm diagnosis	74270

Differential diagnosis:

Incarcerated hernia is best differentiated by ultrasound and surgical consultations because diagnosis may be difficult.

Testicular torsion is best differentiated by ultrasound and surgical consultations because diagnosis may be difficult.

Acute gastroenteritis is differentiated by the presence of symptoms not present in intussusception, such as nausea, vomiting, and lymphocytosis.

Intestinal obstruction and appendicitis are differentiated by ultrasound; patient should be referred to the surgeon for a definitive diagnosis.

Treatment: Refer patient for hospitalization and medical intervention (hydrostatic reduction). Refer for surgical intervention in the following cases: clinical signs of peritonitis or shock or likelihood of discovery of a pathologic lead point.

Follow-up: After hospitalization, observe for signs of recurrence.

Sequelae: If intussusception is not treated promptly, shock or peritonitis may develop. Death may occur if untreated; mortality rate with treatment is 1% to 2%. Recurrence rate is 3% to 4% after medical intervention—usually recurs within 24 hours.

Prevention/prophylaxis: None.

Referral: Refer patient to pediatrician for medical intervention or to pediatric surgeon for surgical intervention.

Education: Reassure parents that they were not to blame.

MEGACOLON (HIRSCHSPRUNG'S DISEASE)

SIGNAL SYMPTOMS▶ passage of enormous formed stools (occasional)

Megacolon (Hirschsprung's disease) ICD-9 CM: 564.7

Description: Megacolon is an aganglionic segment of variable length (5–20 mm) in the colon. In 75% of cases, the segment involved is the rectosigmoid colon, causing narrowing of the denervated segment with dilation of the proximal ganglionic colon.

Etiology: Failure of retrograde migration of neural crest–derived ganglion cells in the developing colon. Research is being conducted on the gene *SOX10* as a factor.

Occurrence: Accounts for 20% of neonatal intestinal obstruction.

Age: May be diagnosed at birth but obvious symptoms may not be noticed until the child is older.

Ethnicity: Not significant.

Gender: Occurs three times more often in males than females.

Contributing factors: There may be a familial pattern; is associated with Down's syndrome (10–15%).

Signs and symptoms: The child presents with no meconium stools in the first 24 hours of life, vomiting, and reluctance to feed. There is a repeated need for rectal stimulation to induce defecation. Stools are characteristically small and ribbon-like.

Findings may include failure to thrive (obtain height and weight), abdominal distention and prominent veins, and palpation of stool in the abdomen with an empty rectum.

Diagnostic tests:

Test	Results Indicating Disorder	CPT Code
Barium enema	Transition zone between aganglionic segment of bowel and dilated proximal segment	74270
Complete blood count	Presence of anemia	85007
Biopsy of rectum	Absence of ganglionic cells	45100
Lateral radiograph in 24 or 48 hours	Assess passage of barium	74000–74022
Radiographs of abdomen (lateral, erect)	Reveals dilated colonic loops and absence of gas below the pelvic colon	74000–74022
Anorectal manometry	Fails to show internal sphincter relaxation	91122

In normal infants, the barium is passed in 24 hours; in infants with megacolon, the barium is retained and mixed with feces.

Differential diagnosis:

Other causes of neonatal intestinal obstruction (e.g., volvulus, intussusception) should be investigated if radiographs are negative for megacolon.

Retentive constipation with colonic distention is differentiated by age of onset, presence of stool in the rectum, and size of the stool in the distended segment.

Celiac disease, a gastrointestinal cause of failure to thrive, is differentiated by age of onset, chronic diarrhea, wasted skeletal muscle mass, and bowel biopsy.

Enterocolitis is differentiated by fever and diarrhea, which may be coexistent with megacolon and accounts for 30% of the mortality after surgery in infants.

Treatment: Surgical intervention is completed in two stages: first stage, a temporary colostomy or ileostomy to divert the feces; second stage, removal of the aganglionic segment and anastomosis at age 12 to 14 months or, in an older child, 3 to 6 months after the initial procedure.

Follow-up: Immediate postoperative visits. Monitor growth and development to look for signs of failure to thrive.

Sequelae: Poor nourishment with associated anemia resulting from a defect in food assimilation. Anal stenosis is a postsurgical complication in 10% to 15% of cases.

Prevention/prophylaxis: None.

Referral: Immediate referral for surgical intervention.

Education: For the older child, teach parents to implement a low-residue diet and to avoid serving the child milk, fried foods, and highly seasoned food. After surgery, the child will probably go home with instructions to eat a normal diet. Instruct parents in presurgery enema techniques. After surgery, instruct parents in colostomy care and skin care of the stoma.

PEPTIC ULCER DISEASE

SIGNAL SYMPTOMS▶   gnawing epigastric pain

Peptic ulcer disease	ICD-9-CM: 533.9

Description: PUD is a circumscribed ulceration of the mucous membrane penetrating through a muscularis mucosa and occurring in areas exposed to acid and pepsin. There are two main kinds:

- Duodenal—located in the duodenum of the small intestine
- Gastric—located in the stomach

Etiology: PUD is caused by an increased production of gastric acid. *Helicobacter pylori*, a multiflagellate, unipolar, spiral bacterium, is responsible for 50% to 60% of PUD cases. PUD may be associated with the use of drugs such as aspirin, NSAIDs, tolazoline, and aminophylline. There is a breakdown of the normal gastric mucosal defense. Close person-to-person contact has been implicated in the transmission of *H. pylori*.

Occurrence: The incidence of PUD in children is unknown, but it is no longer a rare diagnosis in infants and neonates. The rise in prevalence is related to prolonged survival of critically ill neonates and infants at high risk of acute PUD, such as infants with anoxia, hypotension, trauma, and sepsis.

Age: Occurs in any age group but is more common in children age 12 to 18 years.

Ethnicity: Increased incidence in whites.

Gender: After age 6 years, PUD is more common in males.

Contributing factors: In 25% to 50% of patients, there is a family history of ulcers. Environmental factors, such as crowding, climate, dietary habits, and emotional strain, have been implicated. Associated conditions are pancreatitis, cystic fibrosis, uremia, hyperparathyroidism, multiple endocrine neoplasia syndrome, and bleeding disorders. Consider chronic alcohol ingestion in adolescents.

Signs and symptoms:

Age 0 to 3 years: Anorexia, vomiting, crying after meals, melena, or hematemesis. Hemorrhage or perforation may be the first sign.

Age 3 to 6 years: Vomiting after eating, periumbilical or generalized abdominal pain, melena, hematemesis, and perforation.

Age 6 to 18 years: Less than 50% have typical ulcer symptoms; 50% exhibit melena or hematemesis. Occult bleeding and anemia may be present. There may be some periumbilical or generalized tenderness. Child may be irritable.

Diagnostic tests:

Test	Results Indicating Disorder	CPT Code
Upper gastrointestinal series	Visualize lesion	74246–74249
Gastroduodenoscopy	Visualize lesion; if lesions are multiple in the third or fourth portion of the duodenum or in the jejunum, suspect Zollinger-Ellison syndrome	43234–43235
Complete blood count	Presence of anemia	85057
Stool for occult blood	Presence of gastrointestinal bleeding	82270
H. pylori titer	Presence of organism	86677
Rapid ^{13}C urea breath test	Presence of organism	78267–78268

Differential diagnosis:

GER does not cause the patient to wake up with abdominal pain.

Patients with Meckle's diverticulum present with sharp pain from the periumbilical area to the lower abdomen and painless rectal bleeding and obstruction.

Patients with pancreatitis present with acute left upper quadrant pain, which is constant.

Patients with inflammatory bowel disease present with dull, crampy, intermittent pain, lasting 2 hours.

Appendicitis presents with acute, sharp, steady pain located in the epigastric region, localizing to the right lower quadrant.

Treatment: The goal is suppression of gastric acid.

Nonpharmacologic

The patient should avoid caffeine and foods that cause distress, avoid aspirin and NSAIDs, and eat three meals per day without between-meal snacks.

Pharmacologic

Give antacids, 0.5 to 1 mL/kg 2 to 3 hours before feedings and at bedtime (antacids are used alone in children <2 years old).

Give H$_2$-receptor antagonists, such as ranitidine, 2.5 mg/kg every 12 hours, or cimetidine, 5 mg/kg per dose, before meals and at bedtime.

Give proton-pump inhibitors: omeprazole (Prilosec), in children 2 to 16 years old weighing less than 20 kg, 10 mg daily; in children weighing more than 20 kg, 20 mg daily

Give prokinetic agents.

Metoclopramide, 0.1 mg/kg before meals

Give other agents as needed.

Acetaminophen, 0.1 mg/kg for pain

H. PYLORI TITER POSITIVE

H$_2$-antagonist for 6 to 8 weeks plus oral bismuth preparation, two tablets orally every 6 hours for 3 weeks (1 tablet or liquid for smaller children), and amoxicillin, 40 mg/kg per day divided every 8 hours (maximum 1.5 g per day) for 3 weeks, or

Tetracycline, 40 mg/kg per day divided every 6 hours (maximum 2 g per day) for 3 weeks.

Metronidazole, 20 mg/kg per day divided every 8 hours (maximum 1.5 g per day) for 3 weeks, or

Proton-pump inhibitors, such as omeprazole, 20 mg daily, with clarithromycin (Biaxin), 250 mg two to four times per day for 10 to 14 days (adolescents only).

Follow-up: The patient should return in 2 and 3 weeks, then monthly for 4 to 6 months.

Sequelae: Anemia, perforating peritonitis, or pancreatitis may be long-term sequelae.

Prevention/prophylaxis: Patient should avoid caffeine and foods that cause distress, avoid aspirin and NSAIDs, and eat three meals per day without between-meal snacks.

Referral: If there is no improvement or in cases of gastrointestinal bleeding, weight loss, or signs and symptoms of appendicitis, refer patient to primary care physician or surgeon.

Education: Inform child and parent that there is a possibility of recurrence; instruct regarding dietary and medication restrictions.

PYLORIC STENOSIS

SIGNAL SYMPTOMS▶ projectile vomiting, infants

Pyloric stenosis	ICD-9 CM: 750.5

Description: Pyloric stenosis is an increase in the circular muscle of the pylorus resulting in abdominal distention and prominent gastric peristalsis.

Etiology: Several theories, including absence or immature function of pyloric ganglion cells; elevated gastrin levels; elevated substance P, a neurotransmitter that can produce muscle hypertrophy; and poor or lacking innervation of the pyloric musculature.

Occurrence: Occurs in 1 to 4 cases in 1000 births; more common in twins or in a father and his sons.

Age: Occurs at birth.

Ethnicity: Whites, 2 to 4 cases in 1000 births; Hispanics, 1.8 cases in 1000 births; African-Americans, 0.7 cases in 1000 births.

Gender: More common in males (1 in 150) than females (1 in 750).

Contributing factors: Controversial suggested factors are birth order (increased prevalence in firstborn) and the season of birth (spring and fall).

Signs and symptoms: Infant presents at age 2 to 4 weeks with a history of vomiting, usually projectile; poor weight gain or weight loss; and signs of being hungry, fretful, and constipated.

Poor weight gain or weight loss is verified. An olive-sized mass may be palpated in right upper quadrant, and gastric peristaltic waves from left to right may be observed. There is abdominal distention after feeding.

Diagnostic tests:

Test	Results Indicating Disorder	CPT Code
Unconjugated bilirubin	Elevated in 2–3% of cases	82247–827448
Hemoglobin and hematocrit	Elevated owing to hemoconcentration and potassium depletion	85018, 85104
Barium swallow (more cost-effective)	Delayed gastric emptying, elongated pyloric channel (string sign)	74240–74245
Ultrasound	Muscle thickness of >4 mm and a channel length of >16 mm	76700–76705
Gastric aspirate volume	If <10 mL, suspect GER (86%); if <10 mL, suspect pyloric stenosis (92%)	89130–89141
Serum electrolytes	Alkalosis and hypokalemia present; chloride level most predictive	80051
Radiographs of abdomen (flat plate)	Large stomach bubble is suspected pyloric stenosis	74000–74002

Differential diagnosis:

If there are no gastric contents, suspect esophageal stenosis.

If vomitus contains bile (yellow or green), suspect volvulus or small bowel obstruction.

Urinary tract infections may be checked by urine culture.

Gastroesophageal reflux emesis is nonprojectile, and symptoms are insidious; gastric aspirate of less than 10 mL.

Symptoms subside with change in formula (formula intolerance).

Treatment: If patient is dehydrated, restore fluid and electrolyte balance; surgical intervention for pyloromyotomy.

Follow-up: Monitor weight gain and relief of symptoms.

Sequelae: None, if treated promptly; if not, dehydration may develop.

Prevention/prophylaxis: None.

Referral: Refer patient to a surgeon for appropriate intervention.

Education: Instruct parents in proper feeding technique: holding upright, not propping the bottle, feeding slowly, and burping infant after each ounce of formula. Reassure parents regarding the positive outcome of the surgery.

UMBILICAL HERNIA

SIGNAL SYMPTOMS ▶ protruding navel

| Umbilical hernia | ICD-9 CM: 553.1 |

Description: An umbilical hernia is a soft, bulging mass that is easily reducible and more prominent when a child is crying. Spontaneous closure decreases if the defect is greater than 1.5 cm in diameter or if there is a proboscis-like skin defect. Most spontaneous closure occurs by school age in white children.

Etiology: Congenital hernias are the result of incomplete closure of the fascia of the umbilical ring; acquired hernias are a result of an abnormal tumor or organomegaly.

Occurrence: Estimated one in six children have an umbilical hernia.

Age: Occurs in infancy.

Ethnicity: Affects 40% of African-American children younger than 1 year old.

Gender: Occurs more often in males.

Contributing factors: Occurs more frequently in premature infants and in children with Down's syndrome, hypothyroidism, premature infants, or Hurler's syndrome.

Signs and symptoms: During a well-child visit, the parent comments on the status of the protruding umbilicus and may have even strapped the umbilicus. Findings reveal a soft, bulging, reducible mass at the umbilicus. The umbilical ring may be palpated.

Diagnostic tests: None.

Differential diagnosis: None.

Treatment: Surgical intervention to repair the defect if not closed by school age. Reducing and strapping do not hasten the healing process.

Follow-up: Observe patient at each visit to evaluate the progression of healing. Resume usual well-child visits after the first posthospitalization visit if surgical intervention takes place.

Sequelae: Rarely becomes larger unless there is increased intra-abdominal pressure or ascites. In smaller hernias, incarceration is a possibility. If surgical intervention is done to repair the defect, there are no sequelae.

Prevention/prophylaxis: None.

Referral: Refer patient to a surgeon if hernia persists up to school age or there is associated abdominal pain.

Education: Teach parents the signs and symptoms of incarceration: the hernia cannot be reduced, and abdominal pain is severe enough to cause the child to cry.

VOLVULUS

SIGNAL SYMPTOMS▶ intestinal obstruction; bile-stained vomitus

Volvulus	ICD-9-CM: 560.2

Description: A volvulus is twisting of the bowel that results in arterial obstruction, ischemia, and infarction. In 25% of cases, the patients also have congenital cardiac anomalies.

Etiology: An anomaly of intestinal rotation occurs when the small intestine is not fixed in the abdomen and becomes suspended by a stalk containing the superior mesenteric artery.

Occurrence: Not noted.

Age: Occurs predominantly in infants: 80% within the first week of life and 75% within the first 3 weeks of life.

Ethnicity: Not significant.

Gender: Occurs equally in males and females.

Contributing factors: Failure of the midgut to re-enter the fetal abdomen appropriately.

Signs and symptoms: In the neonate (first 3 weeks), a history of bile-stained vomitus and abdominal distention. In the older infant, a history of diarrhea and vomiting and intermittent abdominal obstruction, with vomiting and postprandial abdominal pain.

In the neonate, examination reveals visible gastric peristaltic waves and epigastric or generalized abdominal distention. In the older infant, there is also abdominal tenderness. In a sigmoid volvulus, a palpable mass is present.

Diagnostic tests:

Test	Results Indicating Disorder	CPT Code
Upper gastrointestinal series	Partial or complete small bowel obstruction	74240
Barium enema	Mobile cecum located in midline	74270
Complete blood count with peripheral smear	Suspect midgut volvulus when there are nucleated red blood cells in the peripheral blood	85014

Differential diagnosis:

Meckel's diverticulum is due in 10% of cases to volvulus or intussusception, and the diagnoses overlap. Characteristically the pain in Meckel's diverticulum is sharp in contrast to the pain of intestinal obstruction, which alternates between cramping (colicky) and painless periods. The pain in volvulus is intermittent and cramping.

Treatment: Refer patient to a surgeon. This condition constitutes a surgical emergency.

Sequelae: Intestinal obstruction, peritonitis, perforation, intestinal necrosis, and death.

Follow-up: As required postoperatively.

Prevention/prophylaxis: None.

Referral: Pediatric surgeon for surgical intervention.

Education: Reassurance to the parents that they did not cause the problem.

REFERENCES

Ascariasis

CDC: 1999 Fact Sheet, Ascaris Infection.

Greenberg, M: Ascariasis. EMed J 3, May 23, 2002.

Weiss, E: *Ascaris lumbricoides*. EMed J Mar 2, 2001.

Encopresis

Borowitz, S, et al: Differences in toileting habits between children with chronic encopresis, asymptomatic siblings, and asymptomatic nonsiblings. J Dev Behav Pediatr 20:145, 1999.

Giarelli, E: Hirschsprung's disease: A component of the familial cancer syndrome multiple neoplasia type 2a. Newborn Infant Nurs Rev 2:4, 2002.

Griffin, G, et al: How to resolve stool retention in a child: Underwear soiling is not a behavior problem. Postgrad Med 105, 1999.

Kuhn, B, et al: Treatment guidelines for primary nonretentive encopresis and stool toileting refusal. Am Fam Physician April 15, 1999.

Pashankar, D, and Bishop, W: Efficacy and optimal dose of daily polyethylene glycol 3350 for treatment of constipation and encopresis in children. J Pediatr 139:428, 2001.

Enterobius (Pinworms)

American Academy of Family Physicians: 2000 Fact Sheet. Pinworms and your child.

Gastritis

Shayne, P: Gastritis and peptic ulcer disease. EMed J 3, July 17, 2002.

Gastroenteritis

Armitage, K, et al: Microbes on the menu: Recognizing foodborne illness. Patient Care Nurse Practitioner 3:33, 2000.

Centers for Disease Control and Prevention: Diagnosis and management of foodborne illnesses: A primer for physicians. MMWR Morb Mortal Wkly Rep 50:1, 2001.

Guerrant, R, et al: Practice guidelines for the management of infectious diarrhea. Clin Infect Dis 32:331, 2001.

Pemachio, D: Diarrhea: Differentiation the acute from the chronic. Patient Care Nurse Practitioner 2002.

Sandu, BK: Rationale for early feeding in childhood gastroenteritis. J Pediatr Gastroentol Nutr 33:S13. 2001.

Gastroesophageal Reflux

Bradley, R: Gastroesophageal reflux in children. ADVANCE for NP 9:40, 2001.

Cynamon, H, and Sachs, M: Gastroesophageal reflux: Just spitting up or something more serious? Pediatr Basics 91:10, 2000.

Levy, J: Gastroesophageal reflux and other causes of abdominal pain. Pediatr Ann 30:42, 2001.

Nelson, S, et al: Prevalence of symptoms of gastroesophageal reflux during childhood. Arch Pediatr Adolesc Med 154:150, 2000.

North American Society for Pediatric Gastroenterology and Nutrition: Recommendations on evaluation and treatment of gastroesophageal reflux in infants and children. J Pediatr Gastroenterol Nutr 32:S2, 2001.

Sutphen, J: Is it colic or is it gastroesophageal reflux? J Pediatr Gastroenterol Nutr 33:110, 2001.

Giardiasis

Nash, T: Treatment of *Giardia lamblia* infections. Pediatr Infect Dis J 20:193, 2001.

Patient notes: Avoiding giardiasis. Postgrad Med 109, June 2001.

Zoat, J, et al: Drugs for treating giardiasis. Issue 2 (Cochrane Review). Cochrane Library 2002.

Inguinal Hernia

George, E, et al: Inguinal hernias containing the uterus, fallopian tube, and ovary in premature female infants. J Pediatr 136:696, 2000.

Katz, D: Evaluation and management of inguinal and umbilical hernias. Pediatr Ann 30:729, 2001.

Zitsman, J, et al: Vaginal bleeding in an infant secondary to sliding inguinal hernia. Obstet Gynecol 89:840, 1997.

Irritable Bowel Syndrome

Ballinger, A, et al: Delayed puberty associated with inflammatory bowel disease. Pediatr Res 53:205, 2003.

Bonamico, M, et al: Irritable bowel syndrome in children: An Italian multicentre study: Collaborating centres. Ital J Gastroenterol 27:13, 1995.

Controlling childhood Crohn's disease requires a multipronged approach. Drug Ther Perspect 17:5, 2001.

Gokhale, R: Chronic abdominal pain: Inflammatory bowel disease and eosinophilic gastroenteropathy. Pediatr Ann 30:49, 2001.

Kline, R, et al: Enteric-coated, pH-dependent peppermint oil capsules for the treatment of irritable bowel syndrome in children. J Pediatr 138:125, 2001.

Lake, A: Chronic abdominal pain in childhood: Diagnosis and management. Am Fam Physician Apr 1999.

Levine, A, et al: Evaluation of oral budesonide for treatment of mild and moderate exacerbations of Crohn's disease in children. J Pediatr 140:75, 2002.

Licht, H: Irritable bowel syndrome: Definitive diagnostic criteria help focus symptomatic treatment. Postgrad Med 107:203, 2000.

Olive-Hemker, M: More than a gut reaction: Extraintestinal complications of IBD. Contemp Pediatr 10:45, 1999.

Pardi, D, and Tremaine, W: Inflammatory bowel disease: Keys to diagnosis and treatment. Consultant Jan:87, 1998.

Rayhorn, N: Understanding inflammatory bowel disease. Nursing 29:57, 1997.

Worley, J: Diagnosis and management of inflammatory bowel disease. J Am Acad NP 11:23, 1999.

Youssef, N, and Di Lorenzo, C: The role of motility in functional abdominal disorders in children. Pediatr Ann 30:24, 2001.

Intussusception

Kombo, L, et al: Intussusception, infection and immunization: Summary of a workshop on rotavirus. Pediatrics 108:e37, 2001.

Kuppermann, N, et al: Predictors of intussusception in young children. Arch Pediatr Adolesc Med 154:250, 2000.

Orenstein, J: Update on intussusception. Contemp Pediatr 2:180, 2000.

Megacolon

Mäkitie, O, et al: Hirschsprung disease associated with severe cartilage-hair hypoplasia. J Pediatr 138:929, 2001.

Peptic Ulcer Disease

Braden, B, et al: New immunoassay in stool provides an accurate noninvasive diagnostic method for *Helicobacter pylori* screening in children. Pediatrics 106:115, 2000.

Gold, B, et al: Medical Position Statement: The North American Society for Pediatric Gastroenterology and Nutrition. *Helicobacter pylori* infection in children: Recommendations for diagnosis and treatment. J Pediatr Gastroenterol Nutr 31:490, 2000.

Gold, B, and Goodman, K: *Helicobacter pylori* infection in children: To test or not to test…what is the evidence? J Pediatr 136, 2000.

Kato, S, et al: Urine-based enzyme-linked immunosorbent assay for the detection of *Helicobacter pylori* infection in children. Pediatrics 107:e87, 2001.

Pyloric Stenosis

Letton, R: Pyloric stenosis. Pediatr Ann 30:745, 2001.

Mandell, GA, et al: Cost-effective imaging approach to the nonbilious vomiting infant. Pediatrics 103:1198, 1999.

Nadel, F, and Weinzimer, S: The case of the missing olive. Pediatr Ann 29:119, 2000.

Umbilical Hernia

Katz, D: Evaluation and management of inguinal and umbilical hernias. Pediatr Ann 30:729, 2001.

Volvulus

Salas, S, et al: Sigmoid volvulus in children and adolescents. J Am Coll Surg 190:717, 2000.

Chapter 8

RENAL AND UROLOGIC DISORDERS

ENURESIS

SIGNAL SYMPTOMS ▶ urinary incontinence

Enuresis	ICD-9 CM: 788.30

Description: Involuntary urinary incontinence occurring in a child age 5 or older is categorized as follows:

- *Primary nocturnal enuresis*—has never been dry at night; wet only at night and during sleep
- *Secondary nocturnal enuresis*—has had bladder control, but now wets at night (continent period of 6–12 months)
- *Diurnal enuresis*—wets during the day; 60% to 80% also wet at night

Etiology: See Table 8–1.

Occurrence: An estimated 5 million to 7 million children in the United States. Primary nocturnal enuresis occurs in 15% to 30% of 6-year-old children. Secondary enuresis occurs in 20% of bed wetters older than 4. Diurnal enuresis occurs in 1% of children 6 to 12 years old; 1% to 2% still wet the bed at age 15.

Table 8–1   Possible Causes of Enuresis

Organic	Nighttime Wetting Nonorganic	Daytime Wetting: Functional
Diminished antidiuretic hormone	Family history of enuresis (usually fathers)	Lazy bladder
Fecal impaction	Genetic causes (chromosome 13)	Bladder muscle instability
Urinary tract infection	Emotional stress	Detrusor sphincter dyssynergia
Neurogenic bladder		Constipation Giggle incontinence Postvoid incontinence

Age: Children older than 5; may extend throughout the pediatric age span.

Ethnicity: Occurs more often in African-American boys.

Gender: Three times more often in males than females. Diurnal enuresis is more prevalent in girls.

Contributing factors: Maturational lag, emotional stress, anxiety, timidity or shyness, family history of bed wetting (usually fathers; if both parents were bed wetters, 77% of children have problems), sleep patterns.

Signs and symptoms: Parents may be reluctant to reveal this problem. Inquiries at routine visits as to toileting habits may lead to identification of the problem.

History may reveal past involuntary urinary incontinence. There may be a history of urinary tract infections (UTIs), bladder spasms, dysuria, hematuria, and increased frequency and constipation and fecal soiling. Talk to the child, and elicit his or her feelings and perceptions of the problem. Ask about recent emotional stressors, such as a recent move, divorce, or school problems. Ask about interventions that the family may have initiated.

Assess the genitalia for signs of sexual abuse. Observe the urinary stream for dribbling and small stream. On palpation of the abdomen, a pelvic mass could indicate a fecal impaction.

Diagnostic tests:

Test	Results Indicating Disorder	CPT Codes
Urinalysis for specific gravity and glucose	May indicate diabetes insipidus or diabetes mellitus	81000
Urine culture and sensitivity (especially in females)	Covert infection, may indicate urinary tract malformations	87088
Voiding cystourethrography Renal utrasonography Intravenous pyelography	May identify urinary tract malformations	74450 76999 74400/ 74415

 Clinical Pearl: Small bladder capacity is classified as 10 mL/kg or 1 ounce per year of age + 2 (3 years old = 3 oz + 2 = 5 oz bladder capacity).

Differential diagnosis:

- Behavioral problems, such as depression and anger; these children most often have diurnal enuresis and void voluntarily
- Diabetes, urinary tract abnormalities, and UTIs
- Emotional problems, such as found in cases of sexual abuse
- Chronic constipation

Treatment: Specific treatment is not recommended for children younger than 6 because of spontaneous remission. For children older than 6 and if the parent or child is concerned, treatment can be instituted.

Nonpharmacologic

Behavioral

NOCTURNAL

The goal is for the child to take a responsible, active role in dealing with the enuresis. The following are recommendations for the child:

Keep a calendar of wet and dry nights.

Urinate immediately before bedtime.

Change wet bed linens and clothing and, if age appropriate, launder them.

The following are recommendations for the parent:

Do not give more than 2 ounces of fluid after dinner.

Provide positive reinforcement for dry nights (gold stars or some prearranged reward, praise).

For children who can read, *Dry All Night,* a book for children, may be of assistance in teaching the child to awaken during the night.

The following are some sources of enuresis alarms:

Wet Stop Alarm: 1-800-346-4488

Nite Train'r Alarm: 1-800-544-4240

Nytone Medical Products: 1-801-973-4090

Bedwetting Store: 1-800-214-9605 or www.bedwettingstore.com

Avoid punishments and angry responses.

Diurnal

Initiate a timed voiding schedule around routine events to increase voids to four times per day.

Measure and keep records of voids and amounts. Goal is to empty bladder 75% of capacity at each void ("lazy bladder").

Bladder Training

For children with urgency incontinence, instruct on how to practice stream-interruption exercises. For children with small bladder capacity, recommend enuresis alarms and bladder stretching exercises.

Dietary

If a probable cause is constipation, initiate dietary modifications.

Foods suspected of contributing to enuresis are caffeine, chocolate, dairy products, and citrus fruits and juices.

Pharmacologic

Give tricyclic antidepressants: imipramine hydrochloride (Tofranil-PM), 25 to 50 mg at bedtime for children aged 6 to 12 and 50 to 75 mg for children older than 12. After 1 month of dryness, decrease dosage by tapering off over a 2 to 4 weeks.

Give anticholinergic agents:

DDAVP (desmopressin acetate), in children age 6 to 17 years, 20 µg, 1 hour before bedtime (10 µg in each nostril) for 1 to 2 weeks; increase 10 mg every 2 weeks; maximum dose 40 µg

The child is classified as a nonresponder if unresponsive to DDAVP after several weeks at a dose of 40 µg.

Oxybutynin chloride (Ditropan), for children age 5 and older, 5 mg two times per day for enuresis

Follow-up: Every 2 to 6 weeks during interventions for progress reports; complete blood counts every 2 to 4 weeks while on imipramine.

Sequelae: The child experiences a decline in self-esteem. Social events, such as parties and sleepovers, become a problem.

Prevention/prophylaxis: Reduction of stress; identification and treatment of organic cause.

Referral: Obtain a urology consultation for children with suspected urinary tract abnormalities. Consider mental health referral in cases of children with daytime wetting and secondary enuresis.

Education: Instruct families that patience is a virtue (15% of children have spontaneous remission after age 6). Assist families in identifying appropriate strategies and interventions. To alleviate their self-blame and guilt, reassure parents as to the cause and prognosis.

GLOMERULONEPHRITIS

SIGNAL SYMPTOMS ▶ blood in urine

Glomerulonephritis	ICD-9-CM: 583.9

Description: Glomerulonephritis is a clinical syndrome of glomerular hematuria associated with hypertension, edema, proteinuria, and decreased urinary output and renal function. Glomerular diseases encountered in childhood may be categorized as follows:

Postinfection glomerulonephritis: Onset is 10 to 14 days after an acute illness, usually streptococcal.

Membranoproliferative glomerulonephritis: The etiology is unknown.

IgA nephropathy: Asymptomatic gross hematuria is present.

Schönlein-Henoch purpura glomerulonephritis: There is varied renal involvement.

Glomerulonephritis of systemic lupus erythematosus: On rare occasions, glomerulonephritis is the first sign of systemic lupus erythematosus.

Hereditary glomerulonephritis (Alport's syndrome): Transmission is autosomal-dominant/X-linked, and there is a family history of end-stage renal disease, especially in young males. This syndrome is sometimes associated with deafness and eye abnormalities.

Etiology: Most common cause is poststreptococcal infection.

Occurrence: Worldwide.

Age: Occurs in any pediatric age group, but usually in school-age children.

Ethnicity: Not significant.

Gender: Occurs slightly more in males than females.

Contributing factors: Additional factors to be considered are a past history of streptococcal infection (impetigo, streptococcal throat infection) and family history of urinary abnormalities (genetics).

Signs and symptoms: Parents describe a history of hematuria and decreased urinary output. Many patients complain of headache or malaise. Obtain a past medical history, particularly including streptococcal infections and family history of renal problems.

Physical examination may reveal periorbital edema. Hypertension may be discovered. The patient usually has no fever. In severe cases, ascites is noted (Fig. 8–1).

Diagnostic tests:

Test	Results Indicating Disorder	CPT Codes
Urinalysis for red blood cell casts, gross hematuria ("coffee or tea-colored" urine)	Renal damage	81000
Serum complement level	Decreased in glomerulonephritis	86162
24-hour urine for creatinine and protein	Immunoglobulin proteinuria/24hr	82570
Throat culture and sensitivity	Presence of pathogens	42999
Complete blood count with differential	Assess for continuing infection, anemia	85007
Glomerular filtration rate	Decreased	81001

Differential diagnosis:

In nephrotic syndrome, there is persistent 4+ proteinuria, hyperlipidemia, and periorbital or pedal edema. On spot urine sample, dipstick 1+ or greater is suspect; confirm by quantitative methods.

Acute renal failure needs to be differentiated.

In Alport's syndrome, there is usually malformation of the ears with sensorineural hearing loss.

In polycystic kidney disease or malignancy such as Wilms' tumor, there is usually a palpable abdominal mass.

Pyelonephritis has flank tenderness.

Treatment: Mild-to-moderate disease should be treated with supportive therapy and restrictions regarding salt and water intake. Treatment for

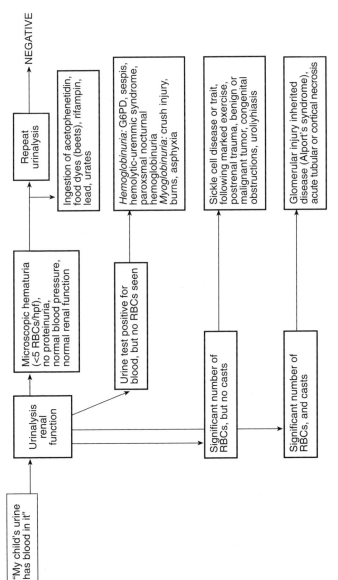

Figure 8–1. Evaluation of hematuria. (G6PD, glucose-6-phosphate dehydrogenase.)

severe disease may include dialysis and renal transplant. Culturing family members and treating asymptomatic carriers may be recommended.

Follow-up: Weekly follow-up for monitoring blood pressure, proteinuria, and edema.

Sequelae: Untreated, glomerulonephritis can result in infection, renal failure, growth failure, anemia, and hypertension.

Prevention/prophylaxis: Adequate treatment of streptococcal infections as a preventive measure.

Referral: Refer child to a pediatric urologist/nephrologist.

Education: Instruct parents in the importance of completion of the antibiotic regimen, the signs and symptoms of renal infection, the methods for monitoring intake and output, and the nutritional requirements and restrictions.

URETHRITIS

SIGNAL SYMPTOMS ▶ urethral discharge

Urethritis	ICD-9-CM: 597.80

Description: Urethritis is an infection of the urethra resulting from contact with a pathogen during sexual contact.

Etiology: Most common bacterial pathogens are *Neisseria gonorrhoeae* and *Chlamydia trachomatis*. *Ureaplasma urealyticum* and *Mycoplasma genitalium* are implicated in possibly one third of nongonococcal urethritis cases.

Occurrence: Common.

Age: Usually occurs in adolescents; 15- to 24-year age group has highest incidence of sexually transmitted diseases.

Ethnicity: Not significant.

Gender: Occurs equally in males and females.

Contributing factors: Multiple sexual partners, failure to use contraceptives, and failure to seek early treatment.

Signs and symptoms: Patients complain of dysuria and urethral discharge. History of sexual activity should be obtained. In females particularly, suspect sexual abuse. Obtain a history related to trauma, sexual abuse, and masturbation. Males may complain of urinary frequency, urgency, and priapism. There may be a clear, white, or purulent discharge from the urethra and suprapubic tenderness. Some infections are asymptomatic.

Diagnostic tests:

Test	Results Indicating Disorder	CPT Codes
First voided urine	At least 10 WBCs/ high-power field	81000
Gram stain urethral secretions	At least 5 WBCs per oil-immersion field	87166
First voided urine	Positive leukocyte esterase test	81099
Pelvic and penile cultures	Identification of specific organism	87999
Culture for N. gonorrhoeae using chocolate agar or Thayer-Martin medium	Identification of specific organism	87166
Culture, enzyme-linked immunoassay or monoclonal antibody	Identification of specific organism	87449
Immunofluorescence test	Identification of Chlamydia	87270

WBCs, white blood cells.

Differential diagnosis:
- Topical irritants
- Pinworms, identified in the discharge

Treatment:

N. gonorrhoeae
For children who weigh less than 45 kg:
    Ceftriaxone, 125 mg intramuscularly (IM) in a single dose
    Alternative: Spectinomycin, 40 mg/kg (maximum 2 g) in a single dose (may not be reliable)
For adults and adolescents:
    Cefixime, 400 mg orally in a single dose or
    Ceftriaxone, 125 mg IM in a single dose or
    Ofloxacin, 400 mg orally in a single dose or
If chlamydial infection is not ruled out:
    Azithromycin, 1 g orally in a single dose or
    Doxycycline, 100 mg orally twice a day for 7 days
Alternative agents:
    Spectinomycin 2 g IM in a single dose or
    Ceftizoxime, 500 mg IM in a single dose or
    Cefotaxime, 500 mg IM in a single dose or
    Cefoxitin, 2 g IM in a single dose with probenicid, 1 g daily

Chlamydia
First-line agents:
    Azithromycin, 1 g orally in a single dose plus
    Doxycycline, 100 mg orally twice a day for 7 days
Alternative agents:
    Erythromycin base, 500 mg orally four times a day for 7 days or
    Erythromycin ethyl succinate, 800 mg orally four times a day for 7 days or

Ofloxacin, 300 mg twice a day for 7 days or
Levofloxacin, 500 mg orally for 7 days

For patients unable to tolerate high doses of erythromycin:

Erythromycin base, 250 mg orally four times a day for 14 days or
Erythromycin ethyl succinate, 400 mg orally four times a day for
14 days

For recurrent or persistent chlamydia:

Metronidazole, 2 mg orally in a single dose plus
Erythromycin, 500 mg orally four times a day for 7 days or
Erythromycin ethyl succinate, 800 mg orally four times a day for
7 days

Follow-up: Return in 1 week for evaluation of therapeutic response.

Sequelae: If untreated or inadequately treated, urethritis can result in cervicitis in females and prostatitis, epididymitis, or orchitis in males.

Prevention/prophylaxis: Preventive measures include practicing safe sex and using appropriate contraceptives. Treatment of both partners is important to prevent reinfection.

Referral: Report sexually transmitted diseases to the local health department.

Education: Emphasize abstinence until both partners have been treated adequately. Teach proper hand-washing technique, and instruct patients to wash hands after voiding.

URINARY TRACT INFECTIONS

SIGNAL SYMPTOMS▶ painful frequent micturition

Urinary tract infection	ICD-9-CM: 599.0

Description: UTIs are caused by the introduction of bacteria or irritants into the urinary tract (bladder or kidneys), resulting in an infection.

Etiology:

Bacterial: Most common organisms are *Escherichia coli, Klebsiella, Proteus,* enterococci, staphylococci (particularly *S. aureus*), and group B streptococcus. In prepubertal girls, a common cause is the novobiocin-resistant, coagulase-negative *Staphylococcus saprophyticus.*

Nonbacterial: Residual urine, foreign bodies, vesicoureteral reflux, and urinary stasis have been implicated.

Occurrence: Most common of the genitourinary problems of childhood: found in 1% of premature infants and newborns, 3% to 7.8% of school-age girls, and 1% to 1.7% of school-age boys.

Age: All age groups.

Ethnicity: Incidence higher in whites.

Gender: During the first months of life, more common in males; from age 2 months to adulthood, more common in females.

Contributing factors: Voiding habits (infrequent, leakage, constipation); anatomic variants such as short urethra in females and congenital defects; environmental factors such as use of bubble baths, colored or perfumed toilet paper, improper wiping after defecating, and too-tight undergarments; sexual activity in females; masturbation; and perianal infection (pinworms).

Signs and symptoms: Presenting symptoms and physical findings depend on age (Fig. 8–2).

- Neonates—feeding problems, diarrhea, vomiting, fever, failure to thrive, hyperbilirubinemia
- 1 month to 2 years—feeding problems, diarrhea, fever of unknown origin, colic, irritability and screaming periods, failure to thrive
- 2 to 6 years—urgency, dysuria, frequency, abdominal pain, strong-smelling urine
- 6 to 18 years—frequency, dysuria, urgency, abdominal or flank pain

Diagnostic tests:

Test	Results Indicating Disorder	CPT Codes
Urinalysis (hematocytometer leukocyte counts have been shown to be more accurate than standard urinalysis)	>5 WBCs/high-power field	8100
Urine culture and sensitivity	10^2 colonies/mL	87088
Radiographic studies Intravenous pyelogram or voiding cystourethrogram Usually 6–8 weeks post-treatment	Evidence of urinary tract malformations	74400 74450

Criteria for conducting such studies are UTI in a male, UTI in the first year of life, and UTI in a female with treatment failure or evidence of pyelonephritis.

Differential diagnosis:

Upper UTIs, as opposed to lower UTIs, show glitter cells and WBC casts; patient has high fever and anatomic abnormalities.

Patients with anatomic abnormalities, such as neurogenic bladder, vesicoureteral reflux, and urinary stasis, initially may present as having a UTI.

Pyelonephritis shows elevated C-reactive protein and high fever.

Treatment:

- Trimethoprim (TMP) and sulfamethoxazole (SMX), 8 mg/kg TMP plus 40 mg/kg SMX per day at bedtime or 5 mg TMP plus 25 mg SMX twice per day ×10 days or
- Nitrofurantoin, 5 to 7 mg/kg per day in divided doses every 6 hours or

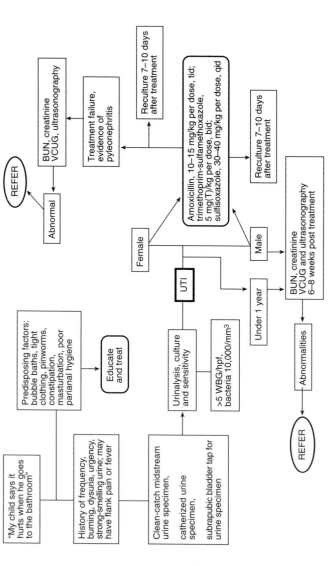

Figure 8–2. Evaluation of urinary tract infection (first episode). (UTI, urinary tract infection; BUN, blood urea nitrogen; CUG, voiding cystourethrogram.)

- Sulfisoxazole, 10 to 20 mg/kg per day in divided doses every 12 hours or
- Methenamine mandelate, 75 mg/kg per day in divided doses every 12 hours

 Clinical Pearl: In children younger than 2 months old, do not use sulfonamide antibiotics or nitrofurantoin because of the risk of displacing bilirubin from albumin.

Follow-up: Follow-up urinalysis in 3 days and again in 10 days to evaluate clinical response. Continue to follow-up every 1 to 2 months until patient is infection-free for 1 year.

Sequelae: If not treated promptly, the infection can result in renal scarring and pyelonephritis.

Prevention/prophylaxis: It has been suggested that newborn circumcision protects male infants from UTIs during the first year of life.

Instruct parent or patient as follows:

Increase water intake to 1 to 2 L per day.

Empty bladder every 3 to 4 hours during the day.

Use improved hygienic measures.

Use white, unscented toilet paper.

Avoid taking bubble baths.

Prescribe suppressive antibiotic therapy for children with recurrent infections or children at high risk for reinfection (e.g., children <5 years old, children with urinary tract abnormalities).

Referral: Refer female patients to an urologist after treatment failure. Treatment failures often suggest an anatomic abnormality. Refer any male with UTI to an urologist.

Education: Teach parents measures to promote a healthy environment, such as avoiding bubble baths, using unscented toilet paper, properly cleansing after voiding, and dressing child in white cotton panties with no aniline dyes. Instruct parents as to the importance of completing the therapeutic regimen.

REFERENCES

Enuresis

Brunell, P, et al: Taking a closer look at nocturnal enuresis. Infect Dis Child May 2001.

Casale, A: Daytime wetting: Getting to the bottom of the issue. Contemp Pediatr 2:107, 2000.

Cendron, M: Primary nocturnal enuresis: Current concepts. Am Fam Physician 153, 1999.

Chandra, M, et al: Giggle incontinence in children: A manifestation of detrusor instability. J Urol 168:2184, 2002.

Hallioglu, O, et al: Brain differences in children with nocturnal enuresis. J Child Neurol 16:714, 2001.

Longstaffe, S, et al: Behavioral and self-concept changes after six months of enuresis treatment: A randomized, controlled study. Pediatrics 105:935, 2000.

Mack, R: Dry All Night. Little, Brown, Boston, 1989.

Neveus, T, et al: Sleep of children with enuresis: A polysomnographic study. Pediatrics 108:206, 2001.

Glomerulonephritis

Cruz, C, and Spitzer, A: When you find protein or blood in the urine. Contemp Pediatr September 1998.

Loghman-Adham, M: Evaluating proteinuria in children. Am Fam Physician 58:1145, 1998.

Stapleton, FB: Acute glomerulonephritis: Impetigo as an etiological factor. J Pediatr 138:783, 2001.

Urethritis

U.S. Department of Health and Human Services, Centers for Disease Control and Prevention: 2002 Guidelines for treatment of sexually transmitted diseases. MMWR Morb Mortal Wkly Rep 51(RR-6), May 10, 2002.

Urinary Tract Infections

Bachur, R, and Harper, M: Reliability of the urinalysis for predicting urinary tract infections in young febrile children. Arch Pediatr Adolesc Med 155:60, 2001.

Committee on Quality Improvement, Subcommittee on Urinary Tract Infection: American Academy of Pediatrics: Practice parameter: The diagnosis, treatment, and evaluation of the initial urinary tract infection in febrile infants and young children. Pediatrics 103:843, 1999.

Downs, S: Diagnostic testing strategies in childhood urinary tract infections. Pediatr Ann 28:670, 1999.

Gorelick, MH, and Shaw KN: Clinical decision rule to identify febrile young girls at risk for urinary tract infection. Arch Pediatr Adolesc Med 154:386, 2000.

Hellerstein, S: The long-term consequences of urinary tract infections: A historic and contemporary perspective. Pediatr Ann 28:695, 1999.

Hoberman, A, and Wald, E: Treatment of urinary tract infections. Pediatr Ann 28:688, 1999.

Honkinen, O, et al: Bacteremic urinary tract infection in children. Pedeatr Infect Dis J 19:630, 2001.

Lin, DS, et al: Comparison of hemocytometer leukocytes counts and standard urinalyses for predicting urinary tract infections in febrile infants. Pediatr Infect Dis J 19:223, 2000.

Pennington, D, and Zerin, JM: Imaging of the urinary tract in children. Pediatr Ann 28:678, 1999.

Plachter, N, et al: Identification and management of urinary tract infections in the preschool child. J Pediatr Health Care 13:268, 1999.

Roberts, K, and Akintemi, O: The epidemiology and clinical presentation of urinary tract infections in children younger than 2 years of age. Pediatr Ann 28:644, 1999.

Schlager, T: The pathogenesis of urinary tact infections. Pediatr Ann 28:639, 1999.

Schoen, E, et al: Newborn circumcision decreases incidence and costs of urinary tract infections during the first year of life. Pediatrics 105:789, 2000.

Steele, R: The epidemiology and clinical presentation of urinary tract infections in children 2 years of age through adolescence. Pediatr Ann 28:653, 1999.

Chapter 9

REPRODUCTIVE SYSTEM DISORDERS

AMENORRHEA

SIGNAL SYMPTOMS ▶ no onset of menses by age 17 three consecutively missed periods

Amenorrhea	ICD-9 CM: 626.0

Description: Amenorrhea, the absence of menses, can occur in either a primary or a secondary form. Primary amenorrhea is diagnosed when the onset of menses has not occurred by age 17. Secondary amenorrhea is diagnosed when menses has not occurred for at least 3 months.

Etiology: There is no genetic predisposition for primary or secondary amenorrhea. Primary amenorrhea may be caused by an imperforate hymen, agenesis of the uterus, Turner's syndrome, or constitutional delay. Secondary amenorrhea may be due to pregnancy, a corpus luteum cyst, menopause, or breast-feeding. Other causes of secondary amenorrhea include diabetes, hypothyroidism or hyperthyroidism, chemotherapy, stress, weight loss, and polycystic ovaries.

Occurrence: Amenorrhea occurs in 3.3% of females.

Age: Amenorrhea can occur from menarche to menopause.

Ethnicity: Not significant.

Gender: Females.

Contributing factors: Strenuous athletic exercise or training, eating disorders including bulimia and anorexia, psychological problems, and emotional crisis may contribute to the incidence of amenorrhea.

Signs and symptoms: In primary amenorrhea, the patient, who is at least 17, reports that she has never had a menstrual period. She may state that this has occurred in other members of her family.

In secondary amenorrhea, the patient may state that it has been a minimum of 3 months since her last menstrual cycle. She may relate signs and symptoms suggestive of pregnancy, including bloating, enlarged and tender breasts, nausea and vomiting at different times of the day (usually in the morning on awakening), and increased lethargy. She may state that she has had unprotected sexual intercourse. Other complaints may include weight gain, polyuria, polydipsia, an emotional crisis, or a recent increase in an athletic training schedule.

Inspection reveals few findings unless the patient is pregnant. In hypothyroidism, the skin may be extremely dry, periorbital edema may be noted, and there may be some apparent voice changes (hoarseness). When a Pap smear and vaginal examination are performed, an imperforate hymen (rare) may be noted. The cervix may be blue or purple, suggestive of changes seen in pregnancy; other changes include breast enlargement and darkened areolae. When constitutional delay is suspected, the nurse practitioner should carefully evaluate breast development and pubic hair distribution to determine the Tanner stage (see Table 1–11).

Palpation and percussion may reveal breast tenderness, increased uterine size, and increased height of the fundus. Thyroid size should be evaluated for enlargement when thyroid disease is suspected (Fig. 9–1).

Diagnostic tests:

Test	Results Indicating Disorder	CPT Code
Serum pregnancy	Positive	84702
Prolactin	Higher than normal	84146
Thyroid-stimulating hormone	Higher than normal	80439
Ultrasound of the ovaries and uterus	Absence of uterus, polycystic ovaries	76805

Differential diagnosis:

Pregnancy is differentiated by a serum pregnancy test.

Overtraining is determined from the history. Menses returns when the training schedule is moderated and there is less physical stress on the body.

Eating disorders are determined from the history but may often be missed by the health care provider, especially during an initial visit; also, subtle changes in weight cannot be known unless the patient shares these facts.

Turner's syndrome is differentiated by physical examination (webbed neck, pectus excavatus, short stature, heart murmur) or genetic screening.

Pituitary diseases and uncontrolled endocrinopathies, which can suppress menses, can be detected by hormonal studies.

Because some medications and medical treatments can suppress menses (e.g., growth hormone–releasing hormone analogue, danazol, medroxyprogesterone acetate [Depo-Provera], chemotherapy), the patient's medication history should be obtained.

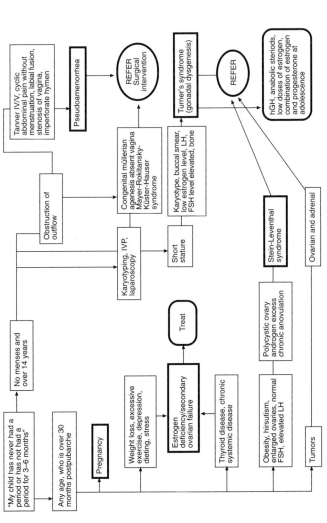

Figure 9–1. Evaluation of amenorrhea. (FSH, follicle-stimulating hormone; LH, luteinizing hormone; hGH, human growth hormone; IVP, intravenous pyelogram.)

Treatment:

Nonpharmacologic

If the patient is overweight or underweight, proper nutritional counseling is needed.

Pharmacologic

If the cause is imperforate hymen, surgery is indicated.

In all cases, hormone replacement therapy is indicated for 6 months to reduce the risk of osteoporosis. Medroxyprogesterone acetate, 5 to 10 mg daily for 5 to 10 days of each month, is a good mode of treatment. Conjugated estrogens, 0.3 to 0.625 mg daily for 21 days, with medroxyprogesterone acetate, 5 to 10 mg daily during the last 7 days of the month, is another treatment modality.

During evaluation and treatment 1500 mg per day of calcium supplement should be given.

Follow-up: Of all cases of secondary amenorrhea, 99% spontaneously resolve; routine health care visits are all that is needed. If the patient is not pregnant and hormone replacement therapy is used, further assessment is suggested in 6 months; the therapy should be stopped and the patient referred if menses does not return spontaneously.

Sequelae: Estrogen-deficiency symptoms, such as hot flashes, vaginal dryness, and signs of osteoporosis, can occur if amenorrhea is prolonged.

Prevention/prophylaxis: Maintenance of proper body weight, moderation in athletic training, and the use of prophylaxis for sexual intercourse can prevent secondary amenorrhea.

Referral: If amenorrhea persists for 6 months after treatment has been instituted, refer to a gynecologist. If pregnancy is suspected or proved by tests and examination, refer immediately to a nurse-midwife or gynecologist. If an endocrine disorder is suspected, refer to an endocrinologist.

Education: The patient must be fully informed of all the findings, including pregnancy. If needed, refer to a gynecologist. The need for regular prenatal care should be stressed. The effects of long-term amenorrhea should be fully explained to the patient. Explain treatment options (e.g., hormonal replacement therapy, lubricants for vaginal dryness, other medication regimens) to the patient, and allow the patient an opportunity to ask questions. As menses returns, offer contraceptive counseling.

CRYPTORCHIDISM

SIGNAL SYMPTOMS▶ maldescended testicles

Cryptochidism	ICD-9 CM: 752.51

Description: Cryptorchidism is the failure of one or both testes to descend into the scrotum.

Etiology: This disorder may be related to some interference with descent of the testes between the seventh and ninth prenatal month. Because it is a congenital defect, the exact cause is unknown.

Occurrence: Found in 3.4% of all newborns and 30% of premature infants. The anomaly is bilateral in 10% of cases, and in 3% to 5% of cases there are no testes. Of patients with cryptorchidism, 10% have an associated upper urinary tract abnormality.

Age: Present at birth.

Ethnicity: Not significant.

Gender: Males.

Contributing factors: Unknown—congenital anomaly.

Signs and symptoms: The parent reports that the scrotal area looks "different" from that of other children or that the sac feels or looks empty. The cremasteric reflex is absent or weak at birth. The testis cannot be palpated in the scrotum. The scrotal sacs appear smaller (bilateral) or asymmetrical (unilateral).

Diagnostic tests:

Test	Results Indicating Disorder	CPT Code
Scrotal sonogram (if defect is bilateral)	Evidence of undescended or absence of testes	76870

Differential diagnosis:

Anorchism is differentiated by sonogram, which shows the absence of one or both testicles.

Retractile testis occurs when one testis remains retracted most of the time but is palpable on examination. It may respond to cold.

Ectopic testis is a testicle that has been diverted from the normal pathway of descent and is found in a superficial inguinal location—the suprapubic, femoral, or perineal site.

Ambiguous genitalia may be confused with bilateral cryptorchidism, but the testes are usually absent, whereas the scrotum is present. Also, female and male genitalia are present.

Treatment: Hormone therapy, which may be instituted by a urologist to facilitate surgery, is followed by an orchiopexy between 6 months and 1 year of age.

Follow-up: By age 1 year, a child with unilateral cryptorchidism should be seen by an urologist. If surgery is performed, the child should be seen at 6-month intervals for 1 to 2 years.

Sequelae: Infertility, atrophy of the testicle, and an increased risk of developing a malignant testicular tumor.

Prevention/prophylaxis: None: congenital abnormality.

Referral: Patients with bilateral or nonpalpable cryptorchidism should be referred to an urologist. Unilateral cryptorchidism should be referred to an urologist by age 1 year.

Education: Parents should be taught to palpate the child's testes so that they can detect any abnormality. Also, they should be shown the difference between a retractile testicle and one that is absent. An open discussion with the child and parent should occur so that all involved are aware of the possible sequelae.

DYSMENORRHEA

SIGNAL SYMPTOMS▶ pain that interferes with daily activities or requires medication and is associated with any part of the menstrual cycle pain in lower abdomen

Dysmenorrhea	ICD-9 CM: 625.3

Description: Dysmenorrhea is painful menstruation characterized by lower abdominal cramping usually occurring during the first few days of bleeding. Dysmenorrhea is divided into two types: primary, which occurs in the absence of any pelvic pathology, and secondary, which is associated with a specific pelvic pathology.

Etiology: Primary dysmenorrhea has no known causative agent, but it is suspected that painful menses occurs when there is an increase of prostaglandin $F_{2\alpha}$ and prostaglanding E_2. Secondary dysmenorrhea is usually caused by pelvic inflammatory disease (PID), endometriosis, uterine myomas, polyps or adhesions, adenomyosis, ovarian cysts or tumors, the presence of an intrauterine device (IUD), cervical stenosis or strictures, or congenital malformations.

Occurrence: Of adolescent girls, 75% experience some pain with menses, 10% to 15% of whom have pain so severe that it limits normal activities.

Age: Dysmenorrhea occurs from about 6 to 12 months after menarche begins to the mid-20s, with a few women experiencing cramping until a more advanced age.

Ethnicity: Not significant.

Gender: Females.

Contributing factors: Underlying pathologies, emotional stress, certain hormonal abnormalities, and familial tendency.

Signs and symptoms: When obtaining a history, ask the following questions.

What is the pain like (sharp, dull, pressure)?
When did you first start having the pain?
Are there associated symptoms, such as nausea and vomiting?
Does the pain cause you to miss school or work?
What remedies have you used, and were they successful?
Is there a maternal or sibling history of painful menses?

The adolescent reports that her first few menstrual cycles were painless, but that recently she experienced lower abdominal and back pain during the first 1 to 3 days of her cycle.

Inspection reveals the patient to be guarding, in pain, and rubbing the abdomen. The skin should be observed for hirsutism, bruising, or petechiae. Palpation and percussion of the abdomen and kidneys should be done to detect masses and tender areas. In primary dysmenorrhea, few findings are noted.

In secondary dysmenorrhea, the history may reveal other symptoms, such as fever (PID); pain that lasts beyond the menstrual cycle (endometriosis); heaviness in the lower abdomen, swelling, or heavy bleeding (cysts or tumors); and a vaginal discharge and odor (sexually transmitted disease [STD]).

Inspection reveals a white-to-brown vaginal discharge with an odor. There may be a string visible if the pain is the result of an IUD. Palpation and percussion may reveal tenderness or a mass in the abdomen or suprapubic area. In the adolescent who is not sexually active, a speculum may not be needed and should not be insisted on for the examination.

Diagnostic tests: Although there are no specific tests needed if under-lying pathology is not suggested by the examination, often the following are performed.

Test	Results Indicating Disorder	CPT Code
Hemoglobin and hematocrit	Lower than normal	83036
Ultrasound of the uterus and ovaries	Presence of ovarian cyst may accompany dysmenorrh	76805

Differential diagnosis:

Abdominal, uterine, or bladder mass is differentiated by sonogram or computed tomography (CT) scan.

STD is differentiated by vaginal cultures or a blood test.

Endometriosis is differentiated by endometrial biopsy.

Treatment:

Nonpharmacologic

Heating pads, mild exercise, and maintenance of a good diet may help to alleviate or decrease the symptoms.

Pharmacologic

Treatment for mild dysmenorrhea includes ibuprofen, aspirin, or aceta-minophen. The most commonly prescribed drug is ibuprofen, 400 mg every 4 to 6 hours for 24 to 72 hours. For moderate-to-severe dysmen-orrhea, nonsteroidal anti-inflammatory drugs (NSAIDs), given for 3 to 4 months, are the treatment of choice:

- Naproxen (Aleve, Naprosyn), 440 mg for the first dose, then 220 mg every 8 to 10 hours or
- Mefenamic acid (Ponstel), 500 mg for the first dose, then 250 mg every 6 hours for 2 to 3 days or
- Naproxen sodium (Anaprox), 550 mg at the first dose, then 550 mg every 12 hours for the duration of the symptoms

If NSAIDs are not effective or if the adolescent is sexually active, low-dose combination oral contraceptives (OCs) should be used. They may be used alone or in combination with the NSAIDs. OCs are about 90% effective in severe dysmenorrhea.

Follow-up: At 3 months, if the symptoms have not worsened, the patient should be seen to evaluate the effectiveness of the treatment. If the patient is sexually active, a yearly Pap smear and examination should be scheduled.

Sequelae: Usually there are no serious physical sequelae; however, adolescents may miss school or work because of severe pain, which results in poor school performance or the loss of a job.

Prevention/prophylaxis: A mild exercise program, good diet, and proper use of medications (NSAIDs and OCs) can prevent serious pain. A menstrual diary may help patients anticipate their menstrual cycle.

Education: Most patients are symptom-free after 3 to 4 months of therapy, so education should include reassurance. The importance of a good diet, mild-to-moderate exercise, and regular use of medications should be stressed.

EPIDIDYMITIS

SIGNAL SYMPTOMS painful swelling of the scrotum

Epididymitis	ICD-9 CM: 604.90

Description: Epididymitis is a painful, acute inflammation of the epididymis.

Etiology: Commonly, epididymitis is caused by *Neisseria gonorrhoeae* and *Chlamydia,* but it also can occur with an infection in the urethra or bladder.

Occurrence: Fairly common; not influenced by seasonality.

Age: Epididymitis is a rare occurrence before puberty, but it can occur any time after a child becomes sexually active. In extremely rare cases, it can occur in children younger than age 2 who have congenital anomalies associated with the urologic system.

Ethnicity: Not significant.

Gender: Occurs only in males.

Contributing factors: Congenital anomalies of the kidney, bladder, or urethra; trauma or irritation; secondary to systemic disease (sarcoidosis, Kawasaki disease, and Henoch-Schönlein purpura); and engaging in unprotected sex.

Signs and symptoms: The child reports painful swelling of the scrotum that can be either acute or insidious. The scrotum is painful to touch and manipulate (Fig. 9–2). Elevation of the scrotum (Prehn's sign) elevates the testicles and usually relieves the discomfort, which differentiates epididymitis from testicular torsion. The cremasteric reflex is present.

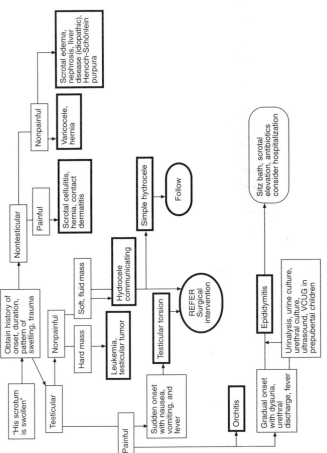

Figure 9–2. Evaluation of scrotal swelling. (VCUG, voiding cystourethrogram.)

The child reports having a fever, dysuria, and increased frequency of urination. The child admits having had unprotected sex within 45 days of the onset of the problem. On inspection, the nurse practitioner notes scrotal swelling and redness; the scrotum feels warm to touch. During palpation of the scrotum, the child reports pain. The epididymis feels hard and enlarged, and tenderness to touch can be elicited. There may be a urethral discharge. A rectal examination, which elicits tenderness of the prostate, can produce urethral discharge.

Diagnostic tests:

Test	Results Indicating Disorder	CPT Code
Urinalysis	Presence of leukocytes and bacteria	81000
Urethral culture and Gram stain	Determines organism	87070
Doppler ultrasound	Increased blood flow in epididymitis and decreased flow in torsion of the testicle	76870
Voiding cystourethrogram (if sexual activity is denied)	Congenital anomalies—urethral-ejaculatory duct reflux	74550

Differential diagnosis:

In testicular torsion, Prehn's sign and the cremasteric reflex are absent, the onset is abrupt, and the urinalysis is usually negative.

Testicular tumors are usually differentiated by ultrasound.

Mumps orchitis has an insidious onset and is associated with fever, malaise, and headache.

Hydrocele is painless swelling of scrotal sac.

Treatment:

Nonpharmacologic

Bed rest is indicated during the acute phase. Elevation of the scrotum above the pubic symphysis is instituted, and ice packs to the area and scrotal support are applied.

 Clinical Pearl: Nonbacterial epididymitis usually requires only supportive therapy.

Pharmacologic

For pain relief, analgesics and NSAIDS are given.

For bacterial based epididymitis, treatment is as follows.

If sexually transmitted, give ceftriaxone, 250 mg intramuscularly one dose, followed by doxycycline, 100 mg twice a day for 10 days. If there is penicillin, tetracycline, or cephalosporin allergy, give ofloxacin, 300 mg twice a day for 10 days.

If non–sexually transmitted, give trimethoprim (TMP)/sulfamethoxazole (SMX) to children older than 2 months, 8 mg/kg TMP/40 mg/kg SMX in two divided doses at 12-hour intervals over 10 days, or give TMP/SMX DS, 1 tablet orally twice a day for 10 days, to children older than 16 years who are able to swallow a pill or ciprofloxacin, 250 twice a day 1 tablet orally for 10 days.

 Clinical Pearl: Ciprofloxacin should not be used in children younger than 16.

Follow-up: If sexual activity is denied, a voiding cystourethrogram should be performed. If no improvement, schedule follow-up visit in 3 to 4 days. Otherwise, no follow-up is necessary if symptoms resolve.

Sequelae: If untreated or incompletely treated, infertility, abscess, or atrophy of the testis can occur.

Referral: If the patient does not have a prompt response to treatment, a referral should be made.

Education: The patient should be taught that unprotected sexual activity is the mode of transmission and that to prevent epididymitis a condom should be worn. Reinfection can occur when sexual partners have not been treated.

GYNECOMASTIA IN MALES

SIGNAL SYMPTOMS ▶ mass in the breast

Gynecomastia	ICD-9 CM: 611.1

Description: Gynecomastia in males is categorized into four groups:

- Type I—benign, self-limiting breast enlargement during Tanner stages II and III; of cases, 20% have bilateral involvement; resolution may take 2 years
- Type II—painful breast enlargement without evidence of a disease process
- Type III—enlargement resulting from generalized obesity
- Type IV—pectoral muscle hypertrophy

Etiology: Testosterone-estrogen imbalance, increased prolactin level, and abnormal serum-binding protein levels are suggested causes of type I gynecomastia.

Occurrence: Occurs in 50% to 60% of males during early adolescence.

Age: Boys aged 12 to 14.

Ethnicity: Not significant.

Gender: Only in males.

Contributing factors: Type I: unknown.

Signs and symptoms: The child is brought to clinic with the complaint, "He is growing breasts." Obtain a history, including time of onset and duration, Tanner staging, family history for familial pattern, and past and present medical history including change in weight. Physical findings include a 1- to 3-cm, round, freely mobile, firm mass immediately beneath the areola.

Diagnostic tests: None. If mass gets larger or does not resolve in 2 years, obtain a thyroid panel, liver function studies, and urinary gonadotropins if indicated.

Differential diagnosis:

Pseudogynecomastia is differentiated by excessive fat tissue (type III) and prominent pectoralis muscles (type 4).

Drug-induced gynecomastia (type II) is caused by ingestion of amphetamines, marijuana, meprobamate, opiates (e.g., codeine, heroin, morphine), prescription drugs (e.g., amitriptyline, cimetidine, diazepam, haloperidol, imipramine, isoniazid, tricyclic antidepressants), hormones, and chemotherapy.

Tumors (e.g., testicular, adrenal, pituitary) are differentiated by elevated prolactin or CT or MRI (type II).

Hypothyroidism or hyperthyroidism is differentiated by a thyroid panel.

Hepatic dysfunction is differentiated by abnormal liver function tests.

Klinefelter's syndrome is differentiated by the clinical picture: tall eunuchoid build, diminished facial hair, normal–to–borderline low IQ, micro-orchidism, and high levels of urinary gonadotropins (type II).

Treatment: None. If condition worsens and associated psychological problems develop, the nurse practitioner may give bromocriptine, a drug that suppresses lactation. Surgical intervention is rarely indicated.

Follow-up: The patient should return to the clinic in 3 months for re-evaluation.

Sequelae: If unresolved, investigate further as to the cause.

Prevention/prophylaxis: None.

Referral: Refer patient to primary care physician if there are any large, hard, or fixed enlargements or masses with any discharge.

Education: Reassure the parent and child that idiopathic gynecomastia is a benign condition that usually resolves within 2 years.

HERPES SIMPLEX VIRUS TYPE 2

SIGNAL SYMPTOMS▶ burning or painful sensation in vaginal or external genital area

Herpes simplex virus (HSV) type 2 ICD-9 CM: 054.9

Description: HSV type 2 causes a vesicular eruption of the skin and mucous membranes that can be a primary or recurrent problem in sexually active individuals. In the young child presenting with these symptoms, sexual abuse should be ruled out.

Etiology: Herpes, which is caused by human herpesvirus, usually affects the skin below the umbilicus. After a primary infection, the virus can remain latent in the cells that are in the area of the original eruption but can become reactivated at various intervals.

Occurrence: Occurs when the patient is sexually active or in contact with another person who has active lesions.

Age: Any age when the patient is sexually active.

Ethnicity: Not significant.

Gender: Occurs equally in males and females.

Contributing factors: Primary infection is due to exposure to a known carrier. Stress (either emotional or physical), fever, or exposure to sun may cause a later eruption.

Signs and symptoms: Mild-to-severe discomfort may be present. If old enough, the patient describes a prodromal phase in which there was some mild paresthesia (e.g., burning, tingling). Dysuria and urinary retention, tenderness of the affected area, dyspareunia, and increasing pain are described. There may be low-grade fever, headache, and malaise. Inguinal lymphadenopathy, maceration in moist areas, and a cluster of blister-like eruptions can be found at the site of infection. In recurrent episodes, the signs tend to be less severe, although eruptions tend to ulcerate.

Inspection of a primary or recurrent episode reveals vesicular eruptions that are fluid-filled, reddened, and tender to palpation. Patients may have frequent or infrequent eruptions.

Diagnostic tests:

Test	Results Indicating Disorder	CPT Code
Tzanck smear	Positive for multinucleated giant cells	87207
Fluorescein antibody test	Positive	87274
HSV culture	Positive culture of vesicular fluid	87207
HSV DNA: PCR	Positive	83898

PCR, polymerase chain reaction.

Differential diagnosis:

Chickenpox is differentiated by vesicular eruptions above and below the umbilicus. Eruptions are widespread over the entire body.

Coxsackievirus and echovirus are differentiated by the appearance of the rash, which is flat, pink, and sometimes lacy in appearance.

Herpangina is not sexually transmitted; it usually occurs in or on the mouth.

Treatment: Pain medication may need to be prescribed. Acetaminophen or ibuprofen for children is appropriate. Viscous lidocaine may be directly applied for relief of symptomatic pain. Oral and topical acyclovir are primary medications in the management of HSV type 2.

Topical acyclovir can be used every 2 hours for the first 2 to 3 days, then every 6 hours. Oral dosing of acyclovir (200/5 mL) should be based on weight (20 mg/kg per dose in four divided doses for 5 days).

Other drugs that may be used with the older child (≥18 years old) for treatment of HSV 2 include valacyclovir (Valtrex), 500 mg every 12 hours given for 3 days, or famciclovir (Famvir) for the treatment of recurrent genital herpes, 125 mg every 12 hours for 5 days (for children >16 years old).

Follow-up: Each exacerbation should be treated, and the patient should be seen in the office by the health care provider. Otherwise, routine health maintenance should be continued.

Sequelae: Spread of the infection to other parts of the body is a frequent problem, which can lead to a generalized eruption of the disease. Secondary bacterial infection (staphylococcus or β-hemolytic streptococcus), which requires appropriate medication, is also a complication of HSV type 2. Immunosuppressed persons are at high risk for contracting the disease, so they should be extremely careful to avoid contact with HSV type 2 patients during the active phase of the disease. If an affected patient becomes pregnant, a cesarean section may be considered for delivery of the infant.

Prevention/prophylaxis: Prevention involves avoidance of contact with persons who have the disease and of open lesions. If any of the lesions are present above the umbilicus (e.g., face, mouth), no direct contact with the person or items used by the person (e.g., drinking cups) should occur. Use of condoms among sexually active persons is crucial in preventing the spread of herpes. If the disease occurs during pregnancy, either as a primary infection or as a recurrent eruption, the obstetrician should be informed so that a decision can be made regarding the mode of delivery (vaginal versus cesarean section).

Referral: Infected immunocompromised patients or patients who do not respond to topical or oral treatment should be referred to an infectious disease specialist. All pregnant females should be referred to an obstetrician or nurse-midwife so that care can be monitored; the fetus also must be carefully monitored.

Education: All patients should be taught that barrier methods of protection, specifically condoms, can reduce the spread of the disease. Herpes patients should begin treatment at the first sign of recurrent eruption of a herpetic lesion.

HYDROCELE

SIGNAL SYMPTOMS ▶ nontender scrotal swelling

| Hydrocele | ICD-9-CM: 603.9 |

Description: A hydrocele is a collection of fluid in the scrotum causing asymptomatic swelling. When the amount of fluid varies, there is communication between the scrotum and the peritoneal cavity. This condition may or may not be accompanied by a hernia; it usually resolves by age 1 year.

Etiology: A congenital hydrocele results from a failure of the processus vaginalis peritonei to close at birth. Acquired hydrocele may result from a trauma or tumor of the scrotum.

Occurrence: Unknown.

Age: May occur at birth if congenital or at any age if related to trauma or tumor.

Ethnicity: Not significant.

Gender: Occurs in males.

Contributing factors: Trauma, tumor, or congenital defect.

Signs and symptoms: The parent states or the nurse practitioner notes that the scrotal sac is enlarged but does not appear discolored or painful. The testes can be palpated in the scrotal sac. There is no discomfort or discoloration associated with the hydrocele. The scrotal sac can be transilluminated.

Inspection reveals a swollen testis that can be transilluminated. Palpation reveals no hardness or tenderness.

Diagnostic tests: None.

Differential diagnosis: Inguinal hernia, neoplasm, infectious process of the testes, trauma, hematoma, hematocele orchitis, and a cystic lesion all should be considered in the differential diagnosis of hydrocele (see Fig. 9–2).

Infectious process is differentiated by laboratory data.

Trauma and hematoma are differentiated by the appearance of bruising or discolorations.

Lesions or masses are differentiated by ultrasound or CT.

Treatment: Monitor patient for 1 year for changes. The hydrocele should resolve within 1 year. If resolution does not occur or if pain, scrotal redness, warmth, or hardness occurs, refer patient to an urologist.

Follow-up: Routine health care visits.

Sequelae: Rare.

Prevention/prophylaxis: None in cases of congenital malformation. Testicular self-examination can be performed each month to detect a mass. Males involved in contact sports should be mandated to wear protective gear to protect the scrotum from injury.

Referral: Refer patient to an urologist if no improvement.

Education: By adolescence, males should be taught how to perform testicular self-examination.

HYPOSPADIAS AND EPISPADIAS

SIGNAL SYMPTOMS displacement of urethral meatus

Hypospadias	male	ICD-9 CM: 752.61
Hypospadias	female	ICD-9 CM: 753.9
Epispadias	male	ICD-9 CM: 752.62
Epispadias	female	ICD-9 CM: 753.8

Description: Hypospadias occurs when the opening for the urethral meatus is on the ventral surface of the penis instead of at the top of the glans penis. The opening most often occurs near the glans but may appear farther along the shaft. This condition is often accompanied by a ventral curvature of the penis (chordae) or a hooded appearance of the penis. Epispadias occurs when the opening of the urethral meatus is placed somewhere along the dorsal side of the penis.

Etiology: There is a familial tendency for these conditions (7%); however, some cases can be related to maternal exposure to progesterone at 8 to 14 weeks' gestation.

Occurrence: Hypospadias occurs in 1 in 250 live male births. Epispadias is a rare occurrence (<1% of live births).

Age: Present at birth.

Ethnicity: Not significant.

Gender: Occurs usually in males.

Contributing factors: Familial tendency (14% recurrence); maternal exposure to progesterone at 8 to 14 weeks' gestation.

Signs and symptoms: Inspection of the penis reveals misplacement of the urethral meatus opening, possibly accompanied by a hooded or curved appearance of the penis. Urethral opening can be seen on either the dorsal or the ventral surface of the penis. Note where along the shaft the opening appears.

Diagnostic tests: None specifically for hypospadias or epispadias, but if other abnormalities are suspected, an ultrasound of the renal organs should be ordered.

Differential diagnosis:

Ambiguous genitalia is identified by inspection.

Treatment: Withhold circumcision. Between 12 and 18 months, refer infant to an urologist for possible surgical repair.

Follow-up: Routine health care visits. If surgery is performed, follow-up is generally at 2 weeks and again at 6 months by the surgeon.

Sequelae: Of boys who have hypospadias, 10% have undescended testes as well. Unrepaired hypospadias may interfere with urination and sexual function and may induce psychological problems related to malformed external genitalia.

Prevention/prophylaxis: None: congenital defect.

Referral: By age 1 year, or no older than 2, the patient should be referred to a urologist.

Education: Parents should be told that this is not a life-threatening condition. At about age 2, surgical repair can be done to correct the defect, and there are no long-term problems.

LABIAL ADHESIONS

SIGNAL SYMPTOMS the labia are adhered and the flow of urine may be impaired or stopped

Labial adhesions	ICD-9 CM: 752.49

Description: Labial adhesions occur when there is partial or complete closure of the external vaginal opening as a result of adhesions of the medial edges of the labia minora. It is an asymptomatic, benign condition seen from age 3 months to 6 years but may occur up until the time of menarche.

Etiology: This condition can be the result of hypoestrogenization, trauma (including rape), inflammation, or an infectious process. In adolescence, as the pH becomes more acidic, this is rarely seen.

Occurrence: Labial adhesions occur in 1.8% of all females.

Age: Labial adhesions can occur in females from infancy to menarche.

Ethnicity: Not significant.

Gender: Females.

Contributing factors: It is believed that when children have low levels of estrogen, there is an increased frequency of labial adhesions. Another factor may be local irritation or scratching, which denudes the thin skin covering the labia, resulting in an adhesion as healing occurs. Sexual abuse must also be considered.

Signs and symptoms: History of trauma, difficulty urinating, or discomfort with urination may be related by the child or parent. Inspection reveals that the labia minora is medially connected by a thin layer of tissue, closing or partially closing the external vaginal opening. Recurrent urinary tract infections may also be a sign of an adhesion.

Diagnostic tests: None.

Differential diagnosis:

Imperforate vagina (rare) is differentiated by physical examination.

Treatment: Often no treatment is indicated because this is a self-limiting problem. When symptomatic, estrogen cream (0.1%, 0.625 mg/g), is topically applied twice a day for 2 to 4 weeks. This regimen is followed by application of the estrogen cream at bedtime only for another 1 to 2 weeks. Vaseline should be applied for 1 to 2 months after adhesion is separated. Mechanical separation should not be done because of the risk of trauma to the area.

Follow-up: Follow-up 2 to 4 weeks after the use of estrogen cream. A routine health care visit schedule should be maintained.

Sequelae: Frequent urinary tract infections and urinary discomfort may result from a labial adhesion.

Prevention/prophylaxis: Improved perineal hygiene and removal of irritants may decrease the incidence of labial adhesions. Discourage scratching the pubic area. Treatment of external genitalia with estrogen creams is recommended.

Referral: When topical application with estrogen is not successful or if severe urinary symptoms exist, surgery is indicated, and the patient should be referred to an urologist.

Education: Parents should be taught to examine child's external genitalia or to be alert for signs and symptoms of urinary difficulty. Because this is a fairly benign and self-limiting condition, inform parents that there are no long-term sequelae.

PELVIC INFLAMMATORY DISEASE

SIGNAL SYMPTOMS▶ mucopurulent vaginal discharge with accompanying pelvic and anal pain and dysuria

Pelvic inflammatory disease	ICD-9 CM: 614.9

Description: PID is an inflammatory disorder of the female upper genital tract that can include salpingitis, endometritis, and pelvic peritonitis. Patients may present as symptomatic or asymptomatic. PID, the result of undetected or inadequately treated STD of the endocervix, is often seen as a complication of common STDs.

Etiology: Generally the etiology is polymicrobial. Sexually transmitted organisms are implicated in most cases. Currently *N. gonorrhoeae, Chlamydia trachomatis, Gardnerella vaginalis,* streptococcus groups A and B, coliform bacteria, and genital tract mycoplasmas should all be suspected as causative agents.

Occurrence: Any age at which a female is sexually active.

Age: PID rate is highest among sexually active adolescents.

Ethnicity: Highest in African-American females.

Gender: Occurs in females.

Contributing factors: Multiple sexual partners, use of douches, or a previous episode of PID.

Signs and symptoms: Patients may present with fever and complaints of lower abdominal pain, vaginal discharge, and irregular bleeding. They are sexually active, and they may have more than one partner. They may also have specific complaints related to the genitourinary system, including dysuria and vaginal discharge (Fig. 9–3 and Table 9–1).

Inspection reveals an affect of discomfort, guarding of the lower abdomen, fever, chills, or sweating. Palpation and percussion reveal tenderness of the lower abdomen, pain on movement of cervix or adnexa,

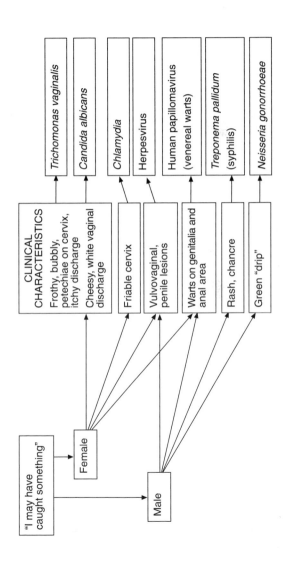

Figure 9–3. Differential diagnosis of sexually transmitted diseases.

Table 9–1 Differential Diagnosis of Sexually Transmitted Diseases

Organism	Laboratory Test	Rule Out
Trichomonas	Wet prep	Candida
Candida	KOH prep	Cervical cancer
Herpesvirus	Viral cultures	
Chlamydia	Viral culture	
Papillomavirus	PAP smear	Melanoma
Neisseria gonorrhoeae	Gram's stain, culture	Nonspecific urethritis
Treponema pallidum	Blood test	

and guarding on palpation. Vital signs should be assessed. When performing the vaginal examination, look for friability or erosion of the cervix, pain on movement of the cervix, or adnexal tenderness.

Diagnostic tests:

Test	Results Indicating Disorder	CPT Code
C-reactive protein	Positive: high	85337
Culture (cervix)	Positive for chlamydia or gonorrhea	88142
Blood culture	Positive for specific bacteria	87081
Complete blood count	Elevated white blood cells >10,500/mL	85031
Erythrocyte sedimentation rate	Elevated	85652

Differential diagnosis:

STDs are differentiated by cultures.

Ectopic pregnancy is confirmed by ultrasound.

Appendicitis is confirmed by examination, pain only in the lower quarter of the abdomen (worse on right side), and ultrasound or CT of abdomen.

Treatment: Treatment is instituted according to symptoms; because the specific organisms are generally not identified, treatment should be broad enough to cover all common causative agents. Prompt initiation of treatment with broad-spectrum antibiotic therapy is indicated to reduce the risk exacerbation of the disease. If the patient fails to respond in 48 hours of outpatient treatment, she should be hospitalized. Advise the patient to abstain from sexual intercourse until treatment is complete. Medications currently suggested include the following (Table 9–2).

For outpatient treatment, give cefoxitin, 2 g intramuscularly once, and probenecid, 1 g orally once, or ceftriaxone, 250 mg intramuscularly once, both followed by doxycycline, 100 mg twice daily for 10 days, or metronidazole (Flagyl), 500 mg orally twice daily for 7 days or 2 g × 1 dose, or oxfloxacin, 400 mg orally twice daily for 14 days.

For inpatient treatment, give intravenous antibiotics, including clindamycin, 900 mg every 8 hours, plus gentamicin, 1.5 mg/kg every 8 hours after a loading dose of 2 mg/kg.

Table 9–2   Summary of Sexually Transmitted Disease Treatment Guidelines, CDC, May 10, 2002

Disease	Recommended Regimens	Alternative Regimens
Chancroid	• Azithromycin 1 g PO in a single dose or • Ceftriaxone 250 mg IM in a single dose or • Ciprofloxacin 500 mg PO bid for 3 days or[1] • Erythromycin base 500 mg PO qid for 7 days	
Genital herpes simplex virus (HSV) First clinical episode	• Acyclovir 400 mg PO tid for 7–10 days or • Acyclovir 200 mg PO 5 × per day for 7–10 days or • Famciclovir 250 mg PO tid for 7–10 days or • Valacyclovir 1 g PO bid for 7–10 days Treatment may be extended if healing is incomplete after 10 days	
Recurrent episodes	• Acyclovir 400 mg PO tid for 5 days or • Acyclovir 200 mg PO 5 × per day for 5 days or • Acyclovir 800 mg PO bid for 5 days or • Famciclovir 125 mg PO bid for 5 days or • Valacyclovir 500 mg PO bid for 3–5 days • Valacyclovir 1 g PO qd	
Severe disease	• Acyclovir 5–10 mg/kg body weight IV q8h for 5–7 days or until clinical resolution	
Granuloma inguinale (donovanosis)	• Trimethoprim-sulfamethoxazole 1 double-strength tablet PO bid for a minimum of 3 weeks or • Doxycycline 100 mg PO bid for a minimum of 3 weeks Add an aminoglycoside (gentamicin 1 mg/kg IV q8h) if lesions do not respond with the first few days of therapy.	• Ciprofloxacin 750 mg PO bid for a minimum of 3 weeks or • Erythromycin base 500 mg PO qid for a minimum of 3 weeks Add an aminoglycoside (gentamicin 1 mg/kg IV q8h) if lesions do not respond with the first few days of therapy. • Azithromycin 1 g qd for 3 weeks

(Continued on the following page)

311

Table 9-2 Summary of Sexually Transmitted Disease Treatment Guidelines, CDC, May 10, 2002 *(Cont'd)*

Disease	Recommended Regimens	Alternative Regimens
Lymphogranuloma venereum syphilis	• Doxycycline 100 mg PO bid for 21 days	• Erythromycin base 500 mg PO qid for 21 days
Primary and secondary syphilis	• Benzathine penicillin G 2.4 million U IM in a single dose	In patients with penicillin allergy • Doxycycline 100 mg PO bid for 2 weeks • Tetracycline 500 mg PO qid for 2 weeks
Latent syphilis	Early latent syphilis • Benzathine penicillin G 2.4 million U IM in a single dose Late latent syphilis • Benzathine penicillin G 7.2 million U total, administered as three doses of 2.4 million U IM each at 1-week intervals	In patients with penicillin allergy • Doxycycline 100 mg PO bid, or • Tetracycline 500 mg PO qid Administer drugs for 2 weeks if the duration of infection is known to have been <1 year; otherwise, administer for 4 weeks
Tertiary syphilis	• Benzathine penicillin G 7.2 million U total, administered as three doses of 2.4 million U IM each at 1-week intervals	
Neurosyphilis	• Aqueous crystalline penicillin G 18–24 million U a day. Administered as 3–4 million U IV q4h for 10–14 days	• Procaine penicillin 2.4 million U IM OD plus probenecid 500 mg PO qid both for 10–14 days
Primary and secondary syphilis in HIV-infected persons	• Benzathine penicillin G 2.4 million U IM in a single dose. Some experts recommend additional doses of three weekly doses	
Latent syphilis in HIV-infected persons	• Benzathine penicillin G 7.2 million U total, administered as three doses of 2.4 million U IM each at 1-week intervals	
Congenital syphilis during first month of life	• Aqueous crystalline penicillin G 100,000–150,000 units/kg per day, administered as 50,000 units/kg per dose IV q12h during the first 7 days of life, and q8h thereafter for a total of 8 days or • Procaine penicillin G 50,000 U/kg per dose IM OD in a single dose for 10 days	

Table 9–2 Summary of Sexually Transmitted Disease Treatment Guidelines, CDC, May 10, 2002

Disease	Recommended Regimens	Alternative Regimens
Urethritis and Cervicitis Nongonococcal urethritis	• Azithromycin 1 g PO in a single dose, or • Doxycycline 100 mg PO bid for 7 days	• Erythromycin base 500 mg PO qid for 7 days or • Erythromycin ethylsuccinate 800 mg PO qid for 7 days or • Ofloxacin 300 mg bid for 7 days For patients who cannot tolerate high doses of erythromycin • Erythromycin base 250 mg PO qid for 14 days or • Erythromycin ethylsuccinate 400 mg PO qid for 14 days
Recurrent and persistent urethritis	• Metronidazole 2 mg PO in a single dose *plus* • Erythromycin base 500 mg PO qid for 7 days or • Erythromycin ethylsuccinate 800 mg PO qid for 7 days	
Chlamydial infection In adults and adolescents	• Azithromycin 1 g PO in a single dose, or • Doxycycline 100 mg PO bid for 7 days	• Erythromycin base 500 mg PO qid for 7 days or • Erythromycin ethylsuccinate 800 mg PO qid for 7 days or • Ofloxacin 300 mg bid for 7 days or • Leuofloxacin 500 mg od × 7 days
In pregnancy	• Erythromycin base 500 mg PO qid for 7 days or • Amoxicillin 500 mg PO tid for 7 days	• Erythromycin base 250 mg PO qid for 14 days or • Erythromycin ethylsuccinate 800 mg PO qid for 7 days or • Erythromycin ethylsuccinate 400 mg PO qid for 14 days or • Azithromycin 1 g PO in a single dose

(Continued on the following page)

Table 9–2 Summary of Sexually Transmitted Disease Treatment Guidelines, CDC, May 10, 2002 *(Cont'd)*

Disease	Recommended Regimens	Alternative Regimens
In infants	• Erythromycin 50 mg/kg per day PO divided in four equal doses daily for 10–14 days	
Infant pneumonia caused by *C. trachomatis*	• Erythromycin base 50 mg/kg per day PO divided in four equal doses daily for 10–14 days	
Infants born to mothers who have a chlamydial infection	Children who weigh <45 kg: • Erythromycin base 50 mg/kg per day PO divided in four equal doses daily for 10–14 days[2] Children who weigh ≥45 kg but are <8 years of age: • Azithromycin 1 g PO in a single dose Children ≥8 years of age: • Azithromycin 1 g PO in a single dose or • Doxycycline 100 mg PO bid for 7 days	
Gonococcal infection		
Uncomplicated gonococcal infections of the cervix, urethra, and rectum	• Cefixime 400 mg PO in a single dose or • Ceftriaxone 125 mg IM in a single dose or • Ofloxacin 400 mg PO in a single dose or • Azithromycin 1 g PO in a single dose or • Doxycycline 100 mg PO bid for 7 days • Ofloxacin 400 mg PO in a single dose	• Spectinomycin 2 g IM in a single dose or • Ceftizoxime 500 mg IM in a single dose or • Cefotaxime 500 mg IM in a single dose or • Cefotetan 1 g IM in a single dose, or • Cefoxitin 2 g IM with probenecid 1 g PO in a single dose • Enoxacin 400 mg PO in a single dose or • Lomefloxacin 400 mg PO in a single dose or • Norfloxacin 800 mg PO in a single dose
Uncomplicated gonococcal infection of the pharynx	• Ceftriaxone 125 mg IM in a single dose or • Ciprofloxacin 500 mg PO in a single dose *plus* • Ofloxacin 400 mg PO in a single dose or • Azithromycin 1 g PO in a single dose or • Doxycycline 100 mg PO bid for 7 days	

Table 9–2 Summary of Sexually Transmitted Disease Treatment Guidelines, CDC, May 10, 2002

Disease	Recommended Regimens	Alternative Regimens
Gonococcal conjunctivitis	• Ceftriaxone 1 g IM in a single dose, and lavage the infected eye with saline solution once	
Disseminated gonococcal infection	• Ceftriaxone 1 g IM or IV E 24h for 24–48 hours after improvement	• Cefotaxime 1 g IV q8h or • Ceftizoxime 1 g IV q8h or For persons allergic to β-lactam drugs: • Ciprofloxacin 500 mg IV q12h, or • Ofloxacin 400 mg IV q12h, or • Spectinomycin 2 g IV q12h. All for 24–48 hours after improvement, at which time may be switched to one of the following regimens to complete a full week of antimicrobial treatment: • Cefixime 400 mg PO bid or • Ciprofloxacin 500 mg PO bid or • Ofloxacin 400 mg PO bid
Gonococcal meningitis or endocarditis	• Ceftriaxone 1–2 g IV q12h for 10–14 days for meningitis and for at least 4 weeks for endocarditis	
Ophthalmia neonatorum caused by N. gonorrhoeae	• Ceftriaxone 25–50 mg/kg IV or IM in a single dose, not to exceed 125 mg	
Disseminated gonococcal infection and gonococcal scalp abscess in newborns	• Ceftriaxone 25–50 mg/kg IV or IM in a single daily dose for 7 days, with a duration of 10–14 days if meningitis is documented or • Cefotaxime 25 mg/kg IV or IM q12h for 7 days, with a duration of 10–14 days if meningitis is documented	
Prophylactic treatment for infants whose mothers have gonococcal infection	• Ceftriaxone 25–50 mg/kg IV or IM in a single dose, not to exceed 125 mg	

(Continued on the following page)

Table 9-2 Summary of Sexually Transmitted Disease Treatment Guidelines, CDC, May 10, 2002 *(Cont'd)*

Disease	Recommended Regimens	Alternative Regimens
Gonococcal infection in children	For children who weigh ≥45 kg: • Use one of the regimens recommended for adults except for quinolones because they are not approved for use in children For children who weigh <45 kg and who have uncomplicated gonococcal vulvovaginitis, cervicitis, urethritis, pharyngitis, or proctitis: • Ceftriaxone 125 mg IM in a single dose For children who weigh <45 kg and who have bacteremia or arthritis: • Ceftriaxone 50 mg/kg (maximum dose: 1 g) IM or IV in a single daily dose for 7 days For children who weigh ≥45 kg and who have bacteremia or arthritis: • Ceftriaxone 50 mg/kg (maximum dose: 2 g) IM or IV in a single daily dose for 10–14 days • Ceftriaxone 25–50 mg/kg IV or IM in a single dose not to exceed 125 mg	• Spectinomycin 40 mg/kg (maximum dose: 2 g) in a single dose but this treatment may be unreliable
Ophthalmia neonatorum prophylaxis	• Silver nitrate (1%) aqueous solution in a single application, or • Erythromycin (0.5%) ophthalmic ointment in a single application, or • Tetracycline ophthalmic ointment (1%) in a single application *Note:* Topical application is adequate and is unnecessary if systemic treatment is administered Treatment should be instilled into both eyes as soon as possible after delivery	

Table 9–2 Summary of Sexually Transmitted Disease Treatment Guidelines, CDC, May 10, 2002

Disease	Recommended Regimens	Alternative Regimens
Bacterial vaginosis Nonpregnant women	• Metronidazole 500 mg PO bid for 7 days or • Clindamycin cream 2%, one full applicator (5 g) intravaginally at bedtime for 7 days or • Metronidazole gel 0.5%, one full applicator (5 g) intravaginally bid for 5 days	• Metronidazole 2 g PO in a single dose • Clindamycin 300 mg PO bid for 7 days
High-risk pregnant women	• Metronidazole 250 mg PO tid for 7 days	• Metronidazole 2 g PO in a single dose • Clindamycin 300 mg PO bid for 7 days
Low-risk pregnant women	• Metronidazole 250 mg PO tid for 7 days	• Metronidazole 2 g PO in a single dose • Clindamycin 300 mg PO bid for 7 days or • Metronidazole gel 0.75% one full applicator (5 g) intravaginally bid for 5 days
Trichomoniasis	• Metronidazole 2 g PO in a single dose	• Metronidazole 500 mg PO bid for 7 days
Vulvovaginitis candidiasis	Intravaginal agents: • Butoconazole 2% 5 g intravaginally for 3 days[3, 4] or • Clotrimazole 1% cream 5 g intravaginally for 7–14 days[3, 4] • Clotrimazole 100 mg vaginal tablet for 7 days[3] or • Clotrimazole 100 mg vaginal tablet, two tablets for 3 days[3] or • Clotrimazole 500 mg vaginal tablet, one tablet in a single application[3] or • Miconazole 2% cream 5 g intravaginally for 7 days[3, 4] or • Miconazole 200 mg vaginal suppository, one suppository for 3 days[3, 4] or	

(Continued on the following page)

Table 9–2 Summary of Sexually Transmitted Disease Treatment Guidelines, CDC, May 10, 2002 *(Cont'd)*

Disease	Recommended Regimens	Alternative Regimens
	• Miconazole 100 mg vaginal suppository, one suppository for 7 days[3, 4] or • Nystatin 100,000-u vaginal tablet, one tablet for 14 days or • Tioconazole 6.5% ointment 5 g intravaginally in a single application[3, 4] or • Terconazole 0.4% cream 5 g intravaginally for 7 days[3] Oral agent: Fluconazole 150 mg PO × 1 dose • Terconazole 0.8% cream 5 g intravaginally for 3 days[3] or • Terconazole 80 mg vaginal suppository, one suppository for 3 days[3] Oral agent: • Fluconazole 150 mg oral tablet, one tablet in single dose	
Pelvic inflammatory disease		
Parenteral regimen A	• Cfotetan 2 g IV q12h or • Cefoxitin 2 g IV q6h *plus* • Doxycycline 100 mg IV or PO q12h Parenteral therapy may be discontinued 24 hours after clinical improvement and then • Doxycycline 100 mg bid should continue for a total of 14 days	• Ofloxacin 400 mg IV q12h *plus* • Metronidazole 500 mg IV q8h or • Ampicillin/sulbactam 3 g IV q6h *plus* • Doxycycline 100 mg IV or PO q12h or • Ciprofloxacin 200 mg IV q12h *plus* • Doxycycline 100 mg IV or PO q12h *plus* • Metronidazole 500 mg IV q8h
Parenteral regimen B	• Clindamycin 900 mg IV q8h *plus* • Gentamicin loading dose IV or IM (2 mg/kg of body weight), followed by a maintenance dose (1.5 mg/kg) q8h. Single daily dosing may be substituted Parenteral therapy may be discontinued 24 hours after clinical improvement and then • Doxycycline 100 mg bid should continue for a total of 14 days or • Clindamycin 450 mg PO qid to complete a total of 14 days of therapy	
Oral regimen A	• Ofloxacin 400 mg PO bid for 14 days or • Metronidazole 500 mg PO bid for 14 days	
Oral regimen B	• Ceftriaxone 250 mg IM once or • Cefoxitin 2 g IM *plus*	

Table 9–2 Summary of Sexually Transmitted Disease Treatment Guidelines, CDC, May 10, 2002

Disease	Recommended Regimens	Alternative Regimens
Epididymitis Most likely caused by gonococcal or chlamydial infection Most likely caused by enteric organisms or for patients allergic to cephalosporins and/or tetracyclines	• Probenecid 1 g PO in a single dose concurrently once or • Other parenteral third-generation cephalosporin (eg ceftizoxime or cefotaxime) *plus* • Doxycycline 100 mg PO bid for 14 days (include this regimen with one of the above regimens) • Ceftriaxone 250 mg IM in a single dose *plus* • Doxycycline 100 mg PO bid for 10 days	
Human papillomavirus infection External genital warts	• Podofilox 0.5% solution or gel. Apply bid to visible genital warts for 3 days, followed by 4 days of no therapy. Repeat as necessary for a total of 4 cycles. Total wart area treated not to exceed 10 cm² and a total volume of podofilox not to exceed 0.5 mL/day or • Imiquimod 5% cream. Apply at bedtime, 3 times per week for as long as 16 weeks. Wash area with mild soap and water 1–10 hours after treatment • Cryotherapy with liquid nitrogen or cryoprobe. Repeat applications every 1 to 2 weeks or • Podophyllin resin 10–25% in a compound tincture of benzoin. Repeat weekly if necessary or	• Intralesional interferon or • Laser surgery

(Continued on the following page)

Table 9-2 Summary of Sexually Transmitted Disease Treatment Guidelines, CDC, May 10, 2002 *(Cont'd)*

Disease	Recommended Regimens	Alternative Regimens
Vaginal warts	• TCA or BCA 80–90%. Apply a small amount to warts and allow to dry, at which time frosting develops; powder with talc or sodium bicarbonate to remove unreacted acid if an excess amount is applied. Repeat weekly if necessary or • Surgical removal either by tangential scissor excision, tangential shave excision, curettage, or electrosurgery • Cryotherapy with liquid nitrogen or • TCA or BCA 80–90%. Apply a small amount to warts and allow to dry, at which time frosting develops; powder with talc or sodium bicarbonate to remove unreacted acid if an excess amount is applied. Repeat weekly if necessary	
Urethral warts	• Podophyllin resin 10–25% in a compound tincture of benzoin applied to a treated area that must be dried before the speculum is removed. Treat with ≤2 cm² per session. Repeat weekly • Cryotherapy with liquid nitrogen or • Benzoin applied to a treated area that must be dried before contact with normal mucosa. Repeat weekly	
Anal warts	• TCA or BCA 80–90%. Apply a small amount to warts and allow to dry, at which time frosting develops; powder with talc or sodium bicarbonate to remove unreacted acid if an excess amount is applied. Repeat weekly if necessary or • Surgical removal	
Oral warts	• Cryotherapy with liquid nitrogen or • Surgical removal	
Proctitis, proctocolitis, and enteritis	• Ceftriaxone 125 mg IM (or another agent effective against anal and genital gonorrhea) *plus* • Doxycycline 100 mg PO bid for 7 days	

Table 9–2 Summary of Sexually Transmitted Disease Treatment Guidelines, CDC, May 10, 2002 *(Continued)*

Disease	Recommended Regimens	Alternative Regimens
Ectoparasitic infections Pediculosis pubic	• Permethrin 1% creme rinse applied to affected areas and washed off after 10 minutes or • Lindane 1% shampoo applied for 4 minutes to the affected area, then thoroughly washed off. This regimen is not recommended for pregnant or lactating women or for children ≤2 years • Pyrethrins with piperonyl butoxide applied to the affected area and washed off after 10 minutes	
Scabies	• Permethrin cream 5% applied to all areas of the body from the neck down and washed off after 8–14 hours	• Lindane 1% precipitated in ointment applied thinly to all areas nightly for 3 nights. Previous applications should be washed off before new applications are applied. Thoroughly wash off 24 hours after the last treatment

1. Contraindicated for pregnant and lactating women and for persons aged <18 years.
2. Effectiveness of treatment is approximately 80%; a second course of therapy may be indicated.
3. Creams and suppositories are oil-based and might weaken latex condoms and diaphragms.
4. Over-the-counter preparations.

Source: U.S. Department of Health and Human Services, Centers for Disease Control and Prevention, Morbidity and Mortality Reports, 2002 Guidelines for Treatment of Sexually Transmitted Diseases. Vol 51. No. RR 6, May 10, 2002

Follow-up: All contacts should be treated, and follow-up cultures should be done in 4 to 6 weeks.

Sequelae: Sterility may result from incomplete or unsuccessful treatment. Chronic pelvic pain or ectopic pregnancy may also result from PID.

Prevention/prophylaxis: The patient should avoid engaging in unprotected sex and having multiple sexual partners. She should not douche after sexual intercourse.

Referral: The patient should be referred to gynecologist if no improvement is seen in 48 hours.

Education: The patient should be educated not to have sexual intercourse until therapy is complete. Partners must be notified and treated. The consequences of PID and modes of transmission should be reviewed. The need to use condoms and the dangers of having multiple sexual partners or unprotected sex should be stressed.

PHIMOSIS/PARAPHIMOSIS

SIGNAL SYMPTOMS▶ inability to retract foreskin behind the sulcus

Phimosis/Paraphimosis	ICD-9 CM: 605.

Description: Phimosis is the inability to retract the prepuce (foreskin) by the age of 3 years. Paraphimosis occurs when the foreskin has been retracted behind the sulcus and cannot be reduced. This condition may warrant immediate surgical intervention (circumcision).

Etiology: Phimosis is either congenital or acquired (i.e., when followed by an inflammation of the foreskin).

Occurrence: Paraphimosis occurs in 0.9% of males; phimosis occurs in approximately 10% of uncircumcised males.

Age: More common in infancy and adolescence.

Ethnicity: Not significant.

Gender: Occurs in males.

Contributing factors: In acquired phimosis, poor hygiene or forceful retraction; body piercing using penile rings.

Signs and symptoms: The parent may report that the child's urinary stream is thin and that he often states that he cannot go to the bathroom.

Phimosis is diagnosed by age 3, when the foreskin still cannot be retracted. It is confirmed when the foreskin cannot be retracted and returned to its original position.

Paraphimosis results in swelling and pain owing to the inability to reduce the foreskin. There is also a possibility of a visibly poor urinary stream. Accumulation of smegma, although not pathologic, is present.

Diagnostic tests: None.

Differential diagnosis:

Traumatic injury to penis is differentiated by the presence of bruising or swelling.

Treatment: Circumcision.

Follow-up: Regular health-care visits.

Sequelae:

- *Phimosis*—interference with sexual and urinary function
- *Paraphimosis*—venous stasis distal to the corona

Prevention/prophylaxis: If congenital, none. If acquired, early treatment of inflammatory infections.

Referral: Refer to surgeon or urologist.

Education: Parents should be told that 90% of all uncircumcised males would be able to retract the foreskin by 2 years of age. Educate parent in the proper care of the uncircumcised and circumcised male infant.

PREGNANCY

SIGNAL SYMPTOMS ▶ amenorrhea after unprotected intercourse; nausea on awakening; tender, enlarged breasts

| Pregnancy | ICD-9 CM: V22.2 |

Description: Pregnancy is a normal physiologic event that spans from conception to birth and lasts approximately 280 days, or 40 weeks. The time between conception and the onset of labor is referred to as the *antepartal period,* whereas the time between conception and the birth of the infant is referred to as the *prenatal period.* The expected date of delivery is calculated by beginning with the first day of the last menstrual period, adding 7 days, then subtracting 3 months. Pregnancy is divided into three trimesters: 0 to 12 weeks, 13 to 28 weeks, and 29 to 40 weeks. Although pregnancy is a normal event, its occurrence in the very young creates a multitude of problems or potential problems. Pregnant children often have school and family problems.

Etiology: Pregnancy results from the fertilization of an ovum by a sperm and the successful implantation of this fertilized egg into the uterus.

Occurrence: Current statistics indicate that the incidence of teenage pregnancy in the United States has decreased slightly in the last 5 years; however, in areas where there is increased poverty and in the African-American population, the teenage pregnancy rate continues to increase.

Age: 8 to greater than 50 years.

Ethnicity: There is a significantly higher incidence of pregnancy in children aged 8 to 16 in the African-American population.

Contributing factors: Poverty, illiteracy, poor access to health care, rape, and incest all contribute to the occurrence of pregnancy in children.

Signs and symptoms: The child presents with a report of a missed period (menstrual suppression); feeling tired; feeling nauseated in the morning (morning sickness) or throughout the day; and other presumptive signs, such as urinary frequency, breast tenderness, dark blue discoloration of the vaginal mucosal membrane (Chadwick's sign), pigmentation of the skin, and abdominal striae.

Probable signs include enlargement of the abdomen, changes in the size and shape of the uterus (Hagar's sign), changes in the cervix, and a positive pregnancy test.

Positive signs include fetal heart sounds, fetal movements felt by the examiner, and ultrasound showing the presence of a fetus.

Diagnostic tests:

Test	Results Indicating Disorder	CPT Code
Serum radioimmunoassay	Positive	84702
Urine human chorionic gonadotropin	Positive	81025
Ultrasound uterus	Presence of fetus	76805

Differential diagnosis:

Amenorrhea, acute infection, pseudocyesis, hyperestrogenism, and STDs can be differentiated by serum human chorionic gonadotropin.

Physical examination can exclude pregnancy by the absence of an enlarged uterus or lack of any other presumptive or suggestive signs.

Treatment: All confirmed pregnancies should be referred to a nurse-midwife or an obstetrician. Pregnant adolescents are at high risk for complications and should be referred as soon as possible to ensure the healthiest outcome for the mother and the infant.

Follow-up: Follow-up is conducted by an obstetrician or nurse-midwife.

Sequelae: Multiple problems may result from a teenager's pregnancy, including alienation from her family, poor fetal outcome, and increased risk to the mother. There is some evidence to support an increased occurrence of neglect and abuse of infants born to young mothers.

Prevention/prophylaxis: One way to decrease the number of unplanned teenage pregnancies is to begin sex education in the early years, preferably during grade school. Other solutions include parental involvement, open communication, development of life goals, and increasing teenagers' knowledge about pregnancy and condoms. With the assistance of parents and schools, children can be educated about the ways to protect themselves from unplanned pregnancies. The regular use of any contraceptive method is essential for success in reducing the teenage pregnancy rate. In conjunction with the use of condoms (to reduce STDs), any of the following methods are acceptable for female teenagers: OCs, medroxyprogesterone acetate injections, and barrier methods. As with any medical regimen, care must be taken to follow up with regularly scheduled visits with a health care provider. The pediatric nurse practitioner is an ideal provider of education and health care supervision for birth control.

Referral: Refer patient to an obstetrician or nurse-midwife.

Education: Teaching methods of safe sex and family planning should be done early by family and schools. The need for early health care to ensure healthy outcomes for the infant and mother should be stressed.

PRIMARY GONOCOCCAL INFECTIONS

SIGNAL SYMPTOMS increased vaginal or urethral discharge accompanied by dysuria in females, abnormal uterine bleeding

Primary gonococcal infections	ICD-9 CM: 098.0

Description: Gonorrhea, an infection of the genitourinary tract, oropharynx, or anorectal tract that may or may not be characterized by pain, is classified as a reportable STD.

 Clinical Pearl: When detected in young children, sexual abuse should be suspected.

Etiology: The bacterium *N. gonorrhoeae*.

Occurrence: Reports show a marked increase in the incidence of gonorrhea; of even more concern, many infections are penicillin resistant, which makes treatment more difficult. The annual incidence in 10- to 14-year-old boys is about 35.7 in 100,000; in girls, it is 1175 in 100,000.

Age: Occurs at any age, even in newborns.

Ethnicity: Not significant.

Gender: Occurs in males and females, but more commonly in females.

Contributing factors: Unprotected sexual intercourse and multiple partners.

Signs and symptoms: In males, urethritis is the most frequent acute presentation. The patient complains of dysuria and frequent urination, and a purulent discharge is present. History may include multiple sexual partners and high-risk or unprotected rectal, oral, or vaginal sexual intercourse. If the contact is a result of orogenital contact, the chief complaint is pharyngitis. With anorectal infection, there is burning in the rectal area, a mucopurulent discharge, and painful defecation. In females, urethritis (with dysuria and frequent urination) is the chief complaint. When salpingitis is present, there is bilateral lower abdominal pain, adnexal tenderness, and tenderness when the cervix is manipulated. In some cases, the patient has an elevated temperature and chills. Occasionally female patients report right upper quadrant pain.

Diagnostic tests:

Test	Results Indicating Disorder	CPT Code
Cervical and urethral Gram stain	Positive for *N. gonorrhoeae*	58999, 50949
Cultures of oral, vaginal, urethral, and anal areas	Positive for *N. gonorrhoeae*	87081
DNA probe	Positive for *N. gonorrhoeae*	83896

Differential diagnosis:

Acute abdominal problems—salpingitis (acute pain) in females and nongonococcal prostatitis in males—are differentiated by examination.

Urinary tract infection is differentiated by urinalysis and culture.

Treatment: Drugs of choice used in the treatment of gonorrhea are the following:

- Ceftriaxone, 125 mg in single intramuscular dose or
- Cefixime, 400 mg orally in single dose or
- Ciprofloxacin, 500 mg in single oral dose or
- Ofloxacin, 400 mg in a single dose *plus*
- A regimen that would be effective for a coinfection with *C. trachomatis* (which is a common occurrence): azithromycin, 1 g orally in a single dose or doxycycline, 100 mg orally twice daily for 7 days

Follow-up: Follow-up cultures should be performed in 7 to 14 days to validate the absence of the disease.

Sequelae: Urethral or rectal strictures may occur. Sterility, although rare, may also result. Other complications include monarticular septic arthritis, disseminated gonococcal infection manifesting primarily as skin lesions, and gonococcal endocarditis.

Prevention/prophylaxis: Stress the use of condoms to all patients who are sexually active. Stress the importance of avoiding all persons suspected of having the disease and reporting all who may have been exposed to the disease so that adequate treatment may be instituted, helping to decrease the spread of the disease.

Referral: Gonorrhea is a reportable STD. Refer patient to a physician if treatment is not effective in 14 days.

Education: Teach patients that the use of condoms can reduce the spread of this disease.

SYPHILIS

SIGNAL SYMPTOMS▶ appearance of lesion in the prepuce or vulva, which changes from a small red papule to a small ulcer and finally a hard chancre

Syphilis	ICD-9 CM: 097.9

Description: Syphilis is a bacterial STD that begins at the primary site and, when untreated, becomes a systemic infection. There are two forms of syphilis. Congenital syphilis results from transplacental transmission, which can occur at any stage of pregnancy but most likely in the third trimester. Acquired syphilis results almost exclusively from unprotected sexual transmission. In acquired syphilis, the signs and symptoms can be divided into three stages: primary, secondary, and tertiary. When seen in young children, sexual abuse should be suspected.

 Clinical Pearl: Syphilis is a reportable disease.

Etiology: Syphilis is caused by *Treponema pallidum,* a bacterial spirochete.

Occurrence: Since 1986, the incidence of acquired and congenital syphilis has decreased dramatically in the United States.

Age: In the pediatric age group, syphilis is most common during adolescence as a result of unprotected sexual practices.

Ethnicity: Syphilis is more prevalent among inner-city and minority populations.

Gender: More prevalent in males (2:1).

Contributing factors: In acquired syphilis, unprotected sexual intercourse.

Signs and symptoms: Congenital syphilis can be an asymptomatic illness, especially during the first weeks of life. If the disease is symptomatic, the symptoms are usually osteitis, hepatitis, lymphadenopathy, pneumonitis, mucocutaneous lesions, anemia, and hemorrhage.

The symptoms of acquired syphilis vary according to stage. In the primary stage, the patient usually presents with one or more painless, indurated ulcers, also known as *chancres,* of the skin and mucous membrane at the site of inoculation. The most common site is the genitalia. The patient relates having had unprotected intercourse or contact with a person who has recently been diagnosed with syphilis.

In the secondary stage, the patient presents with a polymorphic rash, classically on the hands and feet, that is generalized and maculopapular. There may also be lymphadenopathy, fever, malaise, sore throat, headaches, splenomegaly, and arthralgia.

In the tertiary stage, various manifestations of neurosyphilis are seen. This stage takes about 15 years to manifest after the primary infection.

Diagnostic tests:

Test	Results Indicating Disorder	CPT Code
VDRL (darkfield)	Presence of spirochete, *T. pallidum*	86592
Treponemal antibody test (FTA-ABS)	Positive for *T. pallidum*	86781
Lumbar puncture	Presence of venereal antibodies in cerebrospinal fluid	62270
Rapid plasma reagin	Positive	86592–86593
HIV PCR	Should be done for all who test positive for syphilis	83898

VDRL, Venereal Disease Research Laboratory; FTA-ABS, fluorescent treponemal antibody absorption.

Differential diagnosis:

Herpes needs to be differentiated.

Venereal warts and other STDs are differentiated by cultures or serologic testing or both.

Treatment: The preferred treatment is penicillin G benzathine, 2.4 million U intramuscularly. If the patient is penicillin allergic and not pregnant, doxycycline, 100 mg twice daily for 14 days, is given.

 Clinical Pearl: Syphilis is a reportable STD: It should be reported to the state public health department, and all contacts should be identified and treated.

Follow-up: In congenital syphilis, follow-up should continue until nontreponemal serologic tests are negative. In adults, follow-up continues until cultures are negative and quantitative serology is negative.

Sequelae: Untreated, syphilis can affect multiple organs, including the liver, spleen, heart, and skin. In congenital syphilis, teeth are affected with notched or barrel-shaped incisors, abnormal enamel, and tooth destruction. Meningitis can occur in adults and infants. Neurosyphilis and cardiovascular disease resulting in death are complications of this disease.

Prevention/prophylaxis: Early identification of the pregnant female with syphilis assists the health care provider in preparing for treatment of the newborn. Identification of all contacts assists in decreasing the spread of the disease.

Referral: Patients with congenital syphilis should be referred to a pediatrician or local health department. When multiple organs are involved in an adult, the patient should be referred.

Education: Education of adolescents regarding safe-sex practices and barrier methods, such as condoms and foam, is important for preventing the spread of syphilis. Education concerning multiple partners and decreasing the risks of contracting STDs should begin early in childhood.

VARICOCELE

SIGNAL SYMPTOMS▶ presence of elongated, dilated, tortuous spermatic veins

Varicocele	ICD-9-CM: 456.4

Description: Asymptomatic dilated spermatic veins, more often seen on the left side, but may be either side or bilateral.

Etiology: Incompetent and dilated spermatic veins.

Occurrence: Rare before adolescence.

Age: 16% of the age group 10 to 25 years old.

Ethnicity: Not significant.

Gender: Males.

Contributing factors: There may be a familial relationship between fathers and brothers.

Signs and symptoms: Varicocele is usually asymptomatic. The child may complain that the scrotum "feels like a bag of worms."

The veins are larger when standing and smaller when supine. Gradations are as follows:

- Grade III—veins visible and greater than 2 cm in diameter
- Grade II—veins palpable but not visible, 1 to 2 cm in diameter
- Grade I—palpable only with Valsalva maneuver

Diagnostic tests:

Test	Results Indicating Disorder	CPT Code
Doppler ultrasound	Decreased volume indicative of testicular damage	76870

Differential diagnosis:

A thickened spermatic cord resulting from lipoma does not change with position.

Treatment: Usually none. Surgical repair if size variation is 3 mL or greater as measured by ultrasound, if bilateral, or if symptomatic.

Follow-up: Observe at regular visits.

Sequelae: Decreased growth and function of testicle, 20% may experience infertility with persistence into adulthood.

Prevention/prophylaxis: None.

Referral: Refer to urologist if Doppler shows testicular damage or painful scrotum.

Education: None.

VULVOVAGINITIS

SIGNAL SYMPTOMS▶ itching in the genital area vulvar redness vaginal discharge with or without odor

| Vulvovaginitis | ICD-9 CM: 616.10 |

Description: Vulvovaginitis is an inflammation of the vulva and vagina caused by an infection or an irritating substance. It is often accompanied by vaginal discharge.

Etiology: Often the etiology of vulvovaginitis depends on the age of the patient. Maturational factors figure in closely with the causes of this problem. In the prepubertal child, the lack of estrogen causes a thin, atrophic vaginal mucosa. Because of the lack of pubic hair and the thickness of the labia, there is no barrier to protect against irritants or invading organisms. Proximity of the vaginal opening to the anus is another cause of vulvovaginitis. In adolescent girls, vulvovaginitis may be due to normal leukorrhea, bacterial vaginosis, *Trichomonas, Monilia,* β-hemolytic streptococcus, or pinworms. In prepubertal and adolescent girls, foreign bodies should also be considered as a cause.

Occurrence: More prevalent among females who use douches or contraceptive foams and creams; take bubble baths; or have a recent history of antibiotic use, diabetes mellitus, or an immunosuppressive disease.

Age: All ages.

Ethnicity: Usually not significant, but current studies suggest a higher prevalence among African-American females.

Gender: Females.

Contributing factors: Factors that contribute to the manifestation of the disease are emotional stress; poor personal hygiene; multiple sexual partners; and the use of tampons, irritating douches, condoms, contraceptive foams, and creams. Foreign bodies (often tampons) are often responsible for vulvovaginitis in adolescent girls; tissue, toilet paper, or other objects contribute to the occurrence in younger girls. Rape should be considered when this disease is diagnosed.

Signs and symptoms: In prepubertal and adolescent girls, there may be a complaint of genital irritation, itching, pain or redness, and swelling of the labia. There may be a complaint of vaginal discharge. Ask the following questions.

When was this first noted?

How much discharge is present, what color is it, and is there an odor?

What is the consistency of the discharge, and how long has it been present?

Occasionally there is a further complaint of pain on urination. The parent or child may recall the child's recent use of antibiotics. Question the patient about the use of bubble baths and the type of soap used. Also, there may be a complaint of perianal itching, and it should be noted when this symptom is most problematic (e.g., day or night). For the adolescent, a menstrual and sexual history should be obtained and whether there has been a possible exposure to an STD. The recent use of tampons or contraceptive creams or foams should be noted.

For the prepubertal child, use the frog-leg or knee-chest position. Examine not only the external labia and genitalia, but also the anus. If further evaluation is needed, an otoscope may be used to provide a more thorough evaluation of the internal genitalia. Sexually active adolescents should have a complete bimanual pelvic examination, including inspection and palpation.

The type of discharge depends on the causative agent:

- *Normal leukorrhea*—a white-gray, odorless, nonirritating discharge; occurs before puberty
- *Chemical or mechanical vulvovaginitis*—a scant amount of discharge that is clear to yellow, sometimes blood tinged; there is some external inflammation of the genitalia
- *Foreign body, such as toilet paper or other object*—a purulent, foul, brown discharge
- *Bacterial infection (usually streptococcal)*—copious, foul-smelling discharge and bleeding accompanied by a fever and abdominal pain
- *Bacterial vaginosis*—accompanied by a thin, gray-to-clear discharge that has a fishy odor when exposed to a potassium hydroxide test
- *Candidiasis*—a thick, white, curdlike, odorless discharge accompanied by pruritus, dysuria, and dyspareunia.
- *Trichomoniasis*—a foul-smelling, yellow-gray, profuse discharge accompanied by persistent hemorrhagic lesions on the cervix

There may also be irritation caused by itching, and redness and swelling of the external genitalia may be observed.

Diagnostic tests:

Test	Results Indicating Disorder	CPT Code
Vaginal pH	If >4.5, most likely vaginosis or trichonomiasis If < 4.5, most likely candidiasis	84315
Urinalysis	Increased white blood cells, the presence of yeast cells or trichomonads	81000
Wet mount preparation vaginal secretions	Positive for amines (positive whiff test) Presence of flagellated parasite	87210
Pap smear	Trichomoniasis detected	88141–155 88154–167

Differential diagnosis:

Concomitant STDs, cervicitis, PID, and foreign body are determined by cultures and examination.

In the infant or prepubertal child, sexual abuse should be investigated.

Treatment:

Bacterial infections are treated with penicillin, 125 to 250 mg three times a day for 10 days; in penicillin-allergic patients, erythromycin, 30 to 50 mg/kg per day three times daily for 10 days.

Bacterial vaginosis is treated with metronidazole, 2 g orally one time or 500 mg twice a day for 10 days. Another treatment may be clindamycin, 300 mg four times a day for 7 days. In lieu of oral medication, topical clindamycin 2% cream can be used for 7 days at night.

For candidiasis, use a local external medication, such as clotrimazole, miconazole, or butoconazole, which can be applied once or twice daily for 7 days.

Trichomoniasis is treated with oral metronidazole, 2 g orally one time or 500 mg twice daily for 7 days. Partners should always be treated; abstinence from sexual intercourse is required until about 1 to 2 weeks after treatment is completed for both partners.

Follow-up: A follow-up examination is usually not necessary, unless there is a return of symptoms or continued complaints.

Sequelae: In some cases, sterility may result from untreated or fulminating infections. Additionally, secondary infections of the skin may develop, which affect the skin's integrity and result in open wounds.

Prevention/prophylaxis: Condoms may reduce the risk of contracting STDs. Maintaining monogamous relationships can also help decrease one's risk. Patients should be told to urinate after sexual intercourse and to undergo regular examinations if they are sexually active so that if an infection is present, it can be treated early.

Referral: If the symptoms do not resolve or if they recur, after the prescribed therapy, refer the patient. If sexual abuse is suspected, refer the patient immediately to the child protection agency and the police. Often the most effective way to accomplish this is while the child is in the clinic. Call 911, and the police generally send an officer immediately to interview the nurse practitioner, child, and accompanying adult. Erring on the side of protecting the child is much more important than waiting so that no one is embarrassed or angered by your suspicion.

Education: Patients should be told that they are at increased risk for contracting STDs when they engage in unprotected sex or sex with multiple partners. Teaching the patient to urinate after intercourse and to avoid douching may decrease the incidence of STDs further. The importance of treating sexual partners with some of these problems needs to be stressed; the patient should be informed of the risks for reinfection if their partner is not treated. Patients should be taught the importance of completing their prescribed treatment regimens.

REFERENCES

Cryptorchidism

Cortes, D, et al: Testicular neoplasia in cryptorchid boys at primary surgery: Case series. BMJ 319:888, 1999.

Docimo, S, et al: The undescended testicle: Diagnosis and management. Am Fam Physician 62:2037, 2000.

Ferrer, F, and McKenna, P: Current approaches to the undescended testicle. Comtemp Pediatr 3, 2000.

Dysmenorrhea

Baker, S: Menstruation and related problems and concerns. In Youngkin, E, and Davis, S (eds): Women's Health: A Primary Clinical Guide. Appleton & Lange, Stanford, CT, 1998.

Polaneczhy, M, and Slap, G: Dysmenorrhea and dysfunctional uterine bleeding. Pediatr Rev 13:83, 1997.

Siberry, G, and Iannone, R: The Harriet Lane Handbook, ed 15. Mosby, St. Louis, 2001.

Amenorrhea

Lowey, S, et al: Early metabolic abnormalities in adolescent girls with polycystic ovarian syndrome. Southern Medical Journal 94:2, 190–196, 2001.

Marshburn, P: Amenorrhea in a 17 year old. Clin Advisor 1:26, 2000.

Mauldin, M: Amenorrhea in adolescents. Adv Nurse Practitioners 7:45, 2000.

Roche, A, et al: Age of menarche and racial comparisons in U.S. girls. Pediatrics 111:110, 2003.

Epididymitis

Adelman, W, and Joffe, A: The adolescent with a painful scrotum. Contemp Pediatr 3:111, 2000.

Bromberg, W: Managing genitourinary trauma. Clin Advisor 2:42, 1999.

DuFour, J: Assessing and treating epididymitis. Nurse Practit 26:23, 2001.

Galejs, L, and Kass, EJ: Diagnosis and treatment of the acute scrotum. Am Fam Physician 59:817, 1999.

Kadish, H: Painful subject: Pinpointing the cause of acute scrotal swelling. Contemp Pediatr 5:95, 2001.

Raheja, R, et al: Is diagnosis of bacterial "epididymitis" by Doppler scrotal ultra-sonography misleading? Infect Urol 13:121, 2000.

Richman, M, and Bukowsi, T: Pediatric epididymitis: Pathophysiology, diagnosis, and management. Infect Urol 14:31, 2001.

Gynecomastia in Males

Felner, E, and White, P: Prepubertal gynecomastia: Indirect exposure to estrogen cream. Pediatrics 105:e55, 2000.

Johnson, W: Nutritional supplements and the young athlete: What you need to know. Contemp Pediatr 7:632, 2001.

Herpes Simplex Virus Type 2

Johnson, R: Diagnosis and treatment of common sexually transmitted diseases in women. Clinical Cornerstone 4, 2001.

Nadelman, C, and Johnson, V: Herpes simplex virus infections: New treatments make early diagnosis even more important. Postgrad Med 107:189, 2000.

Stockman, J, and Lohr, M: Essence of Office Pediatrics. WB Saunders, Philadelphia, 2001.

Thrall, J, et al: Preferences of Massacchussetts HMO's in providing PAP smears and sexually transmitted disease screening in adolescent females. J Adolesc Health 22:184, 1998.

Hydrocele

Galejs, L, and Kass, EJ: Diagnosis and treatment of the acute scrotum. Am Fam Physician 59:817, 1999.

Kazzi, A, and Rudkin, S: Hydrocele. EMed J 2, 2001.

Hypospadias and Epispadias

Bukowski, T, and Zeman, P: Hypospadias: Of concern but correctable. Contemp Pediatr 2:89, 2001.

Labial Adhesions

Franklin, V: Labial adhesion. Contact: www.medicallibrary.org. Accessed February 8, 2002.

Howard, B: Labial adhesions. In Hoekleman, RA, et al (eds): Primary Pediatric Care. Mosby, St. Louis, 1998.

Stockman, J, and Lohr, M. Essence of Office Pediatrics. WB Saunders, Philadelphia, 2001.

Pelvic Inflammatory Disease

American Academy of Pediatrics, Committee on Child Abuse and Neglect: Gonorrhea in prepubertal children. Pediatrics 101:134, 2002.

Centers for Disease Control and Prevention: Sexually-transmitted diseases treatment guidelines. MMWR Morb Mortal Wkly Rep 51(RR-6), 2002.

Gettes, E, and Irwin, C: Sexually transmitted diseases in adolescents. Pediatr Rev 14:180, 1998.

Rhoads, D, and Elmore, S: Should HPV testing replace the PAP smear? Clin Advisor October:43, 2001.

Shafer, M: Sexually transmitted diseases in adolescents: Prevention, diagnosis and treatment in pediatric practice. Pediatr Rev 13:83, 1998.

Smith, R, et al: Screening for chlamydia in adolescents and young women. Arch Pediatr Adolesc Med 154:1108, 2000.

Phimosis/Paraphimosis

Ashfield, J, et al: Treatment of phimosis with topical steroids in 194 children. J Urol 169:1106, 2003.

Cantu, S: Phimosis and paraphimosis. eMed J 2, 2001.

Choe, J, and Kim, H: Paraphimosis. eMed J 2, 2001.

Pregnancy

American Academy of Pediatrics: Committee on Adolescence: Adolescent pregnancy—current trends and issues: 1998. Pediatrics 103:516, 2000.

D'Ambro, A, and D'Ambro, M: Amenorrhea: Griffith's 5 minute clinical consults. Clin Rev 6:115, 2000.

Dickey, R: Managing Contraceptive Pill Patients. Enis Medical Publishers, Durant, OK, 1998.

Dixon, D, et al: The first prenatal visit. Clin Rev 10:53, 2000.

Vincent, M, and Adeyeles, E: Are you comfortable taking the sexual history? Fam Pract 20:87, 1998.

Primary Gonococcal Infections

American Academy of Pediatrics: Gonorrhea in prepubertal children. Pediatrics 101:134, 1998.

Geishman, K, and Barrow, J: A tale of two sexually transmitted diseases: Prevalence and predictors of chlamydia and gonorrhea in women attending Colorado family planning clinics. Sex Transm Dis 23:481, 1998.

Johnson, R: Diagnosis and treatment of common sexually transmitted diseases in women. Contact: www.ama-assn.org. Accessed February 8, 2002.

Smith, R, et al: Screening for chlamydia in adolescents and young women. Arch Pediatr Adolesc Med 154:1108, 2000.

Syphilis

American Academy of Pediatrics Committee on Child Abuse and Neglect: Gonorrhea in prepubertal children. Pediatrics 101:134, 2001.

Bartlett, J, and Gallant, J: Medical Management of HIV Infection. Johns Hopkins Press, Baltimore, 2001–2002.

Centers for Disease Control and Prevention: Sexually-transmitted diseases treatment guidelines. MMWR Morb Mortal Wkly Rep 51(RR-6), May 10, 2002.

Stockman, J, and Lohr, M: Essence of Office Pediatrics. WB Saunders, Philadelphia, 2001.

Varicocele

Gregory, T: Revisiting the adolescent male genital examination. Patient Care. Feb 2, 2000.

Kerr, R: Consider checking for varicoceles in brothers, sons. Urol Times December, 2001.

Kass, E, and Stork, B: Mitigating the effects of pediatric varicocele. Contemp Urol April, 2001.

Vulvovaginitis

American Academy of Pediatrics Committee on Child Abuse and Neglect: Gonorrhea in prepubertal children. Pediatrics 101:134, 2001.

Maxson, J: New treatment for bacterial vaginosis. Clin Advisor October:39, 2001.

Paek, S, et al: Pruritus vulva in the prepubertal child. J Acad Dermatol 44:795, 2001.

U.S. Department of Health and Human Services, Centers for Disease Control and Prevention: Sexually transmitted diseases treatment guidelines. MMWR Morb Mortal Wkly Rep 51:6, May 10, 2002.

Chapter *10*
MUSCULOSKELETAL DISORDERS

ANKLE SPRAIN

SIGNAL SYMPTOMS ▶ pain with or without swelling of ankle

Ankle sprain	ICD-9 CM: 845.00

Description: Sprain is a stretching of a ligament, whereas a strain is a stretch of a muscle or tendon. Acute ankle sprains may be classified as follows:

- Grade I—caused by low-level activity, such as stepping off a curb
- Grade II—caused by higher level activity, such as a misstep while running
- Grade III—caused by vigorous exertion of force during a foot stroke while the ankle is pliantly flexed and internally rotated

Etiology: Trauma to the ligament, muscle, or tendon and associated ligamental laxity.

Occurrence: Constitutes 5% of all athletic injuries.

Age: All age groups.

Ethnicity: Not significant.

Gender: Occurs equally in males and females.

Contributing factors: Running, jumping, and other sports activities.

Signs and symptoms: The child presents to the clinic because of pain or discomfort in the ankle after walking or running. Have the child describe the circumstances leading to the injury, the site of pain, when the swelling began (immediate swelling may indicate a fracture), and whether weight bearing is possible. Ask what has been done for the injury (e.g., ice, elevation). Ask whether this is a new injury or a reinjury.

Examine ankle for swelling and ecchymosis, crepitus or pain, and limitation of motion. Palpate the ankle, starting with the nontender area first (Table 10–1).

Table 10–1 Categorization of Ankle Sprains

Category	Functional Deficit	Physical Findings	Clinical Implications
Grade I	Little, can walk with no limp, can hop on ankle	Swelling and tenderness over the ATL	Indicative of a partial rupture of the ATL
Grade II	Limping, some functional loss	Localized swelling and tenderness around the ATL	Possible rupture of the ATL and tearing of the calcaneofibular ligament
Grade III	Crutch walking preferred	Diffuse pain and swelling	Complete rupture of the ATL and anterior and bilateral laxity

ATL, anterior talofibular ligament.

Diagnostic tests:

Test	Results Indicating Disorder	CPT Code
Radiographs: anterorposterior, oblique, lateral views in neutral and in internal rotation	Negative for fractures, joint incongruity, and degenerative disease	73600

 Clinical Pearl: Because edema can mask a fracture, radiographic views are more satisfactory if done after swelling has subsided.

Radiographic studies are often recommended in cases of severe pain, in cases with a history of previous injury, or for a child who is still growing.

Differential diagnosis:

Fractures—physeal, osteochondral, lateral and posterior process of the talus, anterior process of the calcaneus, fifth metatarsal base (dancer's fracture), and fifth metatarsal at the metaphyseal-diaphyseal junction (Jones fracture)—can be seen on radiographic film unless the fracture is cartilaginous; magnetic resonance imaging (MRI) provides more definitive evaluation.

Dislocation is an obvious bony deformity seen on radiographic films.

In ligament tear, external rotation of the foot and tibiofibular compression of the calf cause pain in the ankle.

In tendon tear, patient has a history of chronic instability that is not responding to treatment.

Treatment:

Nonpharmacologic

First stage: Treatment is rest, ice, modified Jones compression dressing, and elevation (RICE) to reduce swelling, inflammation, and pain. Grade I and II, prescribe partial weight bearing with crutches. Grade III, immobilize with a U-shaped splint, elevate, use ice, and prescribe crutches (prohibit weight bearing) (Fig. 10–1).

Second stage: For restoration of function, begin active range-of-motion exercises while sitting or lying down (using foot, "inscribe" letters ["alphabet exercises"] in the air) and gait training after swelling has subsided. Weight bearing after 72 hours lessens swelling, reduces pain, and resolves edema.

Third stage: Tape the ankle or use an ankle support or wrap, and begin neuromuscular training and peroneal strengthening. Surgical intervention may be indicated for grade III injuries.

Pharmacologic

For pain, give acetaminophen, 10 to 15 mg/kg per dose or 400 to 480 mg every 4 hours, or ibuprofen, 4 to 10 mg/kg per dose every 6 to 8 hours.

Follow-up: Evaluate swelling, inflammation, and pain in 24, 48, and 72 hours, and at 2 weeks, evaluate weight bearing.

Sequelae: Approximately 10% to 20% of persons with ankle sprains develop chronic functional instability (i.e., episodes in which the ankle "gives way"). This mechanical instability can predispose patients to further injury, functional instability, peroneal tendon weakness, or subluxation.

Prevention/prophylaxis: Properly fitted shoes and proper walking techniques can be preventive. In athletes, although taping provides some protection, the use of semirigid ankle stabilizers has show effectiveness in preventing ankle injuries.

Referral: Refer patients who have gross instability of the ankle or who do not improve within 12 weeks to an orthopedist.

Education: Instruct parent and child in the correct use of crutches, if indicated; in proper shoe fit; in correct walking technique; and in exercises that help an injured ankle. The following are basic guidelines for ankle exercises.

Exercise in stocking or bare feet.

Perform each exercise 10 times and increase by 5 each day to a maximum of 30 repetitions.

Do not continue any exercise that causes pain.

Perform exercises three times per day.

APOPHYSEAL INJURIES

SIGNAL SYMPTOMS ▶ pain and inflammation at tendon insertion site

Sever's disease	ICD-9-CM: 732.5
Osgood-Schlatter disease	ICD-9-CM: 732.4
Sinding-Larsen-Johansson disease	ICD-9-CM: 732.4
Apophysis of the hip	ICD-9-CM: 732.7
Medial epicondylitis	ICD-9-CM: 726.31

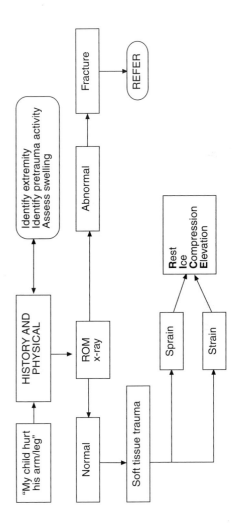

Figure 10–1. Sprains and strains. (ROM, range of motion.)

Description: Apophyseal injuries are characterized by periarticular pain, with inflammation at the site of major tendon insertion at the point of active growth, usually at the heel, knee, hip, and elbow; patients may present with bilateral injuries.

Etiology:

- *Sever's disease (heel)*—repetitive microtrauma with inflammatory changes
- *Osgood-Schlatter disease*—trauma-induced apophyseal injury to the tibia tuberosity
- *Sinding-Larsen-Johansson disease*—multiple episodes of microtrauma to the inferior pole of the patella
- *Apophysitis of the hip*—traction on a growing area of bone, usually at the anterior superior and the anterior inferior iliac spine, the iliac crests, and the ischial tuberosities
- *Medial epicondylitis*—skeletal immaturity of the medial epicondylar apophysis

Occurrence: Fairly common.

Age: Occur in 8- to 15-year-old athletes (average age 11 years).

- *Sever's disease*—8 to 13 years.
- *Osgood-Schlatter disease*—Males, 10 to 15 years; females, 8 to 13 years.
- *Sinding-Larsen-Johansson disease*—10 to 13 years.
- *Apophysitis of the hip*—9 to 13 years.
- *Medial epicondylitis*—9 to 13 years.

Ethnicity: Not significant.

Gender: Occur in males and females (Sever's disease, males; Osgood-Schlatter disease, males and females; Sinding-Larsen-Johansson disease, males; apophysitis of the hip, males; medial epicondylitis, males).

Contributing factors:

- *Sever's disease*—associated with growth, tight heel cords, or other biomechanical abnormalities; participation in soccer and running.
- *Osgood-Schlatter disease*—weakened and inflexible quadriceps muscle; participation in sports requiring running.
- *Sinding-Larsen-Johansson disease*—participation in sports involving running and jumping (e.g., soccer).
- *Apophysitis of the hip*—associated with muscle-tendon imbalance and growth spurts; implicated activities are distance running and dancing.
- *Medial epicondylitis*—skeletal immaturity, overuse phenomenon, participation in sports activities requiring repeated overhead arm motion, such as pitching (baseball) and serving (tennis).

Signs and symptoms: The child is brought to the clinic with pain in one of the following areas: heel, anterior knee, hip (a dull ache), or elbow (tenderness). Physical findings vary by diagnosis:

Sever's disease: There is tenderness at the insertion of the Achilles tendon on the calcaneus.

Osgood-Schlatter disease: There is pain and swelling over the tibia tubercle with worsening of the pain during running, jumping, and ascending or descending stairs; resisted extension of the knee at 90° of flexion causes pain, whereas resisted straight-leg raising does not. Tenderness and erythema are noted over the tibia tuberosity.

Sinding-Larsen-Johansson disease: Pain occurs over the inferior pole of the patella and is worse with running or stair climbing. Palpation of the inferior pole of the patella is positive for tenderness.

Apophysitis of the hip: Dull pain is related to activity located near the hip.

Medial epicondylitis: There is tenderness over the medial condyle and pain with resisted flexion of the wrist.

Diagnostic tests:

Test	Results Indicating Disorder	CPT Codes
Radiographs of heel	Partial fragmentation and increased density of os calcis: Sever's disease	73650
Radiographs of tibia	Enlarged, fragmented, and irregular tibial tuberosity: Osgood-Schlatter disease	73590
Bone age	Normal	76020
Radiographs of patella	Normal to calcification of the inferior pole of the patella: Sindig-Larsen-Johansson disease	735560
Radiographs of elbow	Fragmentation of medial epicondyle: medial epicondylitis	73070–73080
Radiographs of hip(if injury result of traumatic event with pain)	Apophysitis	73500–73520

Differential diagnosis:

Osteosarcoma has positive radiographic studies; gait disturbances are noted.

A child with patellar tendinitis exhibits pain on running and climbing stairs.

Osteomyelitis usually affects a single bone; the child may experience an acute illness or a subacute illness with fever, severe pain at the affected site, erythema, and swelling. Radiographic studies may be normal in the first 10 to 14 days of the illness.

Slipped capital femoral epiphysis has physeal abnormalities and skeletal maturation anomalies.

Treatment:

Nonpharmacologic

> *Sever's disease:* Activity reduction, RICE, use of heel cups, massage, and stretching of the muscle involved. In rare cases, the patient may need crutches for 2 to 3 weeks.

> *Osgood-Schlatter disease and Sinding-Larsen-Johansson disease:* Wearing of a knee support and reducing or modifying athletic activity to reach a pain-free level. Initiate a program of stretching and strengthening with resisted straight-leg raises. The patient may need a trial of crutches for 2 to 3 weeks. Use RICE (apply ice for 20 minutes three times per day) protocol.

> *Apophysitis of the hip:* Initiate a program of stretching and strengthening of the abdominal and hip muscles; recommend a slow return to activity, as tolerated. Use RICE (apply ice for 20 minutes three times per day) protocol.

> *Medial epicondylitis:* Initiate a program of stretching and strengthening of the forearm muscles; recommend a slow return to throwing, as tolerated. Use RICE (apply ice for 20 minutes three times per day) protocol. A long arm splint may be required to reduce ulnar nerve irritation.

Pharmacologic

Naproxen (Aleve), 27.5 mg twice daily or 220 mg every 8 to 10 hours up to 10 days, or ibuprofen, 30 to 40 mg/kg four times daily, is given for 2 to 3 days for relief of pain and inflammation.

Follow-up: The patient should return every 2 weeks for evaluation of therapeutic response.

Sequelae: None, if properly diagnosed and managed.

With medial and lateral epicondylitis, ulnar nerve compression is present in 60% of patients and may require surgical intervention if splinting does not reduce the ulnar nerve irritation.

Prevention/prophylaxis: To help prevent these types of injuries from occurring as well as from becoming chronic, a program of stretching and strengthening should be initiated, focusing on the muscles involved in the activity. Proper equipment may also be a factor (e.g., the proper size grip on the tennis racquet, a larger head to produce fewer bad hits, a graphite or composite racquet rather than a wooden or metal one, and a racquet strung less tightly [<55 lb]).

Referral: Refer patient to orthopedist if there is no improvement after 3 weeks. Refer to a physical therapist for a program of stretching and strengthening exercises.

Education: Increase patient's awareness of overuse injuries and the importance of preparticipation physical conditioning.

ASEPTIC NECROSIS OF THE HIP
(LEGG-CALVÉ-PERTHES DISEASE)

SIGNAL SYMPTOMS limp with pain in thigh and knee

Aseptic Necrosis of the Hip	ICD-9 CM: 732.1

Description: Aseptic necrosis of the hip is an interruption of the vascular supply to the capital femur with necrosis. There are four stages of the disease:

- Prenecrosis or vascular occlusion from trauma, hypercoagulation, emboli, or increased intra-articular pressure
- Necrosis accompanied by involvement of the femoral epiphysis, metaphysis, or bone marrow and resulting in fracture or cyst formation (3–6 months from onset)
- Revascularization with resorption of dead bone and deformation of the softened femoral head (6–12 months from onset)
- Reossification of the deformed femoral head and acetabulum (18–36 months from onset)

Etiology: A disturbance in circulation to the femoral capital epiphysis after trauma or infection. Thrombolytic and hypofibrinolytic disorders are being investigated that may predispose the interruption of blood flow, including factor V Leiden gene.

Occurrence: Unknown.

Age: Occurs at ages 2 to 12 with peak age of 4 to 8.

Ethnicity: Occurs most frequently in whites (10:1) and Chinese; rare in blacks and Native Americans.

Gender: Occurs more frequently in males (5:1).

Contributing factors: Low birth weight, abnormal birth presentation, older mother, lower socioeconomic class, and delayed bone maturation have been suggested as risk factors. Decreased levels of somatomedin C and increased level of thyroxine and triiodothyronine have been reported in children with Legg-Calvé-Perthes disease.

Signs and symptoms: The child presents with hip pain referred to the knee and anterior thigh or groin and a limp. Examination reveals limitation of movement, disturbance in gait, and thigh atrophy (Figs. 10–2 and 10–3).

Clinical Pearl: Any 4- to 9-year-old child who presents with a limp that has failed to improve for 7 to 10 days is highly suspect for Legg-Calvé-Perthes disease.

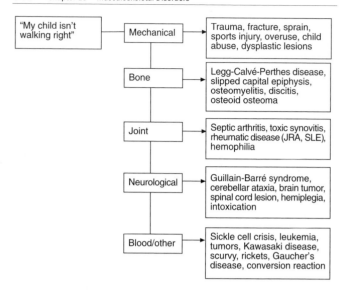

Figure 10–2. Classification of gait disturbance. (JRA, juvenile rheumatoid arthritis; SLE, systemic lupus erythematosus.)

Diagnostic tests:

Test	Results Indicating Disorder	CPT Codes
Radiographs of hip: anteroposterior and frog-leg lateral positions; radiographs of the pelvis	Effusion of the joint, slight widening of the joint space; progressive decreased bone density, alternating areas of rarefaction versus relative density of the epiphysis, fractures	73500–73520, 73540
Joint aspirates	Normal	20600
Bone age	Delay: 75% males, 25% females	76020

Differential diagnosis:

Inflammatory or infectious synovitis is usually transient after about 10 days.

Joint aspirate cultures are positive in septic arthritis.

Slipped capital femoral epiphysis occurs in obese adolescent boys.

Meyer's dysplasia is rare and most often bilateral; it affects the femoral epiphysis in young children. Bone scans are normal.

Treatment: Protection of the affected joint by maintaining abduction and internal rotation, use of crutches, physical therapy for range of motion, Petrie casts, and abduction bracing. Surgery may be indicated, particularly in severe cases.

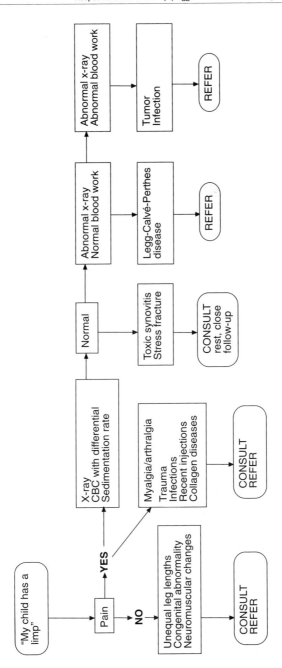

Figure 10–3. Differential diagnosis of limp.

Follow-up: The patient should return for evaluation at least every 3 months.

Sequelae: Sequelae depend on the degree of involvement and the amount of deformity. The prognosis for full return of function is poorer when there is greater involvement of the femoral head and when the disease started later in life.

Prevention/prophylaxis: None.

Referral: In suspected cases, refer patients to an orthopedist for full evaluation.

Education: Teach parents the importance of the child's wearing the brace. Counsel parents regarding the long-term effects of the disease.

DEVELOPMENTAL DYSPLASIA OF THE HIP

SIGNAL SYMPTOMS hip instability, inequality of leg length, delayed walking with gait disturbance

Developmental dysplasia of the hip	ICD-9 CM: 755.63
Dislocated	ICD-9 CM: 754.30

Description: Developmental dysplasia of the hip, formerly called *congenital dislocated hip,* is a misalignment of the femoral head with the acetabulum. There are three types.

Dislocated: The femoral head is located outside of the acetabulum.

Dislocatable: The femoral head is in the acetabulum, but when displaced by the examiner, the femoral head spontaneously returns to its normal position.

Subluxation: The femoral head can be partially moved out of the acetabulum.

The left hip is most often involved (60%), followed by the right hip (20%) and both hips (20%).

Etiology: The etiology is multifactorial:

- Mechanical—birth presentation, postnatal strapping of an infant's hips in extension by Native American parents
- Physiologic—ligamentous laxity in female infants influenced by maternal hormones estrogen and relaxin
- Genetic—family histories and twin studies

Occurrence: Dislocated hip, 1.3 per 1000 births; dislocatable hip, 2.5 per 1000 births; subluxatable hip, 14 per 1000 births. Occurs more often in siblings of infants who have had the condition or twins.

Age: At birth or later.

Ethnicity: More common in Lapps and Native Americans and less common in blacks, Koreans, and Chinese.

Gender: Females 6 times as often than males.

Contributing factors: Hormonal, congenital, and mechanical factors as well as breech births.

Signs and symptoms: Child is asymptomatic until older and walking, then he or she develops a limp. Clinical signs depend on age.

- *Newborn*—hip instability
- *Older infant*—asymmetrical thigh folds, inequality of leg length (Allis sign)
- *Older child*—gait abnormality (waddling), painful limp, and lurch to affected side (Trendelenburg sign)

 Clinical Pearl: In infants, newborn to 2 years old, the thighs can be abducted to touch the examining table; if they cannot be brought to within 25° to 30° of the table, radiographic studies should be obtained.

Diagnostic tests: The following maneuvers should be done during the first 6 months at each well-baby visit to assess hip stability:

- Barlow maneuver (dislocation test)—done during the newborn period; positive if the hip is dislocatable
- Ortolani maneuver (reduction test)—a maneuver that would be positive at 4 to 6 weeks of age but becomes negative by 3 to 5 months; there is a feeling of slipping (a "clunk") as the femoral head is relocated
- Galeazzi sign—asymmetrical skin folds in the groin and apparent femoral shortening with uneven knee heights (>2 months old)
- Allis sign—with the hips and knees flexed, the knees are at unequal heights, with the dislocated side lower

Test	Results Indicating Disorder	CPT Codes
Radiographs of hips	Negative in neonatal period After 6 weeks: lateral displacement of femoral head (maintain films for comparison)	73500–73520
Ultrasound of hips (less accurate after 4–6 months of age)	Documents the cartilaginous components of the proximal femur and acetabulum	76885–76886

Differential diagnosis:

Congenital short femur is differentiated by radiographs.

Treatment:

Most subluxatable hips stabilize by 6 weeks of age.

Use of double or triple diapers is not effective.

Apply splints such as the Pavlik, Ilfield, or Rosen harness to maintain flexion and abduction of the hip.

Follow-up: The patient should return monthly to the clinic for evaluation of progress, at 1 year old, then yearly until skeletal maturity is achieved.

Sequelae: Flexion contractures contribute to marked lordosis, resulting in gait problems. Limited abduction results in limp and gluteal muscle weakness. The most serious complication is avascular necrosis of the hip. Arthritis of the hip in adolescence and adulthood has been reported.

Prevention/prophylaxis: None.

Referral: Refer to orthopedist for confirmation and treatment. Best results are achieved when diagnosis and intervention occur before age 6 months. Ideally the problem should be identified in the nursery.

Education: Educate the parent in the proper application of the harness and the importance of follow-up evaluations.

DISLOCATIONS

SIGNAL SYMPTOMS ▶ painful displacement of joint

Dislocations	ICD-9-CM: 839.8

Description: Dislocation is the displacement of a bony part from its usual site, usually as a result of trauma.

Etiology:

Shoulder: In children, the cause is instability; in adolescents, a tendinitis recurrence or an injury that involves an abduction and external rotation of the shoulder.

Patella: Vigorous quadriceps contraction when the knees are flexed from a valgus position.

Occurrence: Uncommon in children but common in athletes.

Age: Adolescents.

Ethnicity: Not significant.

Gender: Occurs in males, usually athletes; also occurs in females, particularly females with genu valgum.

Contributing factors: Participation in sports-related activities (e.g., jumping), loose-jointedness, and genu valgum (patella dislocation). The third factor contributes to the disorder in females, particularly adolescent girls.

Signs and symptoms: The child presents with the complaint of severe pain in the affected body part. History should include activities preceding the injury, the exact location and distribution of pain, and the quality of the pain. It should also include whether the pain occurs with movement, what limitations or types of weakness there are, and what aggravates and what relieves the pain.

Physical findings depend on type of dislocation.

Patella: The nurse practitioner observes slight flexion of the knee and a bony mass lateral to the knee joint, with a flat area over the normal position for the patella.

Shoulder: The nurse practitioner should inspect for symmetry, swelling, unilateral bony prominences, any changes in skin color, and winging of the scapula. Palpate for tenderness and range of motion, and evaluate the deep tendon reflexes and motor strength.

Diagnostic tests:

Test	Results Indicating Disorder	CPT Code
Patella: radiographs of the knee	Confirmation of dislocation	73560
Shoulder: anteroposterior, transthoracic lateral, and apical oblique	Confirmation of shoulder instability	73030

Differential diagnosis:

Patella: None.

Shoulder: If pain radiates below the elbow, suspect some problem in the cervical spine; any tumors found on x-ray produce pain unrelated to movement.

Treatment:

Nonpharmacologic

Patella: Reduction and immobilization for 3 to 4 weeks; a physical therapy program to strengthen the quadriceps muscle. Surgery may be necessary to tighten the patella capsule.

Shoulder: Immobilization with a sling or shoulder brace or spica wrap; isometric exercises (internal and external rotation) with elbow placed at patient's side.

Pharmacologic

Nonsteroidal anti-inflammatory drugs (NSAIDs) are given for relief of pain and inflammation.

Follow-up: In 3 weeks, then in an additional 3 weeks.

Sequelae:

Patella: If there is repeated damage to the cartilage of the joint, the patient is at high risk for premature degenerative arthritis.

Shoulder: Recurrence rate is high in high school athletes.

Prevention/prophylaxis: None except preparticipation conditioning for persons involved in sports activities.

Referral: Refer patient to a primary care physician or orthopedist for reduction and plan of care.

Education: Emphasize the importance of complying with the regimen, as outlined (immobilization, restriction of athletic activity). Emphasize that the strengthening exercises help to reduce the risk of recurrence.

FLOPPY INFANT

SIGNAL SYMPTOMS ▶ inability to meet motor milestones

Floppy Infant	ICD-9 CM: 781.99

Description: The floppy infant displays a decreased resistance to passive movement with abnormal extensibility of the joints and delay in motor milestones. There are two types:

- *Paralytic group (weakness)*—significant lack of movement against gravity
- *Nonparalytic group*—floppiness without significant paralysis

Etiology: Paralytic causes include the following.

Lesion of the lower motor neuron complex: Infantile progressive spinal muscular atrophy is the most common cause (autosomal recessive).

Neuromuscular junction: Causes include botulism (acquired in infants <1 year old) and myasthenia gravis (12% have a mother with myasthenia gravis).

Muscle disease: Causes include myotonic dystrophy (autosomal dominant).

Nonparalytic causes are as follows:

- Intrauterine or perinatal insults on brain or spinal cord: constitute 75% of cases
- Hypotonia of central nervous system origin: trisomy 21, Marfan's syndrome, Turner's syndrome
- Degenerative disorders: Tay-Sachs disease
- Systemic diseases, malnutrition: cystic fibrosis and celiac disease
- Chronic illness: congenital heart disease, chronic pulmonary disease, metabolic (hypercalcemia) and endocrine (hypothyroid) disorders
- Unknown causes

Occurrence: Common.

Age: Occurs at birth and in older infants.

Ethnicity: Not significant.

Gender: Occurs equally in males and females.

Contributing factors: Prematurity, maternal ingestions, and infections such as poliomyelitis.

Signs and symptoms: The infant is brought to the clinic for an early well-baby visit with the complaint that the "hips are funny." Older infants with the disorder are brought to the clinic when they have not started walking, running, or climbing stairs.

Findings in the newborn nursery include a positive scarf sign (the infant's hands can be pulled across the chest, and the elbows can be pulled past the chin) and a positive hip sign (extended lower extremities can be abducted at the hip >160°). Findings in young infants include the following: The frog-leg position, with arms limp at the sides, is classic; when held horizontally, the infant droops over the hand; when held vertically, it feels as though the infant will slip through the hands; and there is marked head lag. In older infants, there is a delay in achieving motor milestones.

In the paralytic group, the fine motor, personal/social, and language milestones are normal according to results of the Denver Developmental Screening test. There is weakness in the shoulders and hips, tendon reflexes are absent or depressed, and strength is decreased.

In the nonparalytic group, spasticity is present, and reflexes are increased. The Babinski and tonic neck reflexes persist and worsen.

Diagnostic tests:

Test	Results Indicating Disorder	CPT Code
Blood glucose	May indicate hypoglycemia	82947
Blood calcium	May indicate hypercalcemia	82310
Computed tomography of the brain	Determine the presence of abnormalities (lissencephaly) or intracranial hemorrhage	74050
Spinal fluid examination	Rule out meningitis and encephalitis	62270
Creatine kinase	Normal; check for degenerative muscle disorder	82550
Creatinine phosphokinase	Elevated in birth trauma, hypoxia, or ischemia	82552
Electromyography	Abnormal in hypotonias of peripheral origin	51785
Muscle biopsy	Decrease in voluntary motor activity	20200
Gene karyotyping	Deletion of the proximal part of the long arm of chromosome 15, labeled q11-q13, paternally derived (Prader-Willi syndrome) Deletion of the long arm of chromosome 15, maternally derived (Angelman syndrome, "happy puppet")	88261
Origin-specific DNA methylation (PW 71 probe)	Two copies of maternally derived chromosome 15 and an absent paternal chromosome (maternal disomy)	88729

Differential diagnosis:

> Hypoglycemia or hypocalcemia is excluded on the basis of blood workup.
> Sepsis is excluded on the basis of spinal fluid and blood workup.
> Weakness is excluded as the child matures.

Treatment: Supportive, based on the ultimate diagnosis.

Follow-up: Monthly to assess growth and development.

Sequelae: In cases secondary to Tay-Sachs disease, the prognosis is death. In other forms, such as floppiness secondary to Marfan's syndrome, children mature to lead productive lives. Children with paralytic forms (e.g., secondary to congenital muscular dystrophy) may have mental retardation. Children with spinal cord lesions may be wheelchairbound for life.

Prevention/prophylaxis: Improved prenatal care and delivery techniques as a means of possibly preventing intrauterine and birth problems.

Education: Instruct the family in feeding techniques because these patients sometimes have problems with chewing and swallowing. For diseases with a genetic factor, discuss the implications with the family.

FOOT PROBLEMS

SIGNAL SYMPTOMS▶ feet deviate from normal development

Clubfoot	ICD-9 CM: 754.70
Flatfeet	ICD-9 CM: 754.61

Description: Foot problems are deviations from the normal development of the foot. These problems may be related to posturing, the habitual position of the foot, or to deformity, which is similar to posturing except that the foot cannot be manually repositioned. The following are among the most commonly noted problems.

Calcaneovalgus occurs as a result of uterine restraint.

Metatarsus adductus is probably secondary to uterine restraint.

Clubfoot (talipes equinovarus) in severe cases is attributed to anatomic abnormalities.

Flatfoot (pes planus) is a condition that occurs as a result of ligamental laxity.

Etiology: Most commonly due to position in utero but may result from anatomic abnormalities.

Occurrence: Fairly common.

Age: Infancy through early childhood.

Ethnicity: Higher prevalence of pes planus (flatfeet) in persons of African descent.

Gender: Occurs equally in males and females.

Contributing factors: Position of the feet in utero or congenital abnormalities.

Signs and symptoms: Most often noticed in the newborn nursery; however, the caregiver may bring the infant to the clinic with the comment that the feet "turn in" or "turn out." Older children may complain of foot pain (Fig. 10–4).

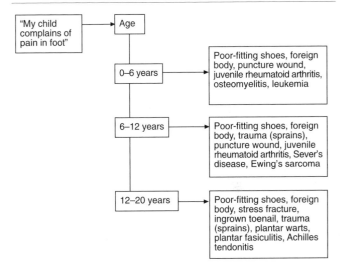

Figure 10–4. Differentiating foot pain.

Calcaneovalgus foot is dorsiflexed at the ankle; bottom of the foot appears convex. The foot may be easily manipulated into normal position.

Clubfoot is a fixed medial deviation of the forefoot, with medial inclination of the heel and downward point of the foot.

In metatarsus adductus, the heel deviates laterally, and the sole of the foot appears to be kidney shaped. The metatarsus adductus angle is measured between axis of heel and axis of third toe.

In flatfoot, the arch does not develop until age 2 to 6; pain usually does not occur before adolescence. To differentiate between flexible flatfoot and rigid flatfoot (congenital vertical talus), have the child stand on tiptoes and observe the arch. The arch reappears in cases of flexible flatfoot.

Diagnostic tests: None. Foot problems are manifested on manipulation of the foot; the inability to return the foot to normal alignment indicates problems.

Differential diagnosis:

Differentiate the calcaneovalgus foot from congenital vertical talus, which is often associated with neurologic disorders.

Deformities associated with metatarsus adductus include developmental dysplasia of the hip.

Treatment:

Metatarsus adductus: Mild, foot exercises; moderate, refer patient for casting when no older than 4 months; after 1 year, surgical intervention is indicated.

Clubfoot: Newborns should have serial casts applied as soon as possible; patients with severe cases usually require surgery.

Flatfoot: Usually a well-fitted tennis shoe.

Follow-up: Monthly until resolution.

Sequelae: Permanent damage to the feet with resulting limited ambulation. Severe cases of clubfoot left untreated can result in a foot that is smaller than the other, a foot that is less mobile, and a leg that is smaller because of muscle involvement resulting in atrophy of the muscle. If not treated, increased stiffening occurs with changes in bone development. The lateral part of the foot has an excess of soft tissue that causes the calf to be thinner.

Prevention/prophylaxis: None.

Referral: Refer patients who do not respond to foot exercises within 2 months to an orthopedist.

Education: Show the parents or caregiver the exercises for remolding the foot. Emphasize the importance of well-fitted shoes for the patient.

FRACTURES

SIGNAL SYMPTOMS ▶ bone pain with loss of function

| Fractures | ICD-9 CM: 829 |
| Stress fractures | ICD-9 CM: 733.16 |

Description: Fractures are disruptions in bone continuity. There are six types.

Simple: Fracture is straight and in good alignment.

Displaced: Ends of the broken bone are not in good alignment.

Greenstick: Fracture is incomplete.

Comminuted: Bone is broken into pieces.

Compressed: Ends of the bone are forced or pressed against each other.

Compound: Bone is broken and is piercing the skin.

Stress fractures are an overuse injury, usually in the weight-bearing bones (legs and feet).

Etiology: Occurs as a result of birth injury (clavicular), wringing of the limb, or major trauma. Stress fractures occur when the muscle transfers the additional stress to the bone, causing a crack.

Occurrence: Common.

Age: Any age group.

Ethnicity: Not significant.

Gender: Occurs equally in boys and girls. Girls have more stress fractures.

Contributing factors: Sports participation, child abuse, and accidents.
Signs and symptoms: The child presents with a history of trauma to a body part and often relates that the bone sounded like it "popped."

Findings usually reveal painful swelling with ecchymoses over the affected part. Make careful notation of pulse and sensation. Evaluate range of motion, noting presence of pain or crepitus and deformity. Observe for variations in posture (clavicular fractures have a characteristic forward drooping of the affected shoulder) and in gait (the short-stance phase [the time that the extremity bears the body weight] and refusal to walk).

Diagnostic tests: Radiographs of the affected part; in cases of suspected child abuse, review films for evidence of old injuries. If the present injury does not appear on the film, do a repeat x-ray in 10 days to determine the presence of new calcifications, proving the presence of a fracture.

A greenstick fracture, a disruption of the cortex on one side of the bone but cleavage plane of opposite side, is not displaced but angulated because bone ends are not separated. It is often missed on first radiographs. Obtain a repeat x-ray in 10 days to determine callus formation.

Stress fractures of the tibia are often missed on the first radiograph. Obtain a repeat x-ray in 10 days to determine callus formation or a bone scan.

Clavicular fractures may be angulated but not displaced.

Epiphysial fractures need to be assessed and classified according to the damage of the growth plate (Fig. 10–5). The Salter-Harris classification categorizes physeal injury by morphology. To determine a meaningful prognosis using this scale, the site of the injury must be taken into account. A type 1 injury to the distal radius causes fewer growth disturbances than the same type of fracture at the distal femoral epiphysis.

Spiral fractures of the femur, suggesting a forceful twist of the extremity, are highly suspicious of child abuse.

Differential diagnosis: None.
Treatment: Because children's bones are less brittle than adults' bones and because they have greater healing power, most fractures can be treated with closed reduction and casting or splinting. Complex fractures caused by major trauma require open reduction, however. Stress fractures are treated with rest and avoidance of the contributing activity for 6 to 8 weeks. Sometimes a cast is applied.
Follow-up:

Greenstick: Follow-up in 7 to 10 days; obtain a repeat x-ray to evaluate alignment.

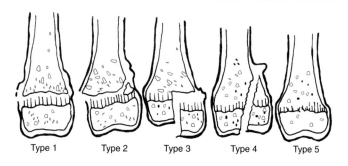

Type 1   Type 2   Type 3   Type 4   Type 5

Figure 10–5. Classification of bone plate injury The Salter-Harris classification categorizes physeal injury by morphology. To determine a meaningful prognosis using this scale, the site of the injury must be taken into account. A type 1 injury to the distal radius caused less growth disturbances than the same type of fracture at the distal femoral epiphysis. (From Salter, RB, and Harris, WH: Injuries involving the epiphyseal plate. J Bone Joint Surg 45A:587, 1963, with permission.)

Clavicular: Apply a figure-of-eight dressing that retracts shoulders and brings clavicle into normal alignment. Healing callus is apparent when consolidation is complete.

For all cases involving casts, patients should return in 48 hours to evaluate status of swelling and cast care, then every 2 weeks. Obtain a repeat x-ray in 1 month to evaluate bone healing.

Sequelae: Deformities secondary to fracture usually are the result of delayed treatment; however, this occurs less often in children than in adults. The callus formation after clavicular fractures may be noticeable for 1 year postinjury. Damage to the blood supply and innervation can lead to disruption in bone growth.

Prevention/prophylaxis: Preventive measures include prevention of child abuse through parent education in parenting skills; safety measures, including using approved car seats and car seatbelts; use of gates for doorways and stairways and guards for windows; and doing preconditioning exercises before sports participation. Have the proper athletic equipment. Eat a diet rich in calcium.

Referral: Refer patient to a primary care physician or orthopedist for definitive diagnosis and treatment.

Education: Counseling and instruction of parents in parenting skills. Instruction in safety measures.

GENU VARUM/GENU VALGUM

SIGNAL SYMPTOMS ▶   gait disturbance; feet turned inward

Genu varum	ICD-9 CM: 736.42
Genu valgum	ICD-9 CM 755.64

Description: Genu varum is a pattern of internal torsion involving the tibia, in which the leg distal to the knee is tilted toward the midline of the body. Bowing is normal until age 2 to 3 years. As growth occurs, genu varum changes to genu valgum (knock-knee), in which the extremity distal to the knee is tilted away from the midline until age 8 to 9 years, when there is a normal straightening with growth.

Etiology: A result of normal intrauterine positioning.

Occurrence: Common.

Age: Occurs at birth to age 8 to 10 years; by age 10 years, adult alignment occurs.

Ethnicity: Not significant.

Gender: Occurs equally in males and females.

Contributing factors:

Genetic factors: Genu varum is seen in achondroplasia, and genu valgum occurs in Hurler's syndrome.

Systemic disease: Anterior bowing of the lower tibia in newborn period or later infancy is seen in neurofibromatosis.

Signs and symptoms: The child is brought to the clinic with the complaint that "the legs are bowed." Findings include an internally rotated tibia about the long axis of the leg. Posterior or anterior bowing occasionally is found.

Diagnostic tests: If the condition does not show improvement in sequential observations, radiographs are indicated. In knee bowing, with the ankles touching, measure the space between the knees; a measurement of more than 5 to 6 inches indicates further evaluation.

Differential diagnosis:

Growth disturbance is evidenced by changes on x-rays.

Rickets involves all growth plates as noted on x-rays.

Treatment: Bracing may be appropriate. Surgical intervention is rarely done, and only children older than 10 years are candidates for surgery. The improvement imparted by wearing special shoes or devices is negligible.

Follow-up: The child should return to the clinic for regular well-baby visits for serial monitoring.

Sequelae: Permanent misalignment is rare.

Prevention/prophylaxis: None.

Referral: The criteria for referral to an orthopedist are persistent bowing beyond age 2, bowing that is increasing, bowing in one leg only, and knock-knee associated with short stature. Refer patient immediately to a primary care physician or orthopedist for posterior or anterior bowing because these conditions usually require surgical intervention.

Education: Teach parents about normal growth and development. Provide reassurance that this is a self-limiting condition.

GROWING PAINS

SIGNAL SYMPTOMS ▶ intermittent limb pain that interrupts normal activity

Growing Pains	ICD-9 CM: 781.99

Description: Growing pains are characterized by recurrent, intermittent limb pain, usually in the calf or thigh, behind the knee, and occasionally in the arms, lasting at least 3 months, that is nonarticular and is severe enough to interrupt normal activities. Pain varies in intensity, but it is usually in the form of a deep ache or a sense of restlessness in the limb.

Etiology: Unknown.

Occurrence: May occur in 15% to 18% of children age 3 to 12 years.

Age: Occurs in children age 3 to 5 or 8 to 12.

Ethnicity: Not significant.

Gender: More common in females.

Contributing factors: Fatigue, infection, emotional factors, and excessive muscle use.

Signs and symptoms: The child presents with a 3-month history of intermittent limb pain. Pain occurs late in the day or awakens the child at night. Pain is not specifically related to joints but interrupts normal activities, such as sleep, and is usually in the legs between the joints. The pain is intense, crampy, and usually lasts 10 to 20 minutes. There is no point tenderness, swelling of joints, or the demonstration of a limp.

Diagnostic tests:

Test	Results Indicating Disorder	CPT Code
Radiographs of tibia	Normal	73590
Erythrocyte sedimentation rate	Normal, indicates no infectious proces	85651

Differential diagnosis:

Osteoid osteoma has bone pain at night that is relieved by aspirin. The pain is characterized as boring and aching.

Patellofemoral pain syndrome occurs in adolescents, affects the knee, and is associated with exercise.

Benign hypermobility syndrome is differentiated by a complaint of leg pain after exercise.

Fibromyalgia most frequently occurs in adolescent girls and is characterized by aches and pains, multiple points of tenderness, stiffness, and chronic fatigue.

Treatment: Measures include reassurance, warm baths, and gentle massage. Ask the child to walk during an attack to show the absence of a limp.

Because the pain lasts only 10 to 20 minutes, an over-the-counter pain reliever is not necessary, as the pain would be over before the drug could take effect.

Follow-up: None.

Sequelae: None.

Prevention/prophylaxis: None.

Referral: None.

Education: Parents should take the child's temperature and check the joints and muscles for redness and swelling. Parents often make the diagnosis before bringing the child in to be examined; they come for validation and reassurance that this is a benign and self-limiting condition.

JUVENILE RHEUMATOID ARTHRITIS

SIGNAL SYMPTOMS▶   pain or stiffness in joints

| Polyarticular | ICD-9 CM: 714.30 |
| Pauciarticular | ICD-9 CM: 714.32 |

Description: Juvenile rheumatoid arthritis (JRA) is characterized by persistent joint pain lasting at least 6 weeks; it occurs in children younger than age 16. There are three types.

Polyarticular JRA (50%): Five or more joints are affected (symmetrical pattern of involvement): small joints of hands and feet; large joints; cervical spine; and temporomandibular, sternoclavicular, and distal interphalangeal joints.

Pauciarticular JRA (40%): Four or fewer joints are involved: large joints such as knees, ankles, and elbows. May be classified based on function:

Class I: Patient can perform all activities.

Class II: Patient performs activities adequately, but with some limitations.

Class III: Patient's activities are limited; can perform self-care only.

Class IV: Patient is wheelchair-bound or bedridden.

Systemic-onset JRA (10%): Number of joints is not relevant; there is remission within 1 year.

Etiology: Unknown.

Occurrence: Affects 100,000 to 250,000 children in the United States.

Age: Occurs in children age 1 to 3 years and in young teenagers.

Ethnicity: Not significant.

Gender: Gender depends on type:

- Polyarticular JRA—females outnumber males
- Pauciarticular JRA—young onset and associated with chronic insidious uveitis in females; older onset and associated with spondyloarthropathy in males
- Systemic-onset JRA—occurs equally in males and females

Contributing factors: Family history of arthritis.

Signs and symptoms: Evaluation of symptoms is done over a 6-month period. The child presents with complaints of joint pain (Fig. 10–6).

The child with systemic-onset JRA is usually younger and may present with a history of initial temperature variations greater than 103°F for 2 weeks. There is usually a small, salmon-colored, macular, pruritic rash, usually on the trunk and extremities, that waxes and wanes with the fluctuations in body temperature.

The younger child (about 2 years old) with pauciarticular JRA is usually female; there is a history of asymptomatic swelling of a joint. The older child (usually >8 years old) is usually male. Systemic signs (e.g., weight loss, anorexia, malaise, diffuse arthralgia) may be present.

The patient with polyarticular JRA presents with no fever or a low-grade fever. Five or more joints are affected (small joints of hands and feet, large joints, cervical spine, temporomandibular joint, sternoclavicular joint, and distal interphalangeal joint).

Physical findings vary according to JRA type:

Polyarticular JRA: There is a symmetrical pattern of joint involvement. Small joints of hands and feet, large joints, cervical spine, temporomandibular joint, sternoclavicular joint, and distal interphalangeal joints are involved. Radiographic changes occur within 1 year of onset. There may be hepatosplenomegaly and chronic uveitis.

Pauciarticular JRA: There is slow development of contractures, and nodules occur over tendons. Joints of the lower extremity (hips, knees, ankles) are usually involved with an asymmetrical pattern. Uveitis, when it occurs (4–81 months after onset), is acute; signs are redness and decreased visual acuity. There is decreased exercise capacity.

Systemic-onset JRA: The number of affected joints is not relevant. There is splenomegaly and lymphadenopathy.

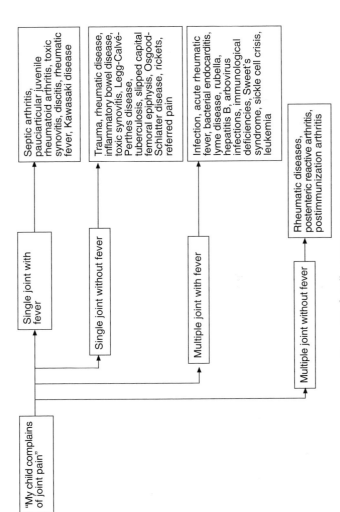

Figure 10–6. Differentiating joint pain.

Diagnostic tests:

Polyarticular JRA

Test	Results Indicating Disorder	CPT Code
Complete blood count	Mild anemia, leukocytosis	85007
Rheumatoid factor	35% seronegative, 5% seropositive	86430
ANA Pauciarticular JRA: 50% of cases in younger children	75% seropositive, 25% seronegative Positive	86038– 86309

ANA, antinuclear antibodies

Pauciarticular JRA
In older children, laboratory tests are normal. Rheumatoid factors and ANA are negative.

Systemic-Onset JRA

Test	Results Indicating Disorder	CPT Code
Complete blood count	Normocytic/normochromic anemia White blood cells elevated with a shift to left Platelet count elevated	85007 85014
Erythrocyte sedimentation rate	Extremely high	85651
Rheumatoid factors	Negative	86430
ANA	Negative	86038-86309

Other
Obtain baseline data on growth and development. Obtain midarm circumference in children in whom inadequate weight gain is observed; less than the 10th percentile is suspected of inadequate weight gain.
    Obtain triceps skinfold measurements to assess deficits in fat stores.
    Iridocyclitis may occur in 30% of cases, especially in girls.

Differential diagnosis:

    Rheumatic fever arthritis has history of streptococcal infection, no morning stiffness, and no eye disease. Rash is an erythema marginatum. ANA and rheumatoid factor are negative.

    Leukemia has no morning stiffness, no rash, and no eye disease; ANA and rheumatoid factor are negative.

    Lyme disease has no morning stiffness. Rash is an erythema chronicum migrans. There is no involvement of the small joints, no eye disease, normal white blood cell count, and increased immune complexes.

Treatment: The goals of treatment are to restore function, relieve pain, restore mobility, and provide adequate nutrition to maintain and restore growth and development.

Nonpharmacologic

Institute a range-of-motion and muscle-strengthening program. Institute occupational and physical therapy to maintain muscle strength and prevent joint contractures. May want to have child sleep in splints.

Meet nutritional needs to address problems ranging from lack of growth to obesity.

Pharmacologic

First-line treatment is with naproxen, 7.5 mg/kg twice daily.

 Clinical Pearl: Fair-skinned children who are given naproxen are at risk for developing pseudoporphyria cutanea tarda, a scarring rash of the face.

Alternative first-line drugs are ibuprofen, 30 to 40 mg/kg four times per day, or tolmetin sodium, 10 mg/kg three times a day.

Second-line treatment is with methotrexate, 5 to 10 mg/m^2 per week. If methotrexate-resistant, try etanercept (a tumor necrosis factor inhibitor) in children 4 to 17 years old, 0.4 mg/kg (to a maximum of 25 mg per dose) twice weekly, subcutaneous injection, 72 to 96 hours apart.

 Clinical Pearl: All immunizations should be current before initiating etanercept. Live vaccines should not be given concurrently. No studies have been done in pregnant women.

For uveitis, give steroid eye drops and dilating agents.

Follow-up: Complete blood count and liver function studies every 1 to 2 months to evaluate decreased hepatic function related to medication use; a routine ophthalmologic examination with slit lamp every 6 months for 4 years to evaluate ocular complications.

Sequelae: Growth retardation (systemic-onset and pauciarticular JRA), pericarditis and myocarditis (systemic-onset JRA), and residual joint damage owing to destructive symmetrical rheumatoid nodules (polyarticular JRA). Patients most likely to have problems are those with unremitting synovitis, hip involvement, or positive rheumatoid factor tests. Macrophage activation syndrome (systemic JRA) has a mortality rate of 15% to 30%.

Prevention/prophylaxis: None.

Referral: Refer patient to an orthopedist or a rheumatologist to delineate plan of care. Refer to an ophthalmologist at the time of diagnosis of JRA for evaluation. Referral to a nutritionist/dietitian may be necessary.

Education: Assist parents and child in coping with chronic illness. Talk with the child and parents about their feelingsregarding the illness. The degree to which the child has to modify activities of daily living depends on his or her functional classification. Use the patient's self-report of functional status. Assist the family in meeting the child's nutritional needs.

OSGOOD-SCHLATTER DISEASE

SIGNAL SYMPTOMS▶ localized swelling tenderness over tibial tuberosity

| Osgood-Schlatter Disease | ICD-9 CM: 732.4 |

Description: Osgood-Schlatter disease is a painful prominence (osteochondrosis) of the tibia tubercle.

Etiology: Chronic trauma to the tibia tuberosity by quadriceps overuse.

Occurrence: Common.

Age: Adolescence.

Ethnicity: Not significant.

Gender: More common in males.

Contributing factors: Participation in strenuous athletic activities, such as football, soccer, or basketball; participation in ballet or gymnastics; or the adolescent growth spurt.

Signs and symptoms: The child presents with a complaint of pain in the knee that worsens with activity and is relieved by rest. Findings include pain and swelling over the tibial tuberosity aggravated by extension of the knee.

Diagnostic tests:

Test	Results Indicating Disorder	CPT Code
Radiograph of knee	Changes in the tibial tuberosity	73560

Radiographic studies may be normal in the first 10 to 14 days of the illness.

Differential diagnosis:

In osteosarcoma, radiographic studies are positive, and gait disturbances are noted.

In patellar tendinitis, the child exhibits pain on running and climbing stairs.

Osteomyelitis usually affects a single bone; the child may experience an acute illness or a subacute illness with fever, severe pain at the affected site, erythema, and swelling.

Treatment:

Nonpharmacologic

Reduce athletic activity and avoid any activity that requires deep knee bending. Institute RICE protocol. A modified knee sleeve with a strap placed inferior to the patella may be used.

Pharmacologic
Give NSAIDs for pain: acetaminophen, 10 to 15 mg/kg per dose or 400 to 480 mg every 4 hours, or ibuprofen, 4 to 10 mg/kg per dose every 6 to 8 hours.

Follow-up: The patient should return at 2-month intervals for evaluation.

Sequelae: If disease is not treated, secondary degenerative arthritis may develop.

Prevention/prophylaxis: Physical therapy to strengthen leg.

Referral: Refer patient to an orthopedist if there is no improvement within 2 months.

Education: Educate parents as to the value of decreasing the child's level of activity. In most cases, the problem resolves spontaneously.

SCOLIOSIS

SIGNAL SYMPTOMS ▶ lateral deviation of the spine

| Congenital scoliosis | ICD-9 CM: 754.2 |
| Acquired/postural scoliosis | ICD-9 CM: 737.30 |

Description: Scoliosis is a lateral curvature of the spine classified by anatomic location (usually thoracic or lumbar); the curvature is accompanied by a secondary curvature to balance the spine. The posterior vertebral elements rotate toward the concavity of the curve, causing the attached ribs on the convex side to rotate posteriorly. Although in most cases the scoliosis stabilizes spontaneously (as shown by the lower incidence in adults), if detected and treated early, the prognosis is excellent. There are three main types.

Congenital: The spinal defects associated with this deformity occur during the first 6 weeks of gestation. The curve is usually a left thoracic curve. These cases should be evaluated for other organic illnesses, such as Klippel-Feil syndrome, Goldenhar syndrome, and Jarcho-Levin syndrome.

Neuromuscular: Most common patients are children with cerebral palsy. This condition is seen in Duchenne and Becker muscular dystrophy, in neurofibromatosis, and in neural defects.

Idiopathic: This is the most common type.

Classification is made based on the degree of the curvature:

- Mild: Less than 20%
- Moderate: 20% to 40%
- Severe: Greater than 40%

Rate of progression is approximately 1° per month.

Etiology: Scoliosis may be due to congenital vertebral anomalies, such as hemivertebra; however, the most common form is idiopathic. Some researchers consider scoliosis as a multigene-dominant condition with a variable phenotypic expression.

Occurrence: Clinically apparent scoliosis (curve of 5%) occurs in 4% of adolescents.

Age: Usually begins between ages 8 and 10 and may progress into adulthood. Rarely seen in infants but may occur in children age 2 to 4 (more common in Great Britain).

Ethnicity: Not significant.

Gender: Scoliosis is more common in females; the ratio ranges from 4 to 5:1 to 7:1.

Contributing factors: Family history is positive in 30% of cases of idiopathic scoliosis. Neuromuscular scoliosis is often associated with cerebral palsy and spina bifida. Congenital scoliosis is associated with a high incidence of renal problems. The presence of lumbar lordosis or thoracic kyphosis is of no value in predicting the prognosis. Females whose scoliosis was noted before the onset of menses are at higher risk for progression.

Signs and symptoms: Adolescents are often asymptomatic, but some may complain of low back pain. Findings reveal a noticeable curvature of the spine when anteriorly flexed from the trunk (forward-bending or Adams test). Positive Scoliometer (Kom Kare Co, Cincinnati, OH) readings of an angle 7° or greater indicates further evaluation. There may be an inequality in hip height, as noted by a difference in the levels of the iliac crests, and elevation of one shoulder with asymmetry in the prominence of the scapula.

Diagnostic Tests:

Test	Results Indicating Disorder	CPT Code
Total spinal x-ray, anteroposterior and lateral, performed with arms extended over the head	Reveal location and extent of the curvature	72069
Platelet calmodulin level	Predictor of progression and severity: 2.83 ng/mg of protein with >100 of progression; 0.06 ng/mg of protein with stable curves of <50 of progression in the previous 12 months	85999

Magnetic resonance imaging is recommended for males and children with atypical curvatures, back or leg pain, neurologic deficits, and rapidly progressive curves.

Differential diagnosis:

Postural compensation resulting from unequal leg length resolves when treated (Fig. 10–7).

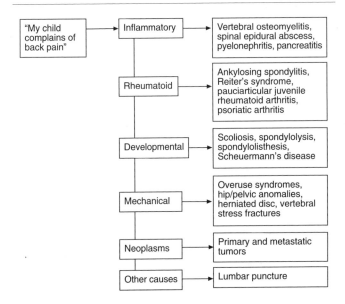

Figure 10–7. Differentiating back pain.

Scoliotic deformity may be secondary to pain in syringomyelia,
tumor, spondylolisthesis, and herniated nucleus pulposus.
Scheuermann's kyphosis is suggested with an accentuated thoracic
kyphosis noticeable on forward flexion.

Treatment: The long-range goal is to halt progression of the curvature.
Treatment options include the following: for mild scoliosis, none; for
moderate, Milwaukee brace or Boston thoracolumbosacral orthosis; and
for severe, surgical procedure for insertion of Herrington or Luque
spinal rods. Compliance with the braces seems to decrease with age:
Younger children are more compliant and teenagers are less compliant.

Follow-up: For curvatures of less than 10°, evaluate yearly; for curvatures of 10° to 20°, evaluate every 6 months until skeletal maturity to
assess progression of the curvature because progression often occurs
during the growth spurt; and for curvatures of 20° to 30°, evaluate every
4 months.

Sequelae: Severe curvatures may result in diminished lung capacity and
low back pain. Thoracic curvatures may progress into adulthood.
Lumbar curvatures may lead to subluxation of the vertebrae and to premature arthritic degeneration of the spine in adulthood.

Prevention/prophylaxis: Routine screening for all children in the
preadolescent and adolescent years. Implementation of appropriate

treatment is recommended. Many states mandate screening as a means of early detection. Parents should receive counseling about genetic transmission and the need for early and periodic screening of children at risk.

Referral: Consult for curvatures of 5% to 7%; refer for curvatures greater than 20% or in cases in which the patient is experiencing symptoms.

Education: Inform parents and school health personnel of the importance of screening and follow-up. If the child must wear a brace, advise the parents in ways to assist the child to use clothing to mask the brace. This helps the child retain his or her self-esteem and positive self-image.

SHIN SPLINTS (MEDIAL TIBIAL STRESS SYNDROME)

SIGNAL SYMPTOMS ▶ pain on anterior tibia

Shin splints	ICD-9 CM: 844.9

Description: Shin splints are microtears at the origins of the anterior and posterior tibial muscles resulting in pain and inflammation along the midshaft or distal third of the tibia.

Etiology: An overuse injury involving microtears at the origins of the anterior and posterior tibial muscles.

Occurrence: Common.

Age: Usually does not occur in children younger than age 10.

Ethnicity: Not significant.

Gender: Occurs equally in males and females.

Contributing factors: Participation in sports that involve running; inadequate preparticipation conditioning.

Signs and symptoms: The child gives a history of pain along the anterior tibia that increases with activity as well as recent involvement in a sports activity.

The anterior surface of the tibia, which is tender to palpation, may be warm to the touch. There is no numbness or tingling in the lower leg or foot, and pain is usually diffuse. Activity may reduce discomfort.

Diagnostic tests: None.

Differential diagnosis:

With tibial stress fracture, repeated activity intensifies the pain, the pain is localized, and it is on the medial border of the distal tibia.

Treatment:

Nonpharmacologic

Rest, elevation, warm compresses, and heel cups may offer relief. Initiate a program of stretching and warm-up exercises to be done before participation in running or jogging activities.

Rehabilitative exercises include the following. Use an exercise band or surgical tubing attached to a stationary object and the foot to be exercised.

Heel raises: In a standing position, raise on your toes, hold for 2 seconds, then slowly lower. Repeat 10 times, and complete two to three sets of 10.

Ankle dorsiflexion: Sitting in a chair, cross affected leg over the unaffected leg. Raise the foot toward you. Repeat 10 times, and complete two to three sets.

Ankle eversion: Sitting in a chair, pull the foot outward. Repeat 10 times, and complete two to three sets.

Ankle inversion: Sitting in a chair with the affected foot close to the stationary object, pull toward the other foot. Repeat 10 times, and complete two to three sets.

Pharmacologic

If analgesics are necessary for pain, the nurse practitioner may give acetaminophen, 10 to 15 mg/kg per dose or 400 to 480 mg every 4 hours, or ibuprofen, 4 to 10 mg/kg per dose every 6 to 8 hours.

Follow-up: Patient should return in 2 weeks to evaluate progress.

Sequelae: None.

Prevention/prophylaxis: Initiate a program of preactivity conditioning exercises (see Table 2–2).

Referral: None.

Education: Instruct children, caregivers, and coaches in the importance of preactivity conditioning. Reassure parents that this condition is self-limiting.

TENDINITIS

SIGNAL SYMPTOMS▶   pain and swelling at tendon site

Tendinitis	ICD-9 CM: 726.90
Achilles tendinitis	ICD-9 CM: 726.71
Patellar tendinitis	ICD-9 CM: 726.74
Shoulder tendinitis	ICD-9 CM: 726.11

Description: Tendinitis is characterized by swelling, pain, and tenderness over the insertion of a tendon, most often involving the Achilles tendon, the patellar inferior pole, or the shoulder.

Etiology: Repetitive mild trauma resulting in inflammation. A shallow bicipital groove allows subluxation of the bicipital tendon (knee); irritation of the avascular portion of the supraspinatus tendon progresses to an inflammatory response (shoulder).

Occurrence: Uncommon in children, but common in athletes.

Age: Usually not before age 10 years and not before participation in sports.

Ethnicity: Not significant.

Gender: Occurs equally in males and females.

Contributing factors: Participation in sports such as basketball and volleyball (knees), running sports and excessive walking (Achilles tendons), and swimming and tennis (shoulders).

Signs and symptoms: Obtain a history of the location and distribution of pain. Note whether the pain is related to movement, whether there is a limitation with movement, what aggravates the tenderness, and what relieves it. Physical findings vary by affected site.

> *Achilles tendon:* Pain occurs on flexion of the foot. There is pain on range of motion and perhaps tightened heel cords.

> *Patella tendon:* Localized tenderness is present at the inferior pole of the patella.

> *Shoulder:* Direct tenderness is present over the involved structure. The examiner elicits a painful arc sign and a Newer impingement sign.

Diagnostic tests:

Test	Results Indicating Disorder	CPT Code
Radiographs of heel (Achilles tendon)	Rule out fracture	73650
Radiographs of shoulder: anteroposterior, transthoracic lateral, and apical oblique views	Reveals shoulder instability	73020–73030, 73050

Differential diagnosis:

> *Achilles tendon:* None.

> *Patella tendon:* In Osgood-Schlatter disease, the pain is related to the tubercle of the tibia rather than the inferior pole of the patella.

> *Shoulder:* Torn rotator cuff is indicated by no improvement in 6 weeks and by radiographic appearance.

Treatment:

Nonpharmacologic

> *Achilles tendon:* Prescribe rest and elevation; in severe cases, casting may be necessary.

> *Patella tendon:* Prescribe rest, elevation, and restriction of athletic activity.

> *Shoulder:* Instruct patient to position the shoulder to avoid pain and maintain motion (keeping arms close to body, elbows in, palms up). Teach patient to externally rotate arm before reaching, to "work low," and to avoid work-related or sport-related activities. Prescribe a sling, but do not immobilize the arm. Initiate Codman (pendulum) exercises; later, have the patient "walk" up a wall with his or her fingers.

Pharmacologic
NSAIDs (usually ibuprofen or acetaminophen) decrease the inflammatory process in and around the joint capsule.

Follow-up: The patient should return in 3 weeks for evaluation of progress and again in 3 weeks.

Sequelae:

Achilles tendon: If associated with plantar fasciitis, there may be a rheumatoid variant. Episodes that last 2 to 3 days and are associated with tenosynovitis may be an early indication of familial hyperlipoproteinemia type II.

Shoulder: If there is no improvement in 6 weeks, order imaging studies to determine presence of a rotator cuff tear.

Prevention/prophylaxis: Proper conditioning before participating in sports that involve running, jumping, and extension of the arm overhead. Patients must learn to pay attention to their bodies and to stop activity before damage occurs.

Referral: If there is no improvement in 6 weeks, refer the patient to a primary care physician or an orthopedist. Refer the patient to a physical therapist for strengthening the rotator cuff and scapular rotators.

Education:

Achilles tendon: Wear proper shoes when walking. Use heel cups.

Patella tendon: During rehabilitation, the patient must comply with the plan of care.

Shoulder: During rehabilitation, the patient must not do overhead work and must restrict sports activity.

TIBIAL TORSION

SIGNAL SYMPTOMS▶ gait disturbance; persistent outward rotation of leg between ankle and knee

Tibial torsion	ICD-9 CM: 732.4

Description: Tibial torsion is the persistent (past age 16 months) rotation of the leg between the ankle and the knee. A growth disturbance of the proximal tibial growth plate is called *Blount disease*.

Etiology: Laxity of the knee ligaments, early or excessive weight bearing; may be due to excessive pressure across the medial aspect of the tibial growth plate.

Occurrence: Common.

Age: Most cases occur between ages 2 and 4 years. Can occur from birth to age 18 months and may occur in middle childhood and adolescence.

Ethnicity: Occurs more often in dark-skinned races.

Gender: Occurs equally in males and females.

Contributing factors: Precocious walking and African ancestry.

Signs and symptoms: The child presents with the complaint of "toeing in." Findings depend on age: At birth to 16 months, the angulation is 20°, but it decreases to neutral rotation by 16 months. Findings of an angulation greater than expected for age should be investigated. In severe bowing, the varus angulation is greater than 20°.

Diagnostic tests:

Test	Results Indicating Disorder	CPT Code
Radiographs of tibia	Medial tibial growth plate reveals a characteristic angular deformity at the proximal tibia	73592
magnetic resonance imaging (advantages over x-ray, no ionizing radiation)	Shape of the ossified and cartilaginous epiphysis is defined as are the meniscal and physeal abnormalities	73718–73720

Differential diagnosis: None.

Treatment: For the most part, no treatment is needed, and rarely are braces prescribed. In some more severe cases, an external rotation splint worn at night or a Brown brace may reverse the process and restore growth.

Follow-up: The patient should return at 2-month intervals for evaluation of bowing.

Sequelae: Without treatment, irreversible damage to the tibial growth plate can occur.

Prevention/prophylaxis: Children usually outgrow the condition by age 16 months.

Referral: Refer patient to an orthopedist if condition continues after age 16 months.

Education: Teach parents the parameters of normal growth and development. Reassure parents that this condition is usually self-limiting but needs regular monitoring.

REFERENCES

Ankle Sprain

Buddecke, D, et al: Is this "just" a sprained ankle? Hosp Med Dec:46, 1998.

Puffer, J: The sprained ankle. Clin Cornerstone 3:38, 2001.

Santarlasci, P: Weekend warriors: Common injuries in recreational athletes. ADVANCE Nurse Practitioners 9:42, 2000.

Thacker, SB, et al: The prevention of ankle sprains in sports: A systematic review of the literature. Am J Sports Med 27:753, 1999.

Wolfe, M, et al: Management of ankle sprains. Am Fam Physician 63:63, 2001.

Apophyseal Injuries

Espejo-Baena, A: A case of apophysistis of the proximal patella. Am J Sports Med 28, 2000.

Meister, K: Injuries to the shoulder in the throwing athlete. Am J Sports Med 28, 2000.

Schmitt, M: Part 2: Common elbow problems. Patient Care Nurse Practitioner 2:40, 1999.

Aseptic Necrosis of the Hip (Legg-Calvé-Perthes Disease)

Adkins, S, and Figler, R: Hip pain in athletes. Am Fam Physician 61:2109, 2000.

Crumrine, P: Gait disorders in children. Emerg Med July:18, 1998.

Eldridge, J, et al: The role of protein C, protein S, and resistance to activated protein C in Legg-Perthes disease. Pediatrics 107:1329, 2001.

Gunner, K, and Scott, A: Evaluation of a child with a limp. J Pediatr Health Care 15:38, 2001.

Harel, L, et al: Meyer dysplasia in the differential diagnosis of hip disease in young children. Arch Pediatr Adolesc Med 153:942, 1999.

Kocher, MS, et al: Differentiating between septic arthritis and transient synovitis of the hip in children: An evidence-based clinical prediction algorithm. J Bone Joint Surg Am 81:1662, 1999.

Leet, A, and Skaggs, D. Evaluation of the acutely limping child. Am Fam Physician 61:1011, 2001.

Roy, D: Current concepts in Legg-Calve-Perthes disease. Pediatr Ann 28:728, 1999.

Developmental Dysplasia of the Hip

American Academy of Pediatrics: Clinical practice guideline: Early detection of developmental dysplasia of the hip. Pediatrics 105:896, 2000.

French, L, and Dietz, F: Screening for developmental dysplasia of the hip. Am Fam Physician 60:177, 1999.

Harei, L, et al: Meyer dysplasia in the differential diagnosis of hip disease in young children. Arch Pediatr Adolesc Med 153:942, 1999.

Hennrikus, W: Developmental dysplasia of the hip: Diagnosis and treatment in children younger than 6 months. Pediatr Ann 28:740, 1999.

Dislocations

Maffulli, N: Sports injuries in children. Medscape Orthop Sports Med eJournal 5, 2001.

Price, D: Dislocations, shoulder. Emedicine April 20, 2001.

Spindler, K, et al: Assessment and management of the painful shoulder. Clin Cornerstone 3:26, 2001.

Floppy Infant

David, WS, and Jones, JR: Electromyography and biopsy correlation with suggested protocol for evaluation of the floppy infant. Muscle Nerves 17:424, 1994.

Mayo, M, and Tunnessen, W: A floppy infant: Making a whale of a diagnosis. Contemp Pediatr June, 1996.

Foot Problems

American Academy of Orthopaedic Surgeons: AAOS Online Service Fact Sheet. Flexible flatfoot in children. Jan 2001.

Garcia-Rodriguez, A, et al: Flexible flat feet in children: A real problem? Pediatrics 103:e84, 1999.

Fractures

American Academy of Orthopaedic Surgeons: Your Orthopaedic Connection. AAOS Fact Sheet. Stress fractures. March 2000.

Brukner, P, et al: Managing common stress fractures: Let risk level guide treatment. Physician Sportsmed 26,1998.

Gillespie, W, and Grant, I: Interventions for preventing and treating stress fractures and stress reactions of bone of the lower limbs in young adults. Cochrane Review Abstracts. Updated: 1/1/2002.

Hoch, A: Stress fractures in female athletes. MCW Health Link January 2001. Contact: http://healthlink.mcw.edu/article/979332792.html.

Growing Pains

Brown, J, et al: Understanding the nature of growing pains. Patient Care April 15, 1998.

Juvenile Rheumatoid Arthritis

American Academy of Pediatrics Section on Rheumatology and Section on Ophthalmology: Guidelines for Ophthalmologic examinations in children with juvenile rheumatoid arthritis (RE9320). Pediatrics 92:295, 1993.

Cuesta, I, et al: Subspecialty referrals for pauciarticular juvenile rheumatoid arthritis. Arch Pediatr Adolesc Med 154:122, 2000.

Gallagher, KT, and Bernstein, B: Juvenile rheumatoid arthritis. Curr Opin Rheumatol 11:372, 1999.

Gottlieb, B, and Ilowite, N: Meeting the challenge of rheumatologic diseases in teens. Contemp Pediatr 12:61, 2000.

Ilowite, N: Current treatment of juvenile rheumatoid arthritis. Pediatrics 109:109, 2002.

Jarvis, J: Juvenile rheumatoid arthritis: A guide for pediatricians. Pediatr Ann 31:437, 2002.

Lovell, D, et al: Etanercept in children with polyarticular juvenile rheumatoid arthritis. N Engl J Med 342:763, 2000.

Kodsi, S, et al: Time of onset of uveitis in children with juvenile rheumatoid arthritis. Journal American Association for Pediatric Ophthalmology and Strabismus 6:373, 2002.

Moore, TL: Immunopathogenesis of juvenile rheumatoid arthritis. Curr Opin Rheumatol 11:377, 1999.

Naidu, S, et al: Small hand joint involvement in juvenile rheumatoid arthritis. J Pediatr 136:134, 2000.

Sharma, S, and Sherry, DD: Joint distribution at presentation in children with pauciarticular arthritis. J Pediatr 134:642, 1999.

Szer, R: Juvenile rheumatoid arthritis and pediatric Sjögren's syndrome. Medscape Conference summaries from the American College of Rheumatology 2000 Annual Scientific Meeting. Medscape 2000.

Wagner-Weiner, L: Laboratory evaluation of children with rheumatic disease. Pediatr Ann 31:362, 2002.

Wright, FV, et al: Development of a self-report functional status index for juvenile rheumatoid arthritis. J Rheumatol 21:536, 1994.

Osgood-Schlatter Disease

Juhn, M: Patellofemoral pain syndrome: A review and guidelines for treatment. Am Fam Physician 60:2012, 1999.

Martin, T, and the Committee on Sports Medicine and Fitness, American Academy of Pediatrics: Technical report: Knee brace use in the young athlete. Pediatrics 108:503, 2001.

Scoliosis

Chin, K, et al: A guide to early detection of scoliosis. Contemp Pediatr 9:77, 2001.

Jeong, G, and Errico, T: Adolescent idiopathic scoliosis. Medscape Orthop Sports Med 6, 2002.

Killian, J, et al: Current concepts in adolescent idiopathic scoliosis. Pediatr Ann 28:755, 1999.

Kindsfater, K, et al: Levels of platelet calmodulin for the prediction of progression and severity of adolescent idiopathic scoliosis. J Bone Joint Surg Am 76:1186, 1994.

Mason, D: Back pain in children. Pediatr Ann 38:727, 1999.

Reamy, B, and Slakey, J. Adolescent idiopathic scoliosis: review and current concepts. Am Fam Physician 64:111, 2001.

Remes, V, et al: Scoliosis in patients with diastrophic dysplasia: A new classification. Spine 26:1689, 2001.

Shin Splints (Medial Tibial Stress Syndrome)

American Academy of Orthopaedic Surgeons: AAOS Online Fact Sheet. Shin splints. Feb 2002.

Koutures, C: An overview of over use injuries. Contemp Pediatr 11:43, 2001.

Tendinitis

Farnsworth, E: Diagnosis and management of repetitive strain injuries. ADVANCE Nurse Practitioner 9:32, 2001.

Koutures, C: An overview of over use injuries. Contemp Pediatr 11:43, 2001.

Mann, R, and Chou, L: Effective intervention for Achilles tendinitis and tendinosis. J Musculoskel Med 15:57, 1998.

Tibial Torsion

American Academy of Orthopaedic Surgeons: AAOS Online Service Fact Sheet. Intoeing. March 2001.

Tibial torsion in infants. Clin Advisor 5:84, 2002.

Chapter 11

CENTRAL AND PERIPHERAL NERVOUS SYSTEM DISORDERS

BELL'S PALSY

SIGNAL SYMPTOMS ▶ obvious drooping of one or both sides of the face to include the inability to close the eyelid completely

Bell's palsy	ICD-9 CM: 351.0
Newborn	ICD-9 CM: 767.5

Description: Bell's palsy is an acute unilateral facial nerve (cranial nerve VII) paralysis not associated with any underlying cranial neuropathy or brainstem dysfunction. This common disorder occurs in infancy. Most cases resolve in 2 weeks, but some take 6 to 8 weeks to resolve. Only about 5% of patients have long-term residual weakness.

Etiology: Bell's palsy is thought to be a postinfectious neuritis that usually develops abruptly within 2 weeks after a systemic viral infection. In about 20% of all reported cases, Epstein-Barr virus caused the preceding infection.

Occurrence: Common in childhood.

Age: Can occur at any age between infancy and adulthood.

Ethnicity: Not significant.

Gender: More frequent in females.

Contributing factors: Infection with a virus, particularly Epstein-Barr.

Signs and symptoms: The patient reports an abrupt loss of sensation on the affected side of the face. The patient is unable to close the eye or mouth, wrinkle the forehead, or puff out the cheek on the affected side. The corner of the mouth droops, and the upper and lower face are paretic. Taste on the anterior two thirds of the tongue is lost on the affected side. Occasionally ear pain is reported. The patient has an open, sometimes tearing eye, drooping of one side of the mouth, and loss of muscle tone on one side of the face. Palpation reveals lack of sensory response on the affected side of the face.

Diagnostic tests: Cranial nerve VII (facial nerve) is assessed by checking the patient's sense of taste of salt and sugar and by asking the patient to smile, grimace, puff cheeks, and raise eyebrows.

Differential diagnosis:

Facial nerve tremors are differentiated by a computed tomography (CT) scan of the head.

Brainstem infarction is differentiated by an arteriogram of the head.

Trauma of the facial nerve is differentiated by bruising, swelling, or other signs of trauma.

Treatment:

Nonpharmacologic

Treatment is symptomatic. Protection of the cornea with eye drops, such as an ocular lubricant, is especially important. Comfort measures, such as using a straw to drink and taping the eye closed at night, are also helpful.

Pharmacologic

Other treatment regimens, such as steroids and surgical decompression of the facial canal, have not proved helpful.

Follow-up: Initial follow-up should take place 2 weeks after the paralysis. Symptoms should resolve between 6 and 8 weeks. Further follow-up is unnecessary in about 85% of all cases.

Sequelae: Of all cases, 85% recover completely and spontaneously. Less than 5% of all patients are left with permanent, severe facial weakness.

Prevention/prophylaxis: None.

Referral: If facial weakness has neither improved nor resolved within 2 weeks, refer the patient to a neurologist.

Education: Instruct the patient and family that care needs to be taken to prevent eye keratoses. Teach measures for taking care of the eye, including the use of lubricants and taping at night. Reassure the patient and family that nearly all cases resolve spontaneously.

CEREBRAL PALSY

SIGNAL SYMPTOMS▶   delayed or missed developmental milestones accompanied by the persistence of primitive neurologic responses.

Cerebral palsy (CP)	ICD-9 CM: 343.9
Spastic CP	ICD-9 CM: 344.89
Athetoid CP	ICD-9 CM: 333.7

Description: CP is an acquired, nonprogressive neurologic problem manifested as a disorder of movement and position resulting from an insult or anomaly of the central nervous system (CNS). CP results in many handicaps related to motor function. Depending on the affected area, handicaps can include mental retardation (75%), seizures (33%), neurosensory disorder, hyperkinesis, speech and learning problems, and emotional problems for the child and family. There are three main types: spastic, athetoid, and ataxic.

> Spastic CP is a severe form of the disease. It has marked motor impairment, which is most often accompanied by mental retardation and a seizure disorder.
>
> Athetoid CP is a rare form of the disease that is identified by hypotonia and poor head control, feeding problems, and tongue thrust.
>
> Ataxic CP is characterized by ataxic movements, tremors, nystagmus, and abnormalities of voluntary movements.

Etiology: In many cases, the etiology of CP is known. A cerebral insult resulting in a period of anoxia may be the underlying cause. About 85% of cases result from an intrauterine or delivery problem. CP is known to result from an injury to the pyramidal or extrapyramidal tract, but the cause is not always discovered.

Occurrence: Occurs in 3 in 1000 live births per year in the United States, which reflects a rise in the incidence despite falling perinatal and neonatal mortality rates.

Age: Most frequently identified in newborns through toddlers.

Ethnicity: Not significant.

Gender: Occurs equally in males and females.

Contributing factors: A maternal trauma (e.g., head trauma, motor vehicle accident, fall), resulting in cerebral anoxia; toxemia and preeclampsia; and fetal problems (e.g., difficult or prolonged deliveries, umbilical cord knots, abnormal presentations, postmaturity, fetal distress).

Signs and symptoms: The parents relate that there were prenatal risk factors or delivery complications and that the infant had a floppy or "rag doll" musculature up to age 6 months. The child may have a history of seizures and feeding problems. Growth is less than expected, developmental milestones are delayed, and there is a persistence of primitive reflexes. Parents may relate that they had difficulty diapering because of scissoring of legs; they may report that the child has a history of head injury or meningitis. On inspection, the child is small for age with hypotonia (especially if <6 months old) or hypertonia (>6 months old). Asymmetrical movement is noted in the arms and legs. Hearing and visual problems (strabismus, nystagmus) may exist. Hydrocephaly and microcephaly are common. Poor muscle tone (<6 months old) and difficult movement (e.g., contractures, scoliosis, hip dislocations) are noted. Deep tendon reflexes are increased. Persistent primitive reflexes are easily elicited syndromes. Oromotor dysfunctions and communication and learning disorders also need to be assessed.

Diagnostic tests:

Test	Results Indicating Disorder	CPT Code
CT of head	Identify brain malformations	70471
Chromosomal studies	Identify single-gene disorders	88280–88289
Metabolic studies	Identify single-gene disorders	88289
EEG	Identify seizure disorder	95819
Denver Developmental Screening Test II	Presence of developmental delays	96100

EEG, electroencephalogram.

Differential diagnosis:

> Prematurity is differentiated by neurologic delays that are not permanent. Milestones are generally met more quickly in premature children than in CP children.
>
> Erb's palsy relates to muscle/nerve compression and affects only one arm.
>
> Spinal cord lesion produces similar symptoms, but in CP the "lesion" is on the brain, not the spinal cord.
>
> Progressive encephalopathy is differentiated by progressive deterioration of neurologic signs.
>
> Muscular dystrophy is a progressive neuromuscular disorder, whereas CP is a nonprogressive disorder.

Treatment:

Nonpharmacologic

There is no specific treatment plan for CP. A multidisciplinary team, including a primary health care provider, a social worker, a dentist, physical and occupational therapists, an ophthalmologist, a developmental psychologist, and educators, should develop an overall plan of care. Treatment is directed toward maximizing function and preventing further handicaps.

Pharmacologic

Although no specific drugs can alter the disease process when severe spasticity is found, baclofen (Lioresal), dantrolene sodium (Dantrium), and diazepam (Valium) may be useful. Surgical intervention, specifically heel cord release, may be appropriate.

Follow-up: Regularly scheduled health care visits should be maintained. Pneumonia and influenza vaccine should be given in addition to routine immunizations. When needed and appropriate, speech, physical, and occupational therapy should be available. A yearly eye and hearing examination should be offered.

Sequelae: Besides their multiple health problems related to the disease process, children with CP may have learning disorders, low self-esteem, and family problems.

Prevention/prophylaxis: Because the etiology often remains obscure, currently the best prevention is early prenatal care and regular health maintenance. Also, early, aggressive intervention for all problems associated with CP should be instituted.

Referral: Refer children with CP to speech, physical, and occupational therapists, as well as a pediatric neurologist, dentist, and ophthalmologist, when first diagnosed and as needed. A regular health care provider can serve as the gatekeeper for these services. Refer the child to a social worker, who can assist the family with obtaining services and benefits, such as Supplemental Security Income (SSI). A nutritionist should also be a part of the team.

Education: Teach parents that children who have CP have a variety of needs and that CP is a nonprogressive, lifelong condition. Assure them that although there are sometimes limitations in potential secondary to the disease, many children with CP lead successful lives. Inform parents of potential problems, such as reflux, which can cause pneumonia; the appearance of seizure symptoms; or other problems that may cause complications. Encourage the family to have a close relationship with the primary health care provider.

ENCEPHALITIS

SIGNAL SYMPTOMS▶ acute illness with accompanying headache, inconsolable crying, and fever

Encephalitis	ICD-9 CM: 323.9

Description: Encephalitis is an inflammation of the brain; diagnosis is made on the basis of neurologic manifestations and epidemiologic information without the assistance of histologic information. True identification of this pathogen can be established only by examination of the brain tissue. Generally the disease is the sequela of another viral illness. Its insidious onset often progresses rapidly to coma and sometimes death.

Etiology: Although only about 25% of all reported cases have established causative agents, it is known that enteroviruses or arboviruses, herpesviruses, and occasionally nonviral agents cause most cases. Some other known causes include mumps, measles, rubella, poxviruses, rabies, parvovirus, influenza types A and B, and adenovirus. Nonviral causes include *Rickettsia, Mycoplasma pneumoniae,* bacterial meningitis, tuberculosis, spirochetes, fungal agents, and certain protozoans.

Occurrence: Most cases occur in summer and fall.

Age: Any age.

Ethnicity: Not significant.

Gender: Occurs equally in males and females.

Signs and symptoms: The history varies from child to child. There is a broad spectrum of clinical manifestations, and the predictability of the pattern of this disease is uncertain. The parent or child may report any or all of the following in the history of this illness.

Acute onset of illness is accompanied by fever, headache, or screaming or inconsolability in infants.

Abdominal pain, nausea, and vomiting may be present. A mild nasopharyngitis is usually noted.

Increasing fever is accompanied by mental confusion, rigidity of the body, seizures, and occasionally incontinence of bladder and bowel. Unprovoked emotional outbursts are also present.

The nurse practitioner should be careful to inquire about recent contact with any persons, animals (specifically horses owing to risk for equine encephalitis), or ticks that may have transmitted the causative organism. Exposure to heavy metals, environmental substances, or pesticides should also be considered.

During inspection, the child appears ill. The skin feels warm or hot, and the abdomen is tender to touch. During the examination, the patient may have difficulty cooperating or following the requests made by the nurse practitioner. There may be occasional emotional outbursts. Some photosensitivity may be noted.

If the patient has a concomitant disease, such as mumps or chickenpox, findings are similar to those of the disease. The abdomen may have hyperactive bowel sounds when vomiting is present, and there may be some tenderness on percussion of the abdomen. If there is a preceding or concomitant upper respiratory disease, adventitious lung sounds may be heard.

Diagnostic tests:

Test	Results Indicating Disorder	CPT Code
Lumbar puncture	In viral encephalitis, the leukocyte count may vary from 0 to several thousand; percentage of polymorphonuclear cells is increased; protein levels are either not or only slightly elevated.	62270
Blood culture	Determines the presence of specific bacteria	87040
Acid-fast bacillus stain and culture on CSF	Determines the presence of specific bacteria, usually microbacteria	88312(stain) 87116 (culture)
Rapid-antigen identification tests on CSF	Presence of bacteria	86652
CT of head	Helps to rule out surgically remedial conditions	70470/70496

CSF, cerebrospinal fluid.

Differential diagnosis:

Exposure to noxious substances (e.g., heavy metals, pesticides) is differentiated by history and blood screening.

Neurologic neoplasm is differentiated by examination.

Brain tumor is differentiated by CT or magnetic resonance imaging (MRI) of the head.

Seizure disorder is differentiated by EEG.

Treatment: If encephalitis is suspected, a physician should dictate and institute all treatment regimens. The child should be admitted to a tertiary care setting with an intensive care unit and available neurologic physicians to oversee care.

Follow-up: Closely supervise the child for months after infection because the sequelae often require supportive services and rehabilitation.

Sequelae: CNS problems, including intellectual, motor, psychiatric, visual, and auditory impairment, may result. There may also be cardiovascular, hepatic, and pulmonary problems. The young infant who contracts encephalitis has a grave prognosis. The child with herpes simplex viral encephalitis has the worst prognosis.

Referral: Refer child immediately to a physician for admittance to a hospital.

Prevention/prophylaxis: Encephalitis secondary to measles, mumps, and rubella has been well controlled since the advent of immunizations for those diseases. For cases of encephalitis caused by arboviruses, there has been less success because of the lack of a vaccine. Control of insect vectors via spraying and the use of pesticides helps control the problem, but eradication has not yet been achieved.

Education: Teach the parents the importance of children receiving immunizations on time.

HEADACHE

SIGNAL SYMPTOMS▶ insidious or sudden onset of pain in the head described as throbbing, pressure, or pain.

Headache	ICD-9 CM: 784.0
Migraine headache	ICD-9 CM: 346.9
Tension headache	ICD-9 CM: 307.81
Cluster headache	ICD-9 CM: 346.2

Description: Headache, a common presenting symptom in the older pediatric group and in febrile children, is a pain in one or more regions of the head. Because a headache may represent a severe underlying pathology, all headaches should be carefully assessed. Children are poor historians and often respond unpredictably to a headache. The nurse practitioner should obtain a history including family history and symptoms, perform a careful examination, and refer when a severe underlying pathology is suspected. Types of headaches include the following:

- Vascular (classic) migraine headache
- Muscular contraction (tension or psychogenic) headache
- Cluster headache

The migraine headache is usually unilateral, but does not always occur on the same side. It is generally preceded by an aura (subjective sensations preceding a migraine), which may be followed by neurologic signs such as tingling and weakness in an extremity. Temporary paralysis may follow a migraine headache. Throbbing gradually increases in intensity to a peak in 1 hour, then the headache pain may gradually diminish in a few hours to several days. Of migraine patients, 80% have a family history of migraines.

Tension headaches are characterized by a dull, aching pain accompanied by occipital pain and tightness across the scalp. Tension headaches are more commonly seen in middle school–age children. These headaches can persist for a long time, with pain often described as a vice-like grip on the head. Tension headaches do not have any associated nausea or vomiting but may often be associated with a period of high tension or emotional distress. There is no aura or neurologic deficit, although patients often state that their scalp is sore during and after a tension headache. The muscles in the posterior neck may be tense and sore.

Cluster headaches are characterized by intense pain associated with rhinorrhea, lacrimation, and flushed skin. These headaches occur at night, are generally localized to one orbit, and last approximately 1 hour. The pain tends to occur in clusters over a period of a few nights to weeks, then usually disappears.

Etiology: The specific etiology of vascular (classic) migraines, muscle contraction (tension or psychogenic) headaches, and cluster headache is unknown.

Occurrence: Headaches occur in 5% to 20% of the pediatric population; prevalence increases proportionally with age.

Age: Headaches have been documented in the literature in 1-year-olds, but they are more common in adolescents.

Gender: During adolescence, headaches occur more in females. In males, onset is generally before age 10.

Ethnicity: Not significant.

Contributing factors: Familial history, environmental irritants, hormonal changes, food allergies, type A personalities, stress, and bright lights may contribute to the occurrence of the three classes of headaches.

Signs and symptoms: A detailed family history, review of symptoms, and a detailed account of the headache needs to be obtained from the patient. The presence or absence of a migraine aura and the frequency, intensity, duration, and location of the pain should be obtained. Age of onset and subsequent course of the headaches should be documented. Treatments that are used to decrease discomfort should be documented. Possible environmental stimulants should be identified (Figs. 11–1 and 11–2).

Inspection may reveal photophobia or phonophobia; if the headache is a migraine, there may be accompanying vomiting or nausea. With a cluster headache, rhinorrhea may be observed. The optic fundus should be observed when the source or type of headache is unknown to rule out eye changes associated with elevated blood pressure, hemorrhage, or glaucoma.

Percussion and palpation of the head does not reveal any significant findings. With a tension headache, there may be some increased sensitivity in the head. There may also be a rise in blood pressure or pulse in response to the pain. Auscultation may reveal cranial bruits.

Diagnostic tests: The diagnosis of a headache, which is a symptom rather than a disease, is often made by history alone because there are no tests or findings that can document a headache. To rule out organic pathology, however, a CT scan of the head, an EEG, and a myelogram are often performed.

Clinical Pearl: A person complaining of "the worst headache of their lives" should be immediately evaluated and become a prime suspect for having a subarachnoid hemmorhage.

Differential diagnosis:

Sinus headache is differentiated by the location of the pain, which is generally over the antrum or around the eyes and most frequently associated with sinus congestion. There is also an accompanying diagnosis of bacterial sinusitis. The sinuses may be tender, and the overlying skin may be sensitive. The headaches often begin at night and intensify with changes in position.

Hypertension headache is differentiated by an accompanying diagnosis of hypertension and the fact that the headaches are generally seen first thing in the morning and are mild to moderate in intensity.

Glaucoma can cause headaches; the pain is located around the orbits and may be associated with nausea and vomiting. The pupils are fixed and semidilated, and the sclerae are injected.

Brain tumor–associated headache does not have a specific characteristic but tends to be a more severe, more deep-seated pain that may come and go and tends to worsen at night. It may awaken the patient. Occasionally, headache may occur in the very early morning hours, also awakening the patient. Usually vomiting accompanies the headache.

Congenital malformations of the head and cervical vertebrae are differentiated by CT scans.

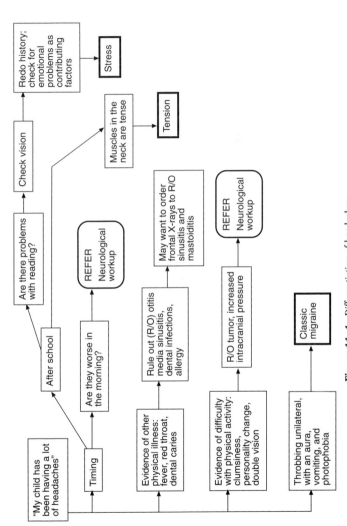

Figure 11–1. Differentiation of headaches.

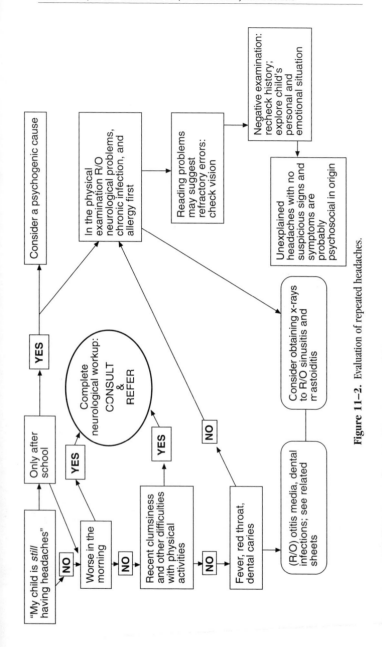

Figure 11–2. Evaluation of repeated headaches.

Table 11-1   Analgesic Drugs for Migraine and Tension Headaches

Drug	Dosage
Acetaminophen	10–15 mg/kg, not to exceed 90
Ibuprofen	5–10 mg/kg per dose (200–800 mg/dose q6–8h; maximum 40 mg/kg per day)
Naprosyn	10 mg/kg per day (250–500 mg bid)
Naproxen (Anaprox)	220–550 mg first dose; maximum dose 825 mg per day
Naproxen (Aleve)	220 mg bid
Butorphanol (Stadol)*	1 spray in one nostril only
Zolmitriptan (Zomig)*	2.5 mg or lower initially; may repeat in 2 hours with maximum of 10 mg per day
Rizatriptan (Maxalt)*	5–10 mg; may repeat in 2 hours if needed, not to exceed 10 mg per day
Naratriptan (Amerge)*	1–2.5 mg; may repeat in 4 hours, not to exceed 5 mg per day

* Not recommended for children <18 years old.

Lead encephalopathy is differentiated by a lead level greater than 50. Dental abscesses are differentiated by signs and symptoms of infection and pain, including fever, swelling, and an elevated white blood cell (WBC) count.

Severe anemia is differentiated by a hemoglobin of less than 7.

Treatment: Specific causes, if known, and identification of exacerbating agents dictate the treatment regimen. Cautious use of medication is mandated in the pediatric population.

Management of an acute headache includes analgesics and antiemetics. Acetaminophen, 5 to 10 mg/kg every 4 to 6 hours, is used if the headache is mild, infrequent, and of short duration. A variety of medications can be given for analgesic and abortive therapy (Tables 11–1, 11–2, and 11–3).

Table 11-2   Abortive Pharmacologic Prophylaxis for Migraine Headaches

Drug	Dosage
Ergotamine tartrate *or*	SL 2 mg
Cafergot	1 mg ergotamine with 100 mg caffeine
Dihydroergotamine (DHE)	0.5–1 mg IM; can be repeated in 1 hour
Metoclopramide (Reglan)	Up to 1 mg/kg
Prochlorperazine (Compazine)	2.5–5 mg*
Promethazine	0.25–1 mg/kg q 4 hours
Sumatriptan	6 mg SC or 100 mg PO

* For young children up to 0.1 mg/kg.
IM, intramuscularly; PO, by mouth; SC, subcutaneously.

Table 11–3   Pharmacologic Prophylaxis for Migraine Headaches

Drug	Dosage	Contraindications
Propranolol	1–2 mg/kg per day bid or tid	Asthma, cardiac arrhythmia, depression, diabetes
Methysergide	Adolescents: 2 mg bid or tid after meals (not to be used for >3 months)	*Not* recommended for children. Use is restricted to *severe* headaches
Amitriptyline	Adolescents: 0.1 mg/kg at bed time (HS) (may be increased every 2 weeks) Children: 0.5–2 mg/kg	*Not* approved for children <12
Cyproheptadine	Children: 0.2–0.4 mg/kg per day in two to three divided doses Adolescents: 4–10 mg/day	None
Nortriptyline	10 mg/day HS	None

Follow-up: Follow-up is generally done about 2 weeks after initiation of treatment regimen; however, the patient should be instructed to come to the office or the emergency department immediately if there is severe pain, paresthesia, or other symptoms. Thereafter, follow-up is done on a semiregular basis (e.g., every 3–6 months) or as symptoms dictate.

Sequelae: Recurrent migraine headaches often result in poor school performance, days missed from school or work, behavioral problems, and depression. Poor self-esteem, difficult peer relationships, and high stress levels may occur.

Prevention/prophylaxis: Avoidance of known irritants or stimuli is the most effective nonpharmacologic prophylaxis. Table 11–3 outlines the drugs used for pharmacologic prophylaxis.

Referral: If the diagnosis is uncertain or the headaches are not controlled with treatment regimens, refer the child to a pediatric neurologist or headache clinic.

Education: Educate children and parents regarding stimuli that are suspected to trigger headaches. Also, teach them to recognize the worsening of signs and symptoms. Children can often be taught relaxation techniques to decrease the severity of the headache symptoms. Stress the use and proper timing of headache medications. Teach children and parents to pay careful attention to the signs and symptoms of depression.

MENINGITIS

SIGNAL SYMPTOMS▶   fever, inconsolable crying, irritability, and lethargy

Meningitis	ICD-9 CM: 322.9

Description: Meningitis is a CNS infection characterized by an inflammation of the brain, specifically the meninges. Early diagnosis and treatment of bacterial meningitis are crucial because all cases of untreated meningitis result in death. Delayed treatment results in serious, permanent neurologic sequelae.

Etiology: *Haemophilus influenzae* type B (HIB), *Neisseria meningitidis, Streptococcus pneumoniae,* β-streptococcus, *Escherichia coli,* and *Listeria monocytogenes* are the most common bacterial causes of meningitis before age 1 month. Aseptic meningitis is caused by an enterovirus. Other rarer forms of meningitis are the sequelae of diseases such as Lyme disease and herpes.

Occurrence: Aseptic meningitis occurs in 1.5 to 4 in 100,000 children per year in the United States, with younger children having the greater incidence. Bacterial meningitis in the neonatal period occurs in 100 in 100,000 live births. The incidence decreases to 45 in 100,000 infants at age 2 months, again peaking to 75 to 80 in 100,000 at age 8 months.

Age: Occurs at any age between the neonatal period and adulthood, with a greater incidence in neonates.

Ethnicity: Not significant.

Gender: Occurs equally in males and females.

Contributing factors: Head trauma involving a fracture of the paranasal sinus or congenital sinus increases the risk of meningitis. These fractures enable bacteria to enter the meninges more easily. Meningitis can occur postoperatively (especially after neurosurgical procedures) if a shunt has been implanted.

Signs and symptoms: The parent may report a recent bout of fever, irritability, lethargy, and poor feeding. Restlessness is reported in all children. If old enough, the child complains of a headache. Sometimes, if the auditory nerve is involved, hearing alterations may be noted. Older children have a recent history of vomiting, along with a variety of other symptoms (e.g., fever, nausea, listlessness, irritability, photophobia, nuchal rigidity, seizures). In infants, the parent reports that the "soft spot" seems enlarged and protruding (bulging fontanel).

 Clinical Pearl: Positive Kernig and Brudzinski signs can also be elicited. Kernig's sign is elicited by flexing the hip, then extending the leg at the knee. If this movement produces pain in the hamstring, the sign is considered positive. Brudzinski's sign is elicited by laying the patient down and flexing the neck. If there is an involuntary flexing of the hip, the sign is positive.

A raised red rash (a potential sign of septic shock) may be seen and palpated. Children may report pain (arthralgia or myalgia) when muscles and joints are palpated. Tachycardia and tachypnea are evident.

Diagnostic tests:

Test	Results Indicating Disorder	CPT Code
Complete blood count	Elevated WBC count >20,000/μL	85031
Blood culture	Presence of specific bacteria	87040
Urine culture	Presence of specific bacteria	87086–87088
EEG	Increased intracranial pressure	95819
Lumbar puncture	Turbid or purulent fluid with elevated WBC count	62270
Counterimmunelectrop horeses of blood, urine, and CSF	Positive for *H. influenzae, S. pneumoniae, N. meningitidis,* or group B streptococci	86185
Latex particle agglutination of blood, urine, and CSF	Positive for *H. influenzae, S. pneumoniae, N. meningiditis,* or group B streptococci	86403–86406
CT of head	Increased intracranial pressure	70470/70496

Differential diagnosis:

Influenza, bacteremia, Kawasaki disease, Rocky Mountain spotted fever, brain tumor, cat-scratch fever, and toxic ingestion (all of which may mimic the signs and symptoms of meningitis) are differentiated by a lumbar puncture.

Brain tumor is differentiated by CT scan of the head along with an MRI.

Treatment: Meningitis is a medical emergency; all treatment should be initiated in a tertiary care setting. As soon as all cultures are obtained, intravenous access should be established and antibiotics initiated.

Antibiotics include the following:

- Ampicillin: Younger than 7 days, 50 mg/kg every 12 hours; older than 7 days, 50 mg/kg every 6 hours
- Aminocaproic acid (Amicar): Younger than 7 days, 10 mg/kg every 12 hours; older than 7 days, 10 mg/kg every 8 hours
- Gentamicin: Younger than 7 days, 2.5 mg/kg every 12 hours; older than 7 days, 2.5 mg/kg every 8 hours
- Cefotaxime: Younger than 7 days, 50 mg/kg every 12 hours; older than 7 days, 50 mg/kg every 8 hours
- Ceftriaxone: 50 to 100 mg/kg every 24 hours in divided doses
- Vancomycin: 40 mg/kg per 24 hours every 6 hours given over at least 1 hour

Children's acetaminophen (Tylenol) or ibuprofen (Advil) can be used for fever and headache (see Tables 3–5 and 3–6). Appropriate anticonvulsants should be given for seizures (see seizures section in this chapter). Phenobarbital is used for seizures. Dexamethasone is also used for bacterial meningitis, specifically *H. influenzae* or pneumococcal meningitis.

Follow-up: Careful audiologic evaluation (yearly) and regularly scheduled checkups should be done to evaluate attainment of developmental milestones. If there are problems with intelligence, development, or seizures, the patient needs to be monitored regularly.

Sequelae: Meningitis can cause serious, irreversible neurologic problems, such as seizures; brain damage (irreversible); and intellectual, motor, visual, and auditory impairment. The severity of these sequelae vary from patient to patient. Damage to the cardiac system and death are other possible sequelae.

Prevention/prophylaxis: Increased use of the HIB series of immunizations for infections has dramatically decreased the incidence of bacterial meningitis in children.

Referral: Refer patient to a physician as soon as meningitis is suspected. Arrange for immediate admission to a tertiary care setting.

Education: Inform parents that although the sequelae vary, many children survive meningitis with few, if any, subsequent problems. Some children do have long-term problems, however, so continued regular health care visits and maintenance of a normal immunization schedule are important parts of their health care. When motor and cognitive impairment has occurred, parents need to stay in close contact with physical therapists, occupational therapists, developmentalists, teachers, and other support personnel as needed.

REYE'S SYNDROME

SIGNAL SYMPTOMS▶   during recovery from another illness, child becomes acutely ill with vomiting and irritability

Reye's syndrome	ICD-9 CM: 331.81

Description: Reye's syndrome is an acute noninflammatory encephalopathy that includes one of the following criteria:

- Fatty changes of the liver confirmed by either biopsy or, in the case of death, autopsy
- Aspartate transaminase (AST), alanine transaminase (ALT), or serum ammonia values three times normal
- Greater than 8 WBCs/mm^3 in the CSF
- No other reasonable explanation for neurologic or hepatic changes

Etiology: Reye's syndrome is associated with *H. influenzae* type A and B infection and is a sequela of chickenpox. Generally, however, the etiology is unknown. Ingestion of aspirin or aspirin-containing drugs may elicit or exacerbate the syndrome.

Occurrence: Incidence is 0.15 in 100,000 children per year in the United States; 16% to 28% of cases are preceded by chickenpox.

Age: Peak incidence is at age 6 years; most cases occur in children between ages 4 and 14.

Ethnicity: Of all cases, 90% occur in whites, 4% in African-Americans, and 6% in other ethnic groups.

Gender: Occurs equally in males and females.

Contributing factors: A history of a recent case of chickenpox or other viral illness.

Signs and symptoms: The parent reports that the child was recovering from an upper respiratory illness, chickenpox, or gastroenteritis when he or she suddenly became acutely ill. The child presents with a history of nausea and vomiting and altered behavior (e.g., irritable, combative, confused, less responsive, lethargic). The child has no focal neurologic signs. Hyperpnea, irregular respirations, and dilated and sluggish pupils are seen. Palpation and percussion reveal mild hepatomegaly. Auscultation reveals increased bowel sounds and hyperventilation. Seizures may be present. In the late stages, stupor, loss of deep tendon reflexes, decerebrate posturing, and possibly coma may occur.

In infants, the signs and symptoms are slightly different: The infant typically presents with an acute onset of respiratory disease (with tachypnea and apnea), followed by seizures and coma.

Diagnostic tests:

Test	Results Indicating Disorder	CPT Code
Serum transaminase	Increased	84460
Serum ammonia level	Increased	82140
Prothrombin time	Increased	85210
Creatinine	Increased	82540
Amino acid levels	Increased	82136
Blood glucose	Decreased	82947
EEG	Slow wave abnormalities	95819

Differential diagnosis:

Meningitis is differentiated by a lumbar puncture showing a WBC count greater than $8/mm^3$ in the CSF; Reye's syndrome does not have this finding.

Septicemia is differentiated by a blood culture.

Salicylate poisoning is differentiated by a salicylate level greater than 25.

Acute hepatitis is differentiated by a hepatitis screen.

Treatment: Immediate referral for admission to a tertiary care setting is crucial. The illness should be staged (Table 11–4). In stages I and II, supportive, symptomatic care is given. Intravenous fluids (10% dextrose

Table 11-4   Staging of Reye's Syndrome

Stage	Symptoms and Signs
I	Subtle central nervous system changes are present, including confusion, lethargy, and apathy. No abnormalities are noted in posture, pain response, or pupillary reaction
II	Delusion, irritability, restlessness, combativeness, and disorientation are all noted. There is normal posture, but pupillary reaction is sluggish
III	Decerebrate posture is seen. There is deep coma and sluggish pupils
IV	Coma, decerebrate posture, sluggish pupils, and inconsistent or absent doll's head phenomenon
V	Coma, flaccidity, nonreactive pupils, and absent doll's head phenomenon

solution) are instituted to decrease lipolysis. Children at later stages are managed in the intensive care unit; treatment may include the administration of mannitol to reduce cerebral edema, vitamin K to alter clotting abnormalities, neomycin sulfate enemas to decrease serum ammonia levels, and plasma in cases of disseminated intravascular coagulation.

Arterial blood gases, glucose, blood urea nitrogen, and hematocrit should be closely monitored to identify problems as they occur. Other treatments may also be given, but they are beyond the scope of the nurse practitioner.

Follow-up: Nonspecific. In children older than age 2 who have had Reye's syndrome, psychological testing should be done because they frequently have resultant learning problems. Otherwise, no other follow-up is necessary.

Sequelae: The mortality rate is approximately 30%; 10% of survivors have severe CNS problems.

Prevention/prophylaxis: Early identification and aggressive treatment often result in a better prognosis. Avoidance of aspirin and aspirin-containing products during the course of a viral illness has greatly reduced the incidence of Reye's syndrome.

Referral: Refer patient to a physician, preferably a pediatric neurologist, as soon as the diagnosis is suspected.

Education: Teach parents not to use aspirin or aspirin-containing products when treating fever or pain in children. Fever-reducing agents such as acetaminophen or ibuprofen should be substituted. Encourage parents not to be overprotective after the illness, but to be alert for subtle and overt signs of brain damage, such as learning, communication, school, or behavioral changes and difficulties.

SEIZURE DISORDER

SIGNAL SYMPTOMS ▶ episode of loss of consciousness or a period observed in which the child appears to be daydreaming and unable to respond; the episode may be accompanied by abnormal motor movements and incontinence

Seizure disorder	
Partial seizure disorder	ICD-9 CM: 345.5
Absence seizure disorder	ICD-9 CM: 345.0
Tonic-clonic seizure disorder	ICD-9 CM: 345.1

Description: A seizure is a misfiring of the neurons resulting in an involuntary paroxysmal disturbance of the brain. This misfiring results in an altered or total loss of consciousness accompanied by abnormal motor behavior and sensory or autonomic dysfunction. Epilepsy can be defined as a condition in which the patient has recurrent seizures not related to any other organic or traumatic causes. Table 11–5 lists three different types of seizures along with more specific information. Seizures are classified as partial or generalized.

Partial seizures include simple partial, motor, sensory, autonomic, psychic, complex partial, or partial seizures with secondary generalization.

Generalized seizures include absence, generalized tonic-clonic, tonic, clonic, myotonic, and atonic seizures, as well as infantile spasms.

Table 11–5   Classification of Seizures

Seizure Type	Age	Associated Symptoms
Partial seizure	All ages	Consciousness is not impaired. Seizure begins locally and can affect any part of the body. Causes include trauma, infection, and tumor. Patient exhibits asynchronous clonic or tonic movements and may have an aura. Seizure lasts 10–20 seconds (simple) or 1 2 minutes (complex partial). EEG is characterized by spikes or sharp waves. Movements tend to involve the face, neck, and extremities (simple); may be accompanying autonomic behaviors (complex)
Generalized seizures (absence)	Ages 4–8 most common	Lasts 5–30 seconds. Patient may have lapses of consciousness. There is no aura or falling, but patient may have hyperventilation preceding the seizure. More common in girls
Infantile spasms	Infancy	Head drops suddenly or there is flexing of the body during the spasm. EEG is abnormal; condition is difficult to treat
Clonic, tonic, tonic-clonic	Any age	Most common seizure types. Grand mal seizures begin with aura and loss of consciousness; 15% of patients are incontinent during the seizure. Characterized by rhythmic clonic contractions alternating with relaxation of all muscle groups. Child may bite tongue during the seizure. Followed by a postictal period lasting 30 minutes to 2 hours, often accompanied by vomiting and severe frontal headache

Etiology: The specific etiology of seizures is unclear; however, anatomic lesions, developmental and genetic factors, pharmacologic agents, and cellular malfunction may be causative factors. Immaturity of the brain is often an underlying cause. Other potential causes are trauma, infections, and biochemical or metabolic alterations.

Occurrence: Of all children, 2% have experienced a type of seizure.

Age: Of all seizures, 75% occur before age 18 years.

Ethnicity: Not significant.

Gender: Seizures occur more frequently in males than females.

Contributing factors: Head trauma, meningitis, and a family history of seizures.

Signs and symptoms: The patient's age, the type and frequency of the seizure, the presence or absence of specific neurologic symptoms, and any events preceding the seizure should be ascertained in the history. Parents should be questioned regarding any underlying disease, such as diabetes, renal disease, or cardiovascular disorder. The parents should be asked whether the child has had any CNS infections or trauma or whether they suspect drug use; the family history must be obtained.

Seizures may be observed along with either of two possible neuro-muscular responses: lip smacking or eye blinking. Focal abnormalities and weakness may also be present. The health care provider should observe for neurocutaneous diseases when the patient presents with café-au-lait spots, facial hemangioma (Sturge-Weber syndrome), ash leaf spots, or adenoma sebaceum (tuberous sclerosis).

Blood pressure may be elevated in cases of concomitant renal disease, and subtle cardiac signs may be found when there is an accompanying cardiovascular disorder (Fig. 11–3).

Diagnostic tests:

Test	Results Indicating Disorder	CPT Code
EEG	Spiked waves or otherwise abnormal results indicative of seizure disorder	95819
CT of head	Tumor or other abnormality may reveal other causes than epilepsy for the seizure	70470
Fasting blood glucose	Discloses that diabetes may have precipitated the seizure	82947

Differential diagnosis:

Behaviors such as daydreaming, breath-holding spells, temper tantrums, and inattentiveness are differentiated by the absence of any neurologic findings.

Syncope is differentiated by changes in blood pressure not associated with seizures and by a normal EEG or CT scan.

Sleep disturbances and apnea are differentiated by sleep studies and a pneumogram, which are negative in seizure disorders.

Migraine headaches are differentiated by the patient's history and by a normal CT scan or EEG.

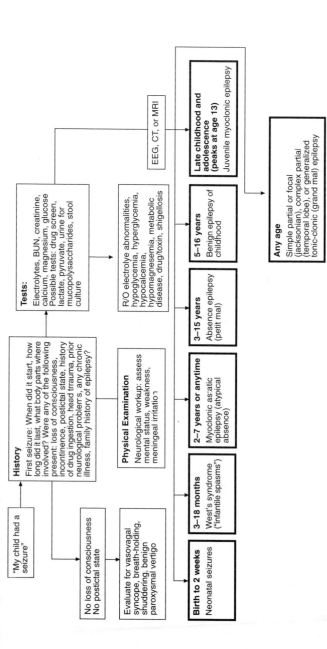

Figure 11–3. Evaluation of nonfebrile seizures (first seizure). (BUN, blood urea nitrogen; CT, computed tomography; EEG, electroencephalogram; MRI, magnetic resonance imaging.)

Intoxication is differentiated by positive blood or urine drug and alcohol screening.

In tics, the movements can be suppressed, whereas in seizures they cannot.

Treatment:

Nonpharmacologic

A ketogenic diet may be used in severe cases of seizures, particularly complex myoclonic epilepsy. This diet restricts carbohydrates and protein and is high in fat. Although the exact mechanism of the diet regimen is unknown, it is suspected that it may inhibit neurotransmission in the brain, decreasing or in some reported cases eliminating seizures.

Pharmacologic

Table 11–6 lists the most common agents used for treatment, the type of seizure for which the agent is used, and the dose. Other treatment regimens include corticotropin (adrenocorticotropic hormone) as the preferred agent for infantile spasms, but this regimen is out of the nurse practitioner's scope of practice. Oral prednisone may be used in place of intramuscular corticotropin.

Follow-up: Children with seizure disorders should be followed closely when first put on medication. Symptoms and blood levels of the medications should be evaluated at least monthly; when the medication level is

Table 11–6   Anticonvulsants of Choice: Maintenance Drugs

Drug	Absence Seizure	Tonic-Clonic Seizure	Simple-Partial Seizure	Complex-Partial Seizure
Phenobarbital: 3–5 mg/kg per day		*	*	*
Phenytoin: 5–10 mg/kg per day		†	†	†
Carbamazepine: 15–30 mg/kg per day: maximum 35 mg/kg per day		†	†	†
Ethosuximide: 20–30 mg/kg per day	†			
Valproic acid: 15–60 mg/kg per day	†	†	*	*
Primidone: 10–25 mg/kg per day		†		*
(Gabapentin) (Neurontin): Children <3 years, 10–15 mg/kg per day			*	*
Topiramate (Topamax): Children >2 years, 1–3 mg/kg per day with a maximum of 25 mg		*	*	

* Second-line adjunct.
† First-line medication.

therapeutic and there are no further seizures, the child can be followed on a regular schedule, with the parents calling or bringing the child in if they suspect that the medication is no longer therapeutic. As a child's body weight increases, medication doses must be increased. Routine examinations should also be performed and immunizations administered. There is, however, a slight disagreement among neurologists with regard to the diphtheria, pertussis, and tetanus (DPT) immunization: Some believe that pertussis should not be included for seizure patients, whereas others believe that its inclusion is still appropriate.

Sequelae: Epilepsy, when poorly controlled, can alter a child's growth and development potential. If well controlled, children have few problems overall. If a grand mal seizure lasts longer than 30 minutes, the patient is at increased risk for brain damage. Overall the mortality rate of seizures is 10% in the United States.

Prevention/prophylaxis: Avoidance of environmental triggers, such as pharmacologic or photic stimuli (e.g., flashing lights, such as those found in discotheques), can prevent the occurrence of seizures. Obtaining adequate rest and guarding against emotional stress may deter the occurrence of a seizure.

Referral: The diagnosis of the specific type of seizure should be determined by a pediatric neurologist. If there is specific cause to suspect a seizure disorder, or results of an EEG or CT scan are abnormal, obtain a neurologic consultation.

Education: Teach families the importance of taking seizure medications on a regular schedule and maintaining a close relationship with a primary care provider. Teach the parents safety precautions in the event of a seizure. Emphasize the importance of precautionary measures, such as avoiding certain stimuli, getting adequate rest, and developing strategies to cope with stress.

REFERENCES

Bell's Palsy

Hickey, J: Bell's palsy: Does anything help? Can Fam Physician 46:1293, 2000.

Murahani, S, et al: Bell's palsy and herpes simplex virus. Ann Intern Med 27:124, 1996.

Salaman, M, and MacGregor, D: Should children with Bell's palsy be treated with corticosteroids? A systematic review. J Child Neurol 16:565, 2001.

Cerebral Palsy

American Academy of Pediatrics, Committee on Children with Disabilities: Screening infants and young children for developmental disabilities. Pediatrics 93:863, 1994.

Damano, D, et al: Should we be testing and training muscle strength in cerebral palsy? Dev Med Child Neurol 44:68, 2002.

Lau, C, and Lao, T: Cerebral palsy and the birth process. Hong Kong Med J 5:251, 1999.

Morton, S, et al: Early feeding problems in children with cerebral palsy: Weight and neurolodevelopmental outcomes. Dev Med Child Neurol 44:40, 2001.

Encephalitis

Johnson, R: The pathogenesis of acute viral encephalitis and post infectious encephalomyelitis. J Infect Dis 180:1738, 1999.

McJunkin, J, et al: Encephalitis in children. N Engl J Med 344:801, 2001.

Headache

Lewis, D, et al: Practice parameter: Evaluation of children and adolescents with recurrent headaches. Neurology 59:490, 2002.

Linder, S, and Winner, P: Pediatric headache. Med Clin North Am 85:1037, 2001.

Lipton, R, et al: Medical consultation for migraine: Results from the American migraine study. Headache 38:87, 1998.

Matcher, D, et al: Toward evidence-based management of migraines. JAMA 284:22, 2001

Maytal, H, et al: The value of brain imaging in children with headaches. Pediatrics 96:413, 1995.

McGrath, P: Chronic daily headache in children and adolescents. Curr Pain Headache Rep 33:230, 2001.

O'Hara, J, and Koch, T: Heading off headaches. Contemp Pediatr 15:97, 1998.

Prensky, A: Childhood migraine headache syndromes. Curr Treatment Options Neurol 3:257, 2001.

Schwartz, B, et al: Epidemiology of tension type headaches. JAMA 279:381, 1998.

Silberstien, S, and Rosenberg, J: Multispecialty consensus on diagnosis and treatment of headache. Neurology 54:1553, 2000.

Waldie, K, and Poulton, R: Physical and psychological correlates of primary headache in young adulthood: A 26 year longitudinal study. J Neurol Neurosurg Psychiatry 72:86, 2002.

Whitley, R: Diagnosis, management, and prevention of viral encephalitis: Herpes simplex, West Nile, and other encephalitis indigenous to the United States. Presented at the New and Emerging Infectious Diseases meetings, Atlanta, June 7–9, 2002.

Meningitis

American Academy of Pediatrics: Recommended childhood and adolescent immunization schedule—United States, 2003. Pediatrics 111:212, 2003.

American Academy of Pediatrics, Committee on Infectious Disease: Meningococcal disease prevention and control strategies for practice based physicians. Pediatrics 106:1500, 2000.

Bedford, H, et al: Meningitis in infancy in England and Wales: Follow up at age 5 years. BMJ 323:533, 2001.

Bruce, M, et al: Risk factors for meningococcal disease in college students. JAMA 286:688, 2001.

Centers for Disease Control and Prevention: Meningococcal disease and college students: Recommendation of the advisory committee on immunization practices. MMWR Morb Mortal Wkly Rep 49:11, 2001.

Colby, C, et al: A 10-week old with meningitis. Clin Pediatr 40:155, 2001.

Dinakaran, S, et al: Retinal hemorrhages in meningococcal septicemia. JAAPOS 6:221, 2002.

Kronmeyer, B: Antibiotic management challenging for meningitis in pediatric patients. Infect Dis 38:77, 2000.

Reye's Syndrome

Meekin, SL, et al: A long term follow-up of cognitive, emotional, and behavioral sequelae to Reye syndrome. Dev Med Child Neurol 41:549, 1999.

Ward, MR: Reye's syndrome: An update. Nurs Pract 22:45, 1997.

Seizures

Curry, W, and Kully, D: Newer epileptic drugs: Gabapentin, iamotrigine, felbatrate, topiramate and fosphenytoin. Am Fam Physician 57:513, 1998.

Gaig, R: (2000) First unprovoked seizure: To treat or not to treat? J Assoc Physicians India 49:590, 2000.

Gill, J, and Gieorn-Kornthals, M: What parents and health care providers need to know about febrile seizures. Contemp Pediatr 139, 2002.

Isselbacher, K, et al: Harrison's Principles of Internal Medicine. McGraw-Hill, New York, 1995.

Klein, P, et al: Onset of epilepsy at time of menarche. Neurology 60:495, 2003.

Kopek, K: New anticonvulsants for use in the pediatric patient. J Pediatr Health Care 15:81, 2001.

Marks, W, and Garcia, J: Management of seizures and epilepsy. Am Fam Physician 57:1589, 1998.

Odell, C, and Shannon, S: Initiation and discontinuation of antiepileptic drugs. Neurol Clin 19:289, 2001.

Reinhold, J, and Benti, A: Pediatric febrile seizures and childhood headaches in primary care. Nurs Clin North Am 35:137, 2000.

Schachter, S, and Gabb, M: (2001) Epilepsy pharmocotherapy: Goals and strategies. Adv Stud Med 1:270, 2001.

Schachter, S: Epilepsy. Neurol Clin 19:22, 2001.

Tich, S, and Peron, Y: Cognitive impairment in childhood epilepsy: The role of antiepileptic drugs. Epilepsy Disorders 2:87, 2001.

Chapter *12*
ENDOCRINE, METABOLIC, AND NUTRITIONAL DISORDERS

ACROMEGALY (GIANTISM)

SIGNAL SYMPTOMS ▶ extreme height or significant or noticeable growth spurt

Acromegaly	ICD-9CM: 253.0

Description: Acromegaly is a condition related to hypersecretion of pituitary hormones (primarily growth hormone [GH]), resulting in abnormal growth mainly of the distal parts of the body. Often this oversecretion affects all portions of the body. The oversecretion of GH results in hyperplasia of the somatotrophs.

Etiology: Acromegaly is most often caused by a pituitary adenoma, but other causes include hypothalamic or pancreatic tumors.

Occurrence: Rare (1 in 4000).

Age: Although it may occur as early as age 2, it is most evident at puberty.

Ethnicity: Not significant.

Gender: Occurs equally in males and females.

Contributing factors: Pituitary or hypothalamic disease, embryologic defects, tumor, or exposure to radiation.

Signs and symptoms: When the tumor occurs in young children, before epiphyseal fusion occurs, parents voice concern at the extreme height of the child and report at least one significant growth spurt (Fig. 12–1). Children may also complain of visual changes or problems related to compression of the optic nerve. In older children, the history may include delayed sexual changes and a sudden onset of menses. The

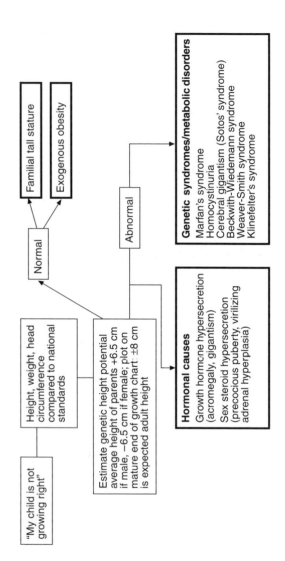

Figure 12–1. Evaluation of excessive growth.

older child may have coarse facial features, protruding jaw, height beyond the norm for age, enlarged hands and feet, and thickened skin. Often the teeth are separated, and dorsal kyphosis is evident. Percussion and palpation may reveal a tumor of the pancreas.

Diagnostic tests:

Test	Results Indicating Disorder	CPT Code
GH levels	Elevated (>10 mg/mL)	83003
Radiographs of skull	Frontal bossing, jutting of chin, and thickening of orbs	70250–70260
CT of head MRI of head	May reveal a pituitary adenoma or a hypothalamic tumor	70470 70496
CT of abdomen	May reveal a tumor of the pancreas	74170–74175

CT, computed tomography; MRI, magnetic resonance imaging.

Serial height and head circumference measurements are taken to document abnormal growth spurts.

Differential diagnosis:

Hereditary tall stature is differentiated by family history.

In precocious puberty, the epiphysis closes early, and stature is ultimately short.

Marfan's syndrome and homocystinuria are differentiated by normal GH levels.

Central nervous system mass is differentiated by CT or MRI of the head.

Treatment: Psychological and genetic counseling should be initiated for the child and parents.

The goal of treatment is to reduce the GH level or, if a tumor is present, to shrink the size of the tumor. Pharmacologic management is with bromocriptine to decrease the size of the tumor. Generally, surgery is performed or radiation therapy instituted by a pediatric endocrinologist.

Follow-up: The patient should maintain regular health care visits. If medications are used, follow-up is weekly or monthly.

Sequelae: Dental problems related to the increased size of the mandible, delayed sexual development, and perhaps arrested development.

Prevention/prophylaxis: Regular screening and health care visits should include a meticulous measurement of height and head circumference. There is no way to prevent acromegaly from occurring.

Referral: As soon as this condition is suspected, refer the patient to a pediatric endocrinologist.

Education: Educate the parents and children as to the nature of this rare disorder. Inform parents of the course of the disease and the treatment regimen; offer counseling. Because children with acromegaly have difficulty with activities that require coordination, parents should be prepared to assist them with these activities and to provide them with safety measures.

CYSTIC FIBROSIS

SIGNAL SYMPTOMS increased diaphoresis noted with a salty taste to the skin in the newborn, inability or difficulty stooling, and all affected stools have a very foul odor increased incidence of respiratory problems often with unusual causative agents found (i.e., *Pseudomonas*)

Cystic fibrosis (CF)   ICD-9 CM: 277

Description: CF, an autosomal-recessive genetic disorder, is found in infants and young children. Characterized by chronic lung problems, pancreatic insufficiency, and abnormally high levels of electrolytes (specifically sodium chloride) in the sweat, the disease is caused by dysfunction of the exocrine glands. The disease affects the pulmonary, gastrointestinal, endocrine/metabolic, and reproductive systems. Transmitted on the seventh chromosome, it is the most common lethal, genetically transferred disease.

Etiology: a single gene defect

Occurrence: 1 in 3300 whites, 1 in 9000 Hispanics, and 1/17,000 African-Americans.

Age: Present at birth, but diagnosis can be made at any age; the oldest recorded age of diagnosis of CF is 65 years.

Ethnicity: CF is more common in whites (1 in 3300); it occurs at a significantly lower rate in African-Americans.

Gender: Occurs equally in males and females.

Contributing factors: Familial history because this disorder is genetically transmitted.

Signs and symptoms: The parent may report that the child sweats heavily and that the skin tastes salty when kissed. The child has a history of chronic lung infections or recurrent bouts of pneumonia or bronchitis caused by unusual organisms, such as *Pseudomonas, Klebsiella,* and *Staphylococcus.* These infections are accompanied by wheezing, coughing, tachypnea, and cyanotic episodes. Chronic constipation may be reported; the stool is foul-smelling, frothy, and pale. The child may have delayed weight gain (compared with failure to thrive in the infant) and delayed growth, and the older child may have delayed appearance of secondary sexual characteristics.

The following questions may help in obtaining a thorough history when CF is suspected.

Does the child have chronic constipation or has there been a need for regular use of suppositories to enable the child to have regular bowel movements?

What does the child's stool look like? Does it have a foul odor?
What is the child's appetite like? Has the child grown as expected?
How often does the child get respiratory infections or have other
    respiratory problems?
Does anyone else in the family have CF, or has anyone had similar
    complaints?

The child, who appears small for his or her age, may have a barrel
chest and cyanosis. There may be a cough and other signs of respiratory
problems, such as tachypnea and dyspnea. Distal clubbing may be noted.
Stool may be palpated in the abdomen, and a prolapsed rectum may be
noted. A significant delay of secondary sexual characteristics in the adolescent may be expected. Bone age is retarded. The skin may be sweaty,
and the parent may report it has a salty taste to it. If a fever is present or
if the child has become overheated, there are signs of dehydration. Nasal
polyps may be visualized on inspection of the nares. The abdomen is distended, is dull to percussion, and has decreased bowel sounds. The liver
is palpable. Decreased sounds at the bases of the lungs are noted when
pneumonia is present. Wheezing may be heard on auscultation of the
lungs, and the lungs are hyperinflated.

Diagnostic tests:

Test	Results Indicating Disorder	CPT Code
Quantitative pilocarpine iontophoresis (sweat chloride test)	Positive	82438
Stool for trypsinogen (for infants <3 months)	Absent or diminished trypsin and chymotrypsin	84488–84490
72-hour fecal fat excretion	Increased fat in stool	82705–82715
Blood albumin	Decreased	82040
Blood for fat-soluble vitamins	Decreased	82725
Respiratory excretions for the presence of *Pseudomonas* (highly suspicious when other symptoms are present)	Positive	89125

Differential diagnosis:

Malabsorption syndrome is differentiated by a negative sweat
    chloride test or genetic screen for CF.
Recurrent reactive airway disease is differentiated by negative sweat
    chloride test and genetic screen for CF.
Infants with failure to thrive (nonorganic) respond to changes in
    nutritional intake.
Congenital lung malformation is differentiated by x-ray of the lungs.
Immune deficiency disease is differentiated by laboratory tests;
    children have a negative sweat chloride test or genetic screen for
    CF.

Treatment:

Nonpharmacologic

Treatment often centers on providing adequate nutritional supervision to foster the child's normal growth and development within his or her limitations. Treatment also concentrates on improving pancreatic function and decreasing the frequency and severity of pulmonary diseases.

For the most part, children with CF are treated on an outpatient basis and are hospitalized only when either the respiratory system is severely compromised or they have a severe infection. The approach should be multidisciplinary, including a specialist with advanced knowledge in the management of CF; a primary health care provider; a nutritionist; a physical therapist, when needed; a social worker, who can assist the family in meeting the needs brought on by a chronic illness; and a respiratory therapist.

The child should be encouraged to engage in regular exercise and to practice good nutrition. The diet should allow liberal use of salt; intake of high-protein, high-calorie (100–150 Kcal/kg per day), and high-fat foods; and daily vitamin supplements.

Postural drainage accompanied by chest physiotherapy should be a part of the child's everyday routine.

Pharmacologic

Pancreatic enzyme replacement, prescribed by the specialist, should be administered on a daily or regular basis; in infants younger than 12 months old, 2000 to 4000 lipase units per 120 mL of formula; in children 1 to 4 years old, 1000 lipase units/kg per meal; and in children older than age 4, 400 lipase units/kg per meal with a maximum of 2500 lipase units per meal. Oxygen for home use should be available. Antibiotics should be given immediately in the presence of an infection to allay exacerbation of the disease (Table 12–1). Human recombinant deoxyribonuclease (DNase), a new aerosolized mucolytic agent, may be used to decrease the viscosity of mucus and improve airway clearance. Enemas may be needed to improve evacuation of the bowel, and at times a bowel-cleaning solution such as GoLYTLEY may be needed. Although not readily available, transplants for the lung, pancreas, and liver may be done.

Although the early use of antibiotics, antivirals, mucolytics, and bronchodilators can reduce the progression of respiratory symptoms, these measures cannot stop the overall progression of the disease. Currently the development of effective antipseudomonal therapy can improve the overall prognosis of the disease, but it should not be presented to parents as a cure for CF because no known cure exists.

Follow-up: Follow-up for the child with CF is continuous. The health care team should maintain a well-formulated plan for the child to achieve the optimal outcome. Ideally the child should be monitored at a CF center at least three times per year. Early intervention for all real or sus-

Table 12-1 Antimicrobial Agents for Lung Infection in Cystic Fibrosis

Route	Organisms	Agents	Dosage (mg/kg per 24 hr)	Doses/ 24 hr
Oral	Staphylococcus aureus	Cloxacillin	50-100	3-4
		Cefaclor	40-60	3
		Clindamycin	20	3-4
		Erythromycin	50-100	3-4
		Amoxicillin/ clavulanate	40	3
	Haemophilus influenzae	Amoxicillin	50-100	3
		Trimethoprim- sulfamethoxazole	20*	2-4
	Pseudomonas	Chloramphenicol	50-100	3-4
	P. aeruginosa	Ciprofloxacin	15-30	3
	Empirical	Tetracycline	50-100	3-4
Intravenous	S. aureus	Oxacillin	150-200	4
	P. aeruginosa	Gentamicin or tobramycin	8-20	1-3
		Amikacin	15-30	2-3
		Netilmicin	6-12	2-3
		Carbenicillin		
		Ticarcillin		
		Piperacillin		
		Mezlocillin or azlocillin	•50-450	4-6
		Ticarcillin/ clavulanate	250-450	4-6
		Imipenem/ cilastatin	45-90	3-4
	P. aeruginosa and P. cepacia	Ceftazidime	150	3
Aerosol	P. aeruginosa	Gentamicin	40-80†	2-4
		Tobramycin	40-80†	
		Carbenicillin	500-1000†	

* Quantity of trimethoprim.
† mg/dose.
Source: Behrman, R: Nelson's Textbook of Pediatrics. WB Saunders, Philadelphia, 1992.

pected infections should be stressed; routine immunizations should be given along with specialized immunizations.

Sequelae: Common sequelae include chronic lung infections, bronchitis, bacterial or viral pneumonia, and *Pseudomonas* infections. Other complications include pneumothorax, hemoptysis, right-sided heart failure, diabetes mellitus, metabolic alkalosis, malnutrition, growth retardation, sterility, intestinal obstructions, biliary cirrhosis, and bleeding esophageal varices. Ultimately, death occurs; the life expectancy of CF patients is a median of 29 years.

Prevention/prophylaxis: Parents should be given adequate genetic counseling so that they can make informed choices regarding future pregnancies. Early intervention is always important. Yearly influenza immunization should be provided. The child also needs adequate protection against measles and pertussis. The child should not receive general anesthesia: Epidural, local, or spinal anesthesia should be used for all surgical procedures. Most important for the child and the family is the maintenance of good teamwork and support for the management of acute and long-term problems associated with the disease.

Referral: When CF is suspected and as soon as the diagnosis is confirmed, refer the patient to a pediatrician and a pediatric endocrinologist, preferably one who specializes in CF.

Education: Teach parents the dietary management of CF. Train them to provide early intervention for infections or other complications. Inform parents and children regarding all of the treatments, therapies, and implications of the disease. Teach them the techniques of chest physiotherapy and respiratory care, and help them recognize the signs of a compromised respiratory system.

HYPOTHYROIDISM

SIGNAL SYMPTOMS ▶ congenital: prolonged jaundice, constipation, feeding difficulties, and increased lethargy acquired: cold intolerance, overly dry skin, hoarseness of voice, slowed growth, decreased school performance, and short stature

Hypothyroidism	
Congenital hypothyroidism (CH)	ICD-9 CM: 243
Acquired hypothyroidism (AH)	ICD-9 CM: 244.9

Description: Hypothyroidism, a deficiency in the production of thyroid hormone or a defect in the receptor, can be acquired or congenital. Establishment of national neonatal screening programs can be credited for the early detection of this potentially fatal disorder.

Etiology: CH is due to thyroid dysgenesis. AH is most commonly caused by lymphocytic thyroiditis.

Occurrence: CH occurs in 1 in 3500 live births. AH occurs in 1 in 500 school-age children.

Age: CH, at birth; AH, any age beyond the newborn period.

Ethnicity: Not significant.

Gender: More prevalent in females (2:1 CH; 2:1 AH).

Contributing factors:

AH: If the child has had a thyroidectomy, has been exposed to a goitrogen (e.g., iodides, antithyroid drugs, or other medications), has an iodine deficiency, or has been exposed to irradiation of the thyroid tissue, there is an increased risk of thyroid disease.

CH: Genetic predisposition and Down's syndrome are contributing factors.

Signs and symptoms: In CH, there is a family history of the disease, prolonged gestation, increased birth weight, delayed first stool, feeding difficulties, constipation, and general lethargy. Physical examination reveals a distended abdomen, a yellow tinge to skin, peripheral cyanosis, macroglossia, and hypotonia. There is delayed closure of the posterior fontanel; cool, dry, scaly skin; poor capillary refill; an umbilical hernia; and possible signs of respiratory distress (e.g., retractions, wheezing, coarse breathing sounds).

In AH, the history is more vague. Parents sometimes note delayed growth. They may report decreased appetite, lethargy, poor school performance, cold intolerance, and delayed puberty. Physical examination may reveal a goiter, delayed dentition, and dry skin. Muscle weakness, tenderness of the anterior neck, and cool, dry skin are also noted (Fig. 12–2).

There is an increased need for sleep in both groups.

Diagnostic tests:

Test	Results Indicating Disorder	CPT Code
Newborn thyroid screen T_4	Low	84437
TSH (if >25 mU/L, do full endocrine workup)	High	84443
Radiographs of the skull	Large fontanels and wide suture lines	70250–70260
Electrocardiography	Enlarged heart	93320–93350
Radiographs of chest	"Beaking" of the ribs (curvature and narrowing at ends of ribs resulting in a beak-like appearance)	71020

T_4, thyroxine; TSH, thyroid-stimulating hormone.

Consultation with a pediatric endocrinologist is needed to make the final diagnosis.

Differential diagnosis:

Transient hypothyroidism is distinguished from thyroid disease because the T_4 and TSH levels return to normal, whereas in AH or CH they do not return to normal.

Sleep apnea is differentiated by an abnormal pneumogram.

Constipation is a transient condition, but in AH and CH it persists despite changes in diet or the use of medication.

Down's syndrome is differentiated by chromosomal testing.

Congenital cardiac defects are differentiated by abnormal cardiac findings that do not generally accompany hypothyroidism.

Short stature is differentiated by failure of thyroid replacement therapy to cause an increase in height.

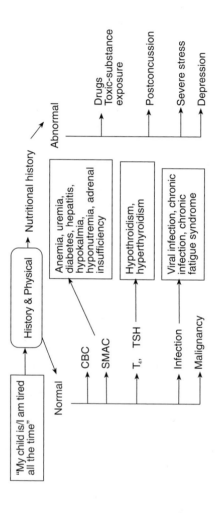

Figure 12–2. Differentiating fatigue. (CBC, complete blood count; SMAC, Sequential Multiple Analyzer Computer; T$_4$, thyroxine; TSH, thyroid-stimulating hormone.)

Treatment:

    CH: Give levothyroxine (Synthroid), 10 to 15 μg/kg per day, to the neonate to maintain T_4 levels within 10 to 15 mg/dL range. At 0 to 1 year, give 8 to 10 μg/kg per day; 1 to 5 years, 6 to 8 μg/kg per day; 6 to 12 years, 5 to 6 μg/kg per day; and older than 12 years, 4 to 5 μg/kg per day. Improvement is noted in 7 to 21 days. Height increases, and skeletal maturation responds rapidly. Thyroid tests (T_4, TSH, and free T_4) should be done every month for the first 6 months, then every other month for 6 to 12 months, then every 3 months. Bone age needs to be determined at the start of therapy, at age 1 year, and about every 1 to 2 years during growth years.

    AH: Give levothyroxine, 8 to 10 μg/kg, up to a maximum of 100 to 150 μg once per day at least 30 minutes before eating. Treatment should start at the lowest levels; TSH levels should be monitored every 2 to 3 months or more often when there are dosage changes or signs of increased hypothyroidism or hyperthyroidism.

Follow-up: The child should keep regularly scheduled health care maintenance appointments besides having TSH level checked every 2 to 3 months.

 Clinical Pearl: TSH greater than 20 uU/L indicates undertreatment or noncompliance; the nurse practitioner first should investigate if the medicine is being taken as ordered and, if so, should increase the dose.

Sequelae: Children's growth expectations are met when hypothyroidism is treated early; however, children with long-standing hypothyroidism may lose 7 cm of predicted adult height.

Prevention/prophylaxis: CH, none; AH, avoidance of goitrogens, adequate iodine in diet, and follow-up after radiation treatment to ensure early detection of a problem.

Referral: If hypothyroidism is suspected, refer patient to a pediatric endocrinologist immediately for confirmation of the diagnosis. Afterward, manage the patient's follow-up.

Education: Teach the parents to give medications each day at the same time to maintain an adequate thyroid level. Signs that the child's levels may be too low include increased fatigue, weight gain, skin and voice changes, and dryness of the skin or hair. Note any of these changes and order an immediate TSH level.

INSULIN-DEPENDENT DIABETES MELLITUS

SIGNAL SYMPTOMS polydipsia, polyuria, polyphagia, and weight loss; sometimes when ketosis is present, a fruity odor (similar to Juicy Fruit gum) is detectable

| Insulin-dependent diabetes mellitus (IDDM) | ICD-9 CM: 250.0 |

Description: IDDM is a common childhood illness. Although its etiology is not completely understood, it is known that this disorder of immune function leads to the destruction of pancreatic islet (β) cells, resulting in an inappropriate use of carbohydrates owing to insulin deficiency. Adequate management of nutritional, medical, behavioral, and emotional aspects of diabetes is important in improving the quality of life and the overall prognosis.

Etiology: Marked lipolysis, proteolysis, and ketone body formation result from decreased synthesis of glycogen, protein, and fat. Serum glucose and ketone levels are elevated, increasing the osmotic level in the kidneys; consequently the kidneys are affected by increased urinary loss and loss of potassium, sodium, and ammonium. There is a genetic predisposition, but tranmission not mendelian in nature. For the most part, IDDM is idiopathic.

Occurrence: IDDM constitutes 97% of cases of childhood diabetes, occurring in 15 in 100,000 children in the United States.

Age: Peak onset is between ages 7 and 13 years.

Ethnicity: Incidence ranges from country to country: The lowest rate is in Korea (0.6 in 100,000), and the highest is in Finland (35 in 100,000). Whites have this disorder much more frequently than blacks.

Gender: Occurs equally in males and females.

Contributing factors: Genetic predisposition is the most significant predictor of IDDM in children, although the process of inheritance is not understood.

Signs and symptoms: The child presents with a recent history of polyuria, polydipsia, and polyphagia accompanied by weight loss. Usually there are no significant findings. There is an increased urinary frequency along with nighttime polyuria and enuresis. Changes in appetite and thirst are also apparent to the parents. Weight loss may be noted. The child may appear dehydrated and may have Kussmaul respirations. A fruity odor to the breath is noted when ketones are present.

Diagnostic tests:

Test	Results Indicating Disorder	CPT Code
Fasting blood glucose	>125 mg/dL	82947
Random blood glucose	>200 mg/dL	82947
Urinalysis	Presence of ketones or glucose	81002

 Clinical Pearl: In children, oral glucose tolerance tests are rarely necessary to confirm the diagnosis. Hemoglobin A, C are not used for diagnosis because of lack of standardization.

Differential diagnosis:

Polydipsia, polyuria, and impaired urinary concentration sometimes occur with hypercalcemia and potassium deficiency, differentiated by serum levels, which reveal increased calcium and decreased potassium in the blood.

Primary renal diseases are differentiated by isotonic urine. In diabetics, hypotonic urine is present.

Psychogenic polydipsia is differentiated by the patient's withholding fluids but failing to produce concentrated urine.

Treatment:

Nonpharmacologic

Early and aggressive management is the key to the successful treatment of IDDM. Long-term goals of treatment include maintaining normal growth and development, regulating glucose metabolism, preventing acute complications, and promoting the patient's acceptance of the disease. Treatment should involve a multidisciplinary team including a diabetes educator, nurse or nurse practitioner, dietitian, social worker, psychologist or therapist, primary health care provider, and pediatric endocrinologist.

Growth should be monitored and growth curves plotted at intervals of 3 to 6 months, depending on the child's age. Blood glucose should be monitored three to five times per day.

Nutritional regimens suggest that the child's diet should consist of 50% to 60% carbohydrates, 12% to 20% protein, and less than 30% fat. Three snacks per day are recommended for children.

Exercise should be regular and moderate; when strenuous exercise is expected, adjustments should be made for the possibility of hypoglycemia.

Pharmacologic

Insulin, the primary agent used in the treatment of IDDM, is initially given at 0.6 to 0.8 U/kg per day in two divided doses: half given before breakfast and half given before dinner. Each dose should be made up of regular (immediate-acting) and NPH (short-acting) insulin (2:1). If there is no ketoacidosis, begin with 0.25 to 0.5 U/kg per day of insulin. When ketoacidosis is present, start with 0.5 to 0.75 U/kg per day. Lantus also can be given once daily at bedtime with a range of 2 to 100 IU adjusted for age and weight to be used as long-acting insulin as needed. When an insulin regimen is established, diabetic children can be managed at about 1 U/kg per day in divided doses. After approximately 3 to 4 months, most children experience a "honeymoon phase," requiring significantly less insulin. Conversely, illness, anxiety, and the onset of puberty increase the requirement for insulin. A physician should institute all changes in insulin. Brand names have slight differences, so a switch in brand may alter the patient's typical reaction to the insulin dose. Lantus, a long-acting (24-hour) insulin, is given to children 6 years and older at night. It is given at approximately 20% of the NPH dose, and can be used alone or in combination with other insulins.

If the dawn phenomenon (morning hyperglycemia) or Somogyi phenomenon (morning hyperglycemia resulting from evening hypoglycemia) occurs, adjustments need to be made in the scheduling of doses. For the dawn phenomenon, the evening dose of intermediate-acting insulin needs to be increased. For the Somogyi phenomenon, the evening dose of intermediate-acting insulin needs to be decreased, or the carbohydrate content of evening snacks may be increased.

For adolescents, changes brought on by puberty may change requirements; 1.5 to 2 U/kg per day should be the dose schedule adhered to in the teenage years.

External infusion pumps are not generally used in young children but should be considered with unstable diabetes or severe, chronic illness.

A protocol acceptable to the child and the health care provider should be established for glucose monitoring. At least a morning blood glucose reading is needed. A range of 80 to 160 mg/dL is considered acceptable. When there are readings above or below this range, the health care provider should be contacted. If the reading is greater than 240 mg/dL, urine should be tested for the presence of ketones.

The health care provider should measure glycosylated hemoglobin (HbA_{1c}) because it indicates degree of adherence to the medication regimen for a 2- to 3-month period preceding the examination. Results of 4% to 6% are normal; 9% to 13% indicates *fair* to *good* control, and greater than 15% indicates *poor* control. HbA_{1c} should be measured every 3 months or in cases of stress or illness.

Follow-up: Routine health care visits should be maintained. Changes in blood glucose levels should be reported to health care providers as they occur.

Sequelae: Diabetes mellitus is a complex disease that has far-reaching consequences when poorly controlled. Problems frequently seen in diabetic children include blindness, learning disorders, emotional problems, and renal and neurologic consequences. Puberty and the development of secondary sexual characteristics are often delayed. Depression and rebellion are commonly seen in adolescent patients, for which quick, effective intervention is required. Long-term complications include peripheral and autonomic neurologic changes, early onset of heart problems, and retinal changes.

Prevention/prophylaxis: Because there is an inherited predisposition to the disease, it cannot be prevented. Good nutrition and weight management may delay onset of diabetes. Exacerbations can be treated and prevented by anticipation of changes in insulin dosage during the honeymoon phase and during illness, stress, exercise, and adolescence. Also, regular measurement of the HgA_{1c} can help validate the child's reports of having been compliant with the medication regimen and can help determine an appropriate plan for the child. An annual eye examination should be scheduled along with regularly scheduled health care visits to the primary care provider for routine health care needs.

Referral: When diabetes is suspected, the child should be referred to a pediatric endocrinologist or diabetes specialist. The team should be contacted to assist in developing a comprehensive, efficacious plan to foster the best outcomes for the child.

Education: With the assistance of a diabetes educator, teach parents, children, and other interested family members the disease process, the signs and symptoms of hyperglycemia and hypoglycemia, and the proper action to take when there are complications. Over time, long-term strategies need to be discussed with the family to decrease complications that may arise.

MILK PROTEIN SENSITIVITY AND LACTOSE INTOLERANCE

SIGNAL SYMPTOMS▶ frequent stomach upset, pain, diarrhea, and cramping after ingestion of milk or milk product; inability to tolerate milk-based formula

Milk protein sensitivity and lactose intolerance	ICD-9 CM: 693.1

Description: Milk sensitivity is an allergic response to whey proteins and casein and is characterized by an intolerance to cow's milk–based products. There may be a crossover allergic response to soy protein products.

Lactose intolerance is the inability to digest carbohydrates (disaccharides, glucose, and galactose).

Etiology:

Milk protein sensitivity: The cause is unknown, but it is thought to be some form of mediated immunologic process.

Lactose intolerance: The most common cause is lactase deficiency. Primary lactose intolerance is a decline in intestinal lactase activity that is genetically determined; secondary lactose intolerance, the most common form, has been associated with infectious processes, such as AIDS, rotavirus, and other infections of the small bowel, and damage to the small bowel, as noted in celiac disease (gluten sensitivity). There may be some genetic variations, such as the lactase-phlorizer (LCT) gene.

Occurrence: Common. Milk protein sensitivity is estimated to be present in 0.5% to 1% of all infants. An estimated 30% of milk protein–sensitive persons are also soy sensitive.

Age: Milk protein sensitivity usually occurs within the first month of life and resolves during the first year. Lactose intolerance occurs in older age groups, usually after age 5 years.

Ethnicity: African-Americans and Mexican-Americans have a higher incidence of lactose intolerance. Other minority groups affected are Native Americans of North, South, and Central America and people of Mediterranean descent. Asian children seem to have a history of earlier onset than do other groups.

Gender: Occurs in girls and boys.

Contributing factors:

Milk protein sensitivity: Family history of allergies may contribute to infant feeding difficulties.

Lactose intolerance: Infections of the gastrointestinal tract and other illness such as celiac disease ("short gut"), which reduces the surface area required for absorption of lactose.

Signs and symptoms:

History

Milk protein sensitivity: The infant is brought to the clinic with the complaint that he or she is not tolerating the present formula. The caregiver relates a history of fussiness, crying, colicky abdominal pain, excessive gas, vomiting, and diarrhea with streaks of blood in the stools. The history may include the presence of skin rashes, clear runny nose, and congestion.

Lactose intolerance: The child is brought to the clinic because of watery diarrhea, complaints of feeling bloated, flatulence, vomiting, and abdominal cramping.

Physical Examination

Milk protein sensitivity: Findings reveal an infant who is not gaining weight appropriately for age. There may be skin rashes, and the diaper area may be more irritated than usual, owing to increased number of stools. There is clear drainage from the nose and some nasal "stuffiness." Blood-streaked stools are consistent with milk protein intolerance in infants.

Lactose intolerance: The findings of the physical examination vary, depending on the severity of the symptoms. Long-term symptoms can lead to dehydration, electrolyte imbalance, and metabolic acidosis.

Diagnostic tests:

Test	Results Indicating Disorder	CPT Code
Total protein	Increased protein	84155
Albumin	Increased albumin	82040
Stool for occult blood	Positive for blood	82270
Breath hydrogen test	Expired hydrogen of 20 pp more than baseline	91065
Skin allergy test	Positive for milk allergy	95010–95099

Differential diagnosis:

CF has a positive sweat chloride test.

Pyloric stenosis has a positive radiograph and characteristic projectile vomiting.

For nonorganic failure to thrive, observe the mother-infant interaction and the feeding technique if neglect and abuse are suspected.

In secondary formula protein intolerance resulting from mucosal injury after a rotavirus infection, a viral antigen in the stool as measured by enzyme-linked immunosorbent assay is confirmatory. Usually resolves in 1 month.

Primary carbohydrate malabsorption resulting from congenital disaccharide deficiency is rare in infancy. The stool contains excessive quantities of carbohydrates.

Treatment: Eliminate the suspected food from the diet. Infants are often placed initially on Enfamil or Similac with Iron; the iron may be a cause of the gastric upset. Try the new formula for a week; if it is not tolerated well, try a different one. Examples of some substitutions are Prosobee or Isomil (soy-based), Nutramigen or Pregestimil (also used with malabsorption disorders), and Alimentum (for infants who cannot tolerate other formulas).

Try Lactofree formula if you suspect lactose intolerance. Improvement of symptoms may occur with the use of milk-containing lactase-producing microorganisms as well as milk pretreated with microbial-derived lactase, such as Dairy Ease (Sterling Health Division of Sterling Winthrop, New York, NY), Lactaid (McNeil Consumer Products Co, Fort Washington, PA) and Lactrase (Schwarz Pharma, Kremeres Urban Co, Milwaukee, WI).

Follow-up: Re-evaluate weekly for weight, feeding pattern, and alleviation of symptoms on the new formula. When formula tolerance has stabilized, resume regularly scheduled visits.

Sequelae: Infants who have extreme milk protein sensitivity and lactose intolerance are at risk for developing failure to thrive and associated growth retardation.

Prevention/prophylaxis:

Milk protein sensitivity: The best method of prevention is for the infant to be breast-fed. Diarrhea in breast-fed infants may be relieved by the elimination of milk from the diet of the mother.

Lactose intolerance: None.

Referral: Normally, none; in severe cases, refer to a pediatric gastroenterologist. The Women, Infant and Children's program is helpful for families who need assistance for special formulas. A written prescription is required for eligible mothers to obtain special formulas.

Education: Instruct patents in proper bottle-feeding techniques and how to read food labels to identify offending substances, such as whey, casein, or lactose. Lactose is frequently used as a filler substance in capsules and tablets; choose medication accordingly.

OBESITY

SIGNAL SYMPTOMS▶ large for age; straie often seen on skin

Obesity	ICD-9 CM: 278.0

Description: Obesity is a condition in which the body weight is 20% above the desired weight for age, gender, height, and body build. Obesity can be related to increased adipose tissue that is typed as either hypertrophy, an increase in the size of the fat cells; or hyperplasia, an increase in the number of fat cells. Although the size of a fat cell can be reduced, the number is not easily decreased; obesity owing to hyperplasia is more difficult to treat.

Etiology: Inadequate activity levels or psychosocial factors that result in a child's turning to food for comfort can contribute to obesity in children. The intake of calories beyond the recommended number, coupled with a decreased level of activity or slowed metabolism, can also result in obesity. There is an interplay between genetic and environmental factors, but this is not understood.

Occurrence: In the United States, 27% of all children and 21% of teenagers are obese. Of these, it is estimated that one third to one half of children and 80% of teenagers will remain obese into adulthood.

Age: Can occur at any age.

Ethnicity: Not significant.

Gender: Occurs equally in males and females.

Contributing factors: Of children diagnosed with Prader-Willi syndrome, Down's syndrome, or spina bifida, 50% are obese. In general, any disorder that reduces energy output, limits mobility, or impinges on the body's metabolism can increase the risk of obesity at any age.

Signs and symptoms: The parent may relate a diagnosis of a disorder or disability that has caused a decreased activity level for the child. The parent may also relate that many members of the family are obese. The child presents with a history of decreased level of activity, intake of an increased amount of calories, and a sense of being "always hungry." Previous attempts at weight reduction may have been unsuccessful. The child's level of activity—time spent in aerobic sports or exercise, time spent reading or watching television, and sleep history—should be evaluated. The pattern of eating and the quality of food consumed in a day should be reviewed.

Height and weight, body frame, and muscle mass should be evaluated. Body mass index (BMI) should be calculated for all suspected of obesity.

BMI is calculated by dividing the weight in kilograms by the height in meters squared. Children with a BMI greater than 85% are at risk for becoming overweight. Children with a BMI of 95% are overweight. In uncomplicated obesity, the only significant finding is weight greater than expected for the height and age of the child. Obesity is diagnosed when triceps skin fold is greater than 85%, and weight for height is greater than the 75th percentile.

In extremely obese patients, it may be difficult to palpate or percuss any organs. Blood pressure should be monitored because it is sometimes elevated in obese persons (Fig. 12–3).

Diagnostic tests: None for uncomplicated obesity.

Differential diagnosis:

Diabetes mellitus is differentiated by elevated blood glucose levels when fasting.

Hypothyroidism is differentiated by TSH level, which is normal in obesity but decreased in thyroid disease.

Hypoparathyroidism is differentiated by laboratory tests to assess the function of the parathyroid gland. The results show decreased levels in this disease but not in obesity.

Inborn errors of metabolism are differentiated by a positive phenylketonuria test and by routine tests for galactosemia or maple syrup urine disease.

Treatment: Although a reduction in the child's caloric intake should be stressed, a "diet" is not an effective approach to the problem of obesity. Rather the child should be encouraged to increase physical activity and eat well-balanced meals. Diets often encourage eating disorders, so they may interfere with normal growth and development.

Evaluate the relationship between the parent and child and the parents' attitudes about eating and food. Positive behavioral techniques centered on improving self-esteem, attitudes, and body image should be taught. The child, parent, and health care provider should set realistic goals to decrease weight.

Children should be taught that they should eat only until they are full and that the old adage of "clean your plate" often leads to obesity. Daily exercise should be stressed, decreased television viewing time should be enforced (<4 hours per day), and positive feedback and praise should be given to the child. Rewards should be incorporated into positive behavioral strategies: All weight loss, improved dietary habits, and increased physical activity should be acknowledged. Consultation with a nutritionist is usually helpful for families.

Follow-up: Weekly weight and monthly height measurements are recommended until optimal weight is achieved.

Sequelae: Obesity increases the likelihood of hypertension, impaired glucose tolerance, low self-esteem, depression, social isolation, and orthopedic problems.

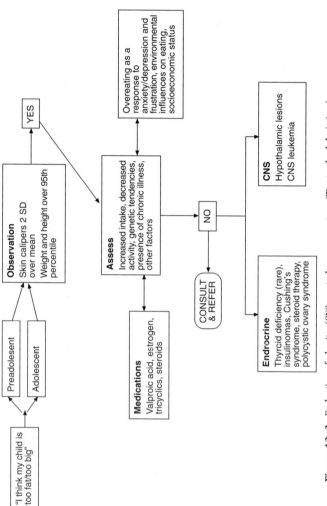

Figure 12–3. Evaluation of obesity. (CNS, central nervous system; SD, standard deviation.)

Prevention/prophylaxis: Good nutritional strategies should be employed in every family. Balanced meals, low-calorie nutritional snacks, and an exercise program should be started early and become part of a family's regular practices.

Referral: If a metabolic disorder is suspected, immediately refer the patient to a pediatric endocrinologist. To assist the child and parent in sound meal and snack planning, refer the child to a nutritionist in conjunction with medical supervision.

Education: Encourage parents to set the example for good nutritional patterns. Although dieting in children is not usually a good method of controlling obesity, teach families to change their eating patterns. Institute positive reinforcement strategies.

SHORT STATURE

SIGNAL SYMPTOMS child appears to be shorter than expected for age; height between third and fifth percentile

Short stature	ICD-9 CM: 783.43

Description: Constitutional (familial) short stature, the most common cause of short stature in children, is an abnormally short stature relative to the age of the child. Pituitary dwarfism is related to insufficient GH. Congenital short stature is caused by hypothyroidism. Primordial short stature is caused by intrauterine growth retardation.

Etiology: No causative agent is noted in constitutional short stature; rather, it is caused by constitutionally delayed growth. Insufficient levels of GH cause pituitary dwarfism. Thyroid insufficiency may cause congenital short stature. Intrauterine growth retardation is the cause of primordial short stature.

Occurrence: Rare (1 in 4000).

Age: Present from birth.

Ethnicity: Not significant.

Gender: Occurs equally in males and females.

Contributing factors: Family history of short stature.

Signs and symptoms: A family history of delayed growth, short stature, and related skeletal and pubertal delays is given by the parent. In cases of pituitary dwarfism, hypothyroid-induced short stature, and primordial short stature, the patient usually has no prior history. In pituitary dwarfism, the birth weight is normal, but there is decreased height at birth with small hands and feet (Fig. 12–4).

Hypothyroid-induced short stature: The patient may report persistent constipation.

Constitutional short stature: Growth curve is at about the third to fifth percentile.

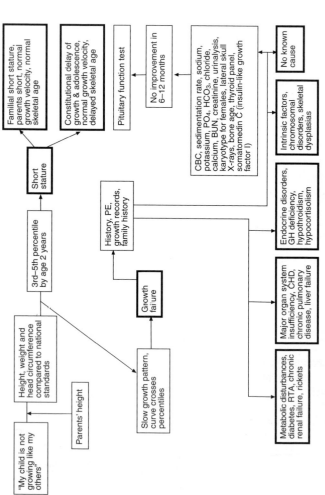

Figure 12–4. Differential diagnosis of growth disturbances. (BUN, blood urea nitrogen; CBC, complete blood count; CHD, coronary heart disease; GH, growth hormone; RTA, renal tubular acidosis; PE, physical examination.)

Pituitary dwarfism: Patient has cherub-like or infantile facial
features with persistent infantile fat distribution, the norm being a
loss of infantile fat and elongating of face with approaching
puberty.

Hypothyroid-induced and primordial short stature reveal no significant findings by inspection except short stature.

Diagnostic tests:

Test	Results Indicating Disorder	CPT Code
GH	Reduced in primary dwarfism	83003
Ultrasound during pregnancy	Intrauterine growth retardation in cases of primordial short stature	76999
Thyroid panel	Altered TSH and T_4 in hypothyroid-induced short stature	80418
Bilirubin	Prolonged hyperbilirubinemia in hypothyroid-induced short stature	82247–82248
Radiographs of long bones	Delayed epiphyseal maturation (pituitary dwarfism)	76040
Bone age	Delayed except in constitutional short stature (>2 standard deviations)	78339

No abnormalities in laboratory tests are found in constitutional short
stature.

Serial height and head circumference measurements are taken for
comparison with the norm.

Differential diagnosis:

Hypothyroidism is differentiated by bilirubin test and by abnormal
TSH and T_4 levels.

Treatment: Pharmacologic treatment, if indicated, includes testosterone for boys starting at age 15 years. The dose is typically 50 to 100
mg intramuscularly per month for 3 to 6 months. For girls, at age 12 to
13.5, low-dose estradiol is administered.

When GH insufficiency is the problem, GH is administered, 0.043
mg/kg per day, beginning early in life (<10 years old). The goal of therapy is to improve growth rates.

Parents and children should receive reassurance and support regarding height expectations. Although some improvement in height is likely,
the child will probably continue to be shorter than his or her classmates.
Psychological counseling, when indicated, should be available.

Follow-up: Serial height and head circumference measurements
should be taken about every 1 to 3 months.

Sequelae: Short stature is associated with psychological or emotional
problems, poor learning and school performance, delayed sexual maturation, and developmental delays.

Prevention/prophylaxis: None.

Referral: As soon as a problem related to stature is suspected, refer the patient to a pediatric endocrinologist.

Education: Counsel families about the emotional problems often encountered with significant short stature (third to fifth percentile). Care should be taken when explaining therapies so that neither the child nor the parent has unrealistic expectations regarding the outcomes.

REFERENCES

Acromegaly (Giantism)
Connaughty, S: Accelerated growth in children. J Pediatr Health Care 6:316, 1992.

Cystic Fibrosis
Gaylor, A, and Reilly, J: Therapy with macrolides in patients with cystic fibrosis. Pharmacotherapy 22:227, 2002.

Herbst, D: Cystic fibrosis and lung transplantation: Ethical concerns. Pediatr Nurs 27:87, 2001.

Reid, D: Iron deficiency linked with cystic fibrosis disease severity. Chest 121:48, 2002.

Weiner, D: Respiratory tract infections in cystic fibrosis. Pediatr Ann 31:116, 2002.

Hypothyroidism
American Academy of Pediatrics, American Thyroid Association: Newborn screening for congenital hypothyroidism: Recommended guidelines. Pediatrics 91:1203, 1993.

Begay, T, et al: When to screen, when to treat thyroid disease. JAAPA 11:72, 2001.

Wiczk, H: Recognizing thyroid disease. Female Patient 23:9, 2002.

Wiersinga, W: Thyroid hormone replacement therapy. Horm Replacement 56:74, 2001.

Insulin-Dependent Diabetes Mellitus
American Diabetes Association: Diabetes mellitus and exercise. Diabetes Care 21:540, 1998.

Barclay, L: Metformin may benefit type I teen diabetics. Diabetes Care 26:138, 2003.

Englebert, D: Focus Drug of the Month. Pharmacy News Capsule 9: 1–4, 2000.

Erick, L: The newly diagnosed child with diabetes. Adv Nurse Pract 4:14, 1996.

Levitsky, L: Diabetes Mellitus Ambulatory Pediatric Care. Lippincott-Raven, Philadelphia, 1999.

Wilkes, D: Diabetes and Insulin Confusion. Pharm Journ 270: 7237, 267, 2003.

Milk Protein Sensitivity and Lactose Intolerance
Host, A: Clinical courses of cow's milk allergy and intolerance. Pediatr Allergy Immunol 9(Suppl 11):48, 1998.

Pongracic, J: Is it food allergy? Contemp Pediatr 12:101, 2000.

Obesity
Biscoas, S: Thyroid function in very preterm infants. Pediatrics 109:222, 2002.

Greger, N, and Edwin, C: (2001) Obesity: A pediatric epidemic. Pediatr Ann 30:694, 2001.

McWhorter, J, et al: The obese child: Maturation as a tool for exercise. J Pediatr Health Care 17:1, 2003.

Nelms, B: Childhood obesity: Taking on the issue. J Pediatr Health Care 15:47, 2001.

Ogden, C, et al: Prevalence and trends in overweight among US children and adolescents, 1999–2000. JAMA 288:1728, 2002.

Stetler, N, et al: Early growth and overweight status. Pediatrics 109:194, 2002.

Sztarna, D, et al: Weight related concerns and behaviors among overweight adolescents. Arch Pediatr 150:171, 2002.

Short Stature

Anhalt, H, and Chin, D: Endocrine treatments for short stature. Pediatr Ann 29:576, 2000.

Hoyme, H: A clinical genetics and dysmorphology approach to growth deficiency. Pediatr Ann 29:549, 2000.

MacGillivray, M: The basics for the diagnosis and management of short stature: A pediatric endocrinologist's approach. Pediatr Ann 29:570, 2000.

Miller, K: Evaluating growth in children: Distinguishing between normal and worrisome. ADVANCES NP 9:42, 2001.

Modan-Moser, D, et al: Stunting growth as a major feature of anorexia nervosa in male adolescents. Pediatrics 111:270, 2003.

Samuel, R, and Cohen, L: Understanding growth patterns in short stature. Contemp Pediatr Arch 6:94, 2001.

Shulman, D: Growth hormone therapy: An update. Contemp Pediatr 15:95, 1998.

Vogratzi, M, and Copeland, K: The short child. Pediatr Rev 19:92, 1998.

Zanzola, L: Revised pediatric growth charts. Available from CDC, AAP News, 7/6, 2000.

Chapter 13
HEMATOLOGIC AND IMMUNOLOGIC DISORDERS

ANEMIA, IRON DEFICIENCY

SIGNAL SYMPTOMS ▶ a noticeable increase in fatigue or pallor, particularly pallor of the mucous membranes

Iron-deficiency anemia (IDA)	ICD-9 CM: 280.9

Description: IDA is a microcytic, hypochromic anemia resulting from an inadequate supply of iron for synthesis of hemoglobin. Anemia reduces the blood's capacity to combine with and transport oxygen to the peripheral tissues.

Etiology: A decreased hemoglobin concentration in red blood cells (RBCs), which reduces the oxygen capacity of the blood, causes IDA. Inadequate stores of iron in the full-term infant can cause this problem in children younger than age 6 months. For some children, periods of rapid growth may precipitate IDA.

Occurrence: The incidence is inversely proportional to socioeconomic status.

Age: IDA occurs in 17% to 44% of children between ages 6 weeks and 3 months; peak prevalence is found in children aged 10 to 15 months (25%).

Ethnicity: IDA is more prevalent among lower socioeconomic groups; more African-American children have IDA than other ethnic groups.

Gender: Not significant until puberty, at which point it is more frequent in females.

Contributing factors: Preterm or low-birth-weight infants are at higher risk. If there has been fetal or perinatal blood loss without replacement, there is an increased likelihood of IDA. Children who consume large amounts of unfortified cow's milk (a low source of iron) or have poor dietary intake are also at risk.

Signs and symptoms: The parent may relate a history of irritability, decreased attention span, lethargy, anorexia, pica, headache, or learning problems (Fig. 13–1).

On physical examination, there is mild-to-severe conjunctival pallor, mucous membranes are pale, poor growth or weight gain is noted, and palmar creases are pale. The child may appear small for age. The nails are flat, ridged, concave, and spoon-shaped, and they split easily. Splenomegaly and hepatomegaly may be noted on palpation or percussion. Auscultation reveals tachycardia and a systolic flow murmur.

Diagnostic tests:

Test	Results Indicating Disorder	CPT Code
Hemoglobin	Decreased	85018
Hematocrit	Decreased	85014
Reticulocyte count	Reticulocyte count increased	85044
Serum iron	Low	82728
Blood ferritin level	Decreased	82728
Blood lead level	Higher than normal	84655
Free erythrocyte protoporphyrin	Increased	87228
Hemoglobin electrophoresis	Helps to determine which type of anemia is present	83020

Differential diagnosis:

Thalassemia is differentiated by hemoglobin electrophoresis.

Lead poisoning is differentiated by a lead level greater than 10.

Immune disorders that induce anemia are differentiated by a positive Coombs' test.

Sickle cell anemia is differentiated by electrophoresis.

Treatment: Supplemental iron, 6 mg/kg per day in two divided doses, is the most common treatment regimen. If this supplementation increases the hemoglobin by at least 1 g/dL in 1 month, this is considered diagnostic of IDA; therapy is continued for at least 3 months. Another drug now used is ICAR pediatric suspension, which is given at a dose of 1/4 teaspoon per day (15 mg) for no longer than 3 months.

Follow-up: Initially, hematocrit and hemoglobin levels should be obtained 1 month after start of treatment start, then every month for no longer than 5 months to avoid iron overload.

Sequelae: Poor growth rate, learning problems, lethargy, and an increased incidence of infection are common. Iron overload can occur if the child is kept on supplemental iron therapy longer than 5 to 6 months.

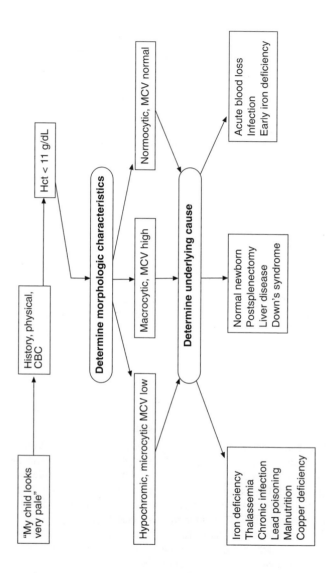

Figure 13–1. Diagnosis of anemia. (Hct, hematocrit; MCV, mean corpuscular volume.)

Prevention/prophylaxis: Routine screening should be done to identify children who have IDA or possibly other anemia. The schedule is as follows:

- Age 6 to 9 months
- Age 1 year, then yearly up to age 12
- Age 13 to 20 years, every 2 to 3 years or if symptoms arise

Referral: If hemoglobin does not increase at least 1 g/dL after 1 month of treatment, refer the child to a physician for further evaluation.

Education: Teach parents that absorption of iron is increased when taken on an empty stomach or given with vitamin C. Nausea, constipation, diarrhea, epigastric pain, and abdominal cramping are common side effects of iron therapy. If these occur, instruct parents to administer iron after a meal. Teach parents safety precautions of iron administration because iron overdose can be fatal. Teach them that iron can turn the stool black. Patients should administer the iron drops by putting the tip of the dropper in the back of the mouth to avoid staining the teeth. Instruct parents to limit milk intake to 16 oz per day; limit empty caloric consumption; and increase age-appropriate, iron-rich foods.

ANEMIA, SICKLE CELL

SIGNAL SYMPTOMS persistently low hemoglobin and hematocrit that is unresponsive to pharmacologic intervention; a painful or vaso-occlusive crisis

Sickle cell anemia   ICD-9 CM: 282.6

Description: *Sickle cell disease* is a term for a group of genetic disorders characterized by production of hemoglobin S (HbS), anemia, and acute and chronic tissue damage secondary to the blockage of blood flow produced by abnormally shaped cells. Sickling of the cells may develop spontaneously or may be precipitated by infection, exposure to cold, dehydration, low oxygen molecular tension acidosis, or localized hypoxia. Today 85% of all persons affected with sickle cell anemia, or hemoglobin SS (HbSS), survive to age 20. The principal cause of death in infants with HbSS is overwhelming infections, cerebrovascular accident, and acute splenic sequestration crisis. Other sickle cell diseases include hemoglobin SC (HbSC) (1 in 835 African-Americans affected) and sickle β-thalassemia (1 in 1667 African-Americans affected).

Etiology: Genetic causes are responsible for SS disease (Table 13–1).

Table 13–1   Genetic Causes of Sickle Cell

Parent Traits	S	s
S	SS	Ss
s	Ss	Ss

SS, sickle cell disease; s, no disease; Ss, carrier of sickle cell trait

For each birth, if the genetic code is trait/carrier, there is a 25% chance of having the disease, 25% chance of not having disease or being a carrier, or 50% chance of being a carrier. If the code is no trait or disease, there is a 50% chance of not being a carrier or 50% chance of being a carrier.

It is recommended that all infants at age 4 months, regardless of racial or ethnic background, be screened for sickle cell disease if they were not screened at birth or if no reliable record of such screening exists. There are three reasons why this screening is necessary:

Prophylactic penicillin can decrease mortality and morbidity.

It is impossible to define accurately a person's heritage by physical appearance or surname.

Screening should benefit all equally.

Screening should be linked to other newborn screening tests, if possible, to facilitate collection, identification, and handling. Clinical manifestations are minimal before age 4 months because of the presence of fetal hemoglobin.

Occurrence: HbSS is the most common type of sickle cell disease, and it is estimated that it affects more than 50,000 Americans.

Age: Present at birth (genetically transmitted).

Ethnicity: Currently, approximately 1 in 375 African-Americans is affected with HbSS. Approximately 8% of the U.S. population have sickle cell trait. HbSS also affects persons from Mediterranean, Caribbean, South and Central American, Arabian, and East Indian descent.

Gender: Occurs equally in males and females.

Contributing factors: Because HbSS is caused by an abnormal recessive mutation by the G-globin gene, the parents' genetic code is the most significant contributing factor.

Signs and symptoms: The primary caregiver reports a history of poor growth with episodes of poor feeding and irritability. The child has a family history of sickle cell disease or trait (Fig. 13–2). There may be periods of pain reported, which varies in severity. The parent also may give a history of frequent bouts of acute upper respiratory or gastrointestinal infections.

The health care provider observes that the child is small for age. There may be pronounced or mild scleral jaundice. Hands and feet may be swollen. The child may appear pale, fatigued, or in pain. Splenomegaly and cardiomegaly (in older children) can be palpated. There may be pain on palpation of joints or abdomen or in the muscles. Severe abdominal pain with rebound may indicate gallbladder disease. When hemoglobin is extremely low, often a murmur is heard. A loose or dry hacking cough or pneumonia may indicate acute chest syndrome.

In a vaso-occlusive crisis, there may be a painful, prolonged erection (priapism). The child may have fast or difficult breathing, chest pain,

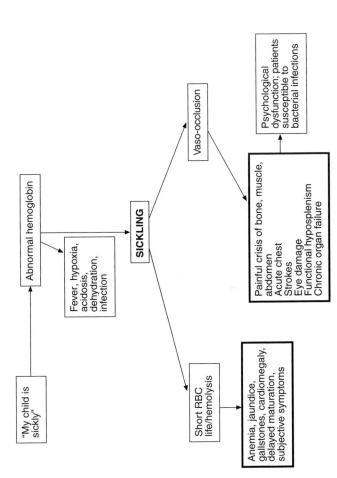

Figure 13–2. Evaluation of sickle cell anemia. (RBC, red blood cell.)

Table 13–2 Signs and Symptoms of Vaso-occlusive Crisis

Area	Signs and Symptoms
Hand-foot syndrome	Patient <5 years, painful swelling of hand and foot
Bone crisis	Painful bones, usually occurs at ages 3–4 years; rule out osteomyelitis
Abdominal crisis	Infarctions in liver, spleen, and lymph nodes
Central nervous system crisis	Convulsions, meningeal signs, cerebral infarction, blindness, vertigo, and acute mental syndrome
Acute chest	Pleuritic chest pain, dyspnea, fever; rule out pneumonitis
Priapism	Predisposing factors: sexual intercourse, masturbation, local trauma, and impotence
Hematuria	Mild, painless
Interhepatic crisis	Sudden onset of painful, enlarged liver; increase in bilirubin and liver enzyme levels

fever, rales, and decreased breath sounds. There may be loss of consciousness or dysfunction of an extremity (painful or not); for example, the child may drag a foot or stop using a hand. The median age for stroke in these children is 7 years (Table 13–2).

Diagnostic tests:

Test	Result Indicating Disorder	CPT Code
Hemoglobin electrophoresis	90% HbS, normal HbA_2, 10% HbF	83020
Complete blood count	Increased WBCs, increased platelets, decreased hematocrit and hemoglobin	85007
Reticulocyte count	5–15%	85044
Peripheral smear	Contains target and sickled cells	85060
Hemoglobin	Results between 5 and 9	85021
Erythrocyte sedimentation rate	Slow	85652

WBCs, white blood cells.

Differential diagnosis:

Rheumatoid arthritis produces an elevated anti–streptolysin O titer.
Anemia (macrocytic or microcytic) is differentiated by complete blood count.
Thalassemia is differentiated by hemoglobin electrophoresis.
Pneumonia is seen on x-ray and not accompanied by other signs of sickle cell anemia.

Treatment:

Nonpharmacologic

For children with sickle cell anemia, well-child care should be provided on the same schedule as for disease-free patients; take each visit as an opportunity to reinforce previous teaching. Office visits are scheduled every other month for the first year of life, then quarterly for the second year of life; the schedule after this depends on the severity of the disease.

Clinical Pearl: Children with sickle cell disease are often zinc deficient. Consider 10 mg per day of elemental zinc daily to avoid growth deficits and delayed development.

Pharmacologic
Penicillin prophylaxis should begin by age 2 months for infants suspected of having definitive sickle cell disease ($<$3 years old, 125 mg twice daily; $>$3 years old, 250 mg twice daily). This therapy is usually discontinued by age 6. Folic acid should also be given for life, 1 μg per day.

 Clinical Pearl: Fever in infants with sickle cell disease should be treated as an emergency. Parents should avoid giving aspirin because it may increase acidosis; acetaminophen should be used.

Hydroxyurea, an antineoplastic drug, is currently being investigated for the palliative treatment of sickle cell disease. It is thought that because hydroxyurea increases the production of HbF, it would inhibit the polymerization of HbS.

Treatment of complications, specifically a vaso-occlusive crisis, includes the following.

Acute chest syndrome: Hospitalization, hydration, oxygen, antibiotics, and transfusions are indicated.

Stroke: Periodic RBC transfusions are the best therapy for preventing recurrence of stroke. Neurologic workup should include magnetic resonance imaging and transcranial ultrasound, if possible.

Hand-and-foot syndrome: Analgesics and hydration with application of warm compresses, massage, or warm baths may provide relief.

Priapism: Hospitalization is indicated, with possible evacuation of pooled blood.

Severe abdominal pain: Hydration, analgesia, gallbadder x-ray, and hospitalization are indicated.

Acute splenic sequestration crisis: Treatment is immediate restoration of blood volume by RBC transfusion and possible splenectomy (after age 2 years).

Aplastic anemia: Treatment is RBC transfusion.

Follow-up: Regular scheduled health care should be maintained, with all episodes of pain and fever being reported to the health care provider.
Sequelae: Short stature or delayed physical growth and sexual maturation, stroke, pain, gallbladder disease, and multiple crises.

Acute splenic sequestration crisis: Sudden entrapment of a large portion of the blood volume in the spleen occurs with cardiovascular compromise similar to hypovolemia (peak age, 6 months to 2 years).

Aplastic crisis: Temporary arrest of RBC production in the bone marrow occurs, usually caused by a parvovirus infection (this is transient).

Prevention/prophylaxis: None. This is a congenital, genetic disease.

Referral: Refer patient to a pediatric hematologist or the local sickle cell clinic for overall maintenance and during times of severe crisis. Otherwise, for routine care, the nurse practitioner can oversee the child's health regimen.

Education: Teach caregivers to recognize the signs and symptoms of the disease and to manage treatment on their own, provided that the child is afebrile. Specific instructions should be given with regard to oral fluid therapy, analgesics, and antipyretics. Teach caregivers the following precautions to minimize vaso-occlusive episodes: (1) Prevent dehydration (especially in warm weather); (2) shield child from the cold (slows circulation and increases stasis); and (3) make sure child avoids immersion in cold water, dresses warmly, gets adequate rest, and avoids wearing constrictive clothes.

CAT-SCRATCH FEVER

SIGNAL SYMPTOMS▶   scratch embellished by papule or vesicle

Cat-scratch fever	ICD-9 CM: 078.3

Description: Cat-scratch fever is characterized by regional lymphadenopathy after contact with cats or kittens that harbor the bacteria responsible for the disease. The nodes usually affected are the parotid, preauricular, axillary, epitrochlear, and inguinal. From the initial scratch to the primary cutaneous lesion to lymphadenopathy, there is a median incubation period of 12 days or in some cases 50 days.

Etiology: A scratch from a cat harboring the causative agent *Bartonella henselae* (formerly called *Rochalimaea henselae* or *Afipier felis*). The cat flea, *Ctenocephalides felis felis,* is responsible for cat-to-cat transmission.

Occurrence: Approximately 20,000 cases occur in the United States each year. Occurs more frequently in fall and winter.

Age: Occurs primarily in children and persons younger than age 20.

Ethnicity: Not significant.

Gender: Occurs equally in males and females.

Contributing factors: Contact with a cat.

Signs and symptoms: The child presents with malaise, fatigue, and a low-grade fever. The parent or child provides information regarding contact with a cat or kittens within the known incubation period.

Physical examination reveals a crusted papule, vesiculopustule, or ulcer at the site of the scratch or inoculation. There are enlarged, tender, single or multiple lymph nodes proximal to the scratch site. The most serious scratch sites involve the eyelid or conjunctiva. Atypical presentations, such as acute encephalopathy, Perinaud's oculoglandular syndrome, or acute facial nerve paralysis, occur in 11% of children.

Diagnostic tests:

Test	Results Indicating Disorder	CPT Code
Cat-scratch skin test (antigen may be difficult to obtain)	Test is positive	87229
Aspiration of node and use of Warthin-Starry silver stain (not usually done)	Identification of causative agent	38542
Erythrocyte sedimentation rate	Elevated	85651
ELISA for *B. henselae* titers	Positive	87449

ELISA, enzyme-linked immunosorbent assay.

 Clinical Pearl: An incision and drainage of the lesion should not be done because of the risk of chronic draining sinus.

Differential diagnosis:

Infectious mononucleosis has presence of soft palate petechiae and enlargement of posterior and anterior cervical nodes.

Treatment: Trimethoprim-sulfamethoxazole, 20 to 40 mg/kg per day for 7 days, may be helpful; routine treatment is not recommended.

Follow-up: Return in 1 week for evaluation of enlarged nodes and the primary lesion.

Sequelae: Rare complications include encephalitis, osteolytic lesions, hepatitis, and chronic systemic illness.

Prevention/prophylaxis: Avoid situations in which children could be scratched. Keep cats free from fleas. Immunosuppressed children should avoid contact with kittens less than 1 year old. All cat scratches should be cleansed thoroughly to decrease the risk of infection.

Referral: None, unless the progression of the recovery is not timely or the signs and symptoms of complications are observed.

Education: Teach children how to handle pets properly to reduce the risk of being scratched.

CYTOMEGALOVIRUS

SIGNAL SYMPTOMS fever, hepatomegaly, splenomegaly, motor retardation

Cytomegalovirus (CMV)	ICD-9 CM: 078.5

Description: CMV is a human herpesvirus transmitted by intrauterine transfer, maternal milk, secretions in the birth canal (incubation period 2–6 weeks), saliva of playmates, sexual partners, transfusions (incubation period 2–4 weeks), and transplanted organs. Infection may range from acute, severe illness to a mild, self-limiting illness. CMV is harbored in the body and may be reactivated.

Etiology: Infection through intrauterine or milk transfer or contact with secretions harboring the virus, such as saliva and urine.

Occurrence: Estimated congenital infection is 1% to 2% of all newborns; 10% of these are symptomatic, and an estimated 75% of children in day care centers are viral excreters.

Age: The infection may occur during the perinatal period; it can be found in newborns, older children, adolescents, and immunosuppressed children.

Ethnicity: Not significant.

Gender: Occurs equally in males and females.

Contributing factors: Infection of the mother during the first half of pregnancy, infection in the birth canal, viral shedding in maternal milk, blood transfusions, contact with secretions of infected children.

Signs and symptoms:

Congenital infections: Hepatosplenomegaly, jaundice, purpura, microcephaly, cerebral calcifications, chorioretinitis, petechial rash with splenomegaly on first day of life, spasticity, and hypertonia.

Acquired infections: Pneumonia; paroxysmal, nonproductive cough; no chest pain; and fatigue, myalgia, and headache.

Diagnostic tests:

Newborn

Test	Results Indicating Disorder	CPT Code
Complete blood count	Anemia, thrombocytopenia, lymphocytosis	85007
Spinal tap	Elevated protein and pleocytosis	62270
Culture of urine, saliva, stool, and spinal fluid	Identification of organism	87999
IgM antibody titer	Elevated	82657
Radiographs of skull	Microcephaly and periventricular calcification	70250
Radiographs of long bones	"Celery stick" pattern	73592
Radiographs of chest	Interstitial pneumonia	71010–71035

Infants and Children

Test	Results Indicating Disorder	CPT Code
Complete blood count	Anemia, atypical lymphocytes, thrombocytopenia	85007
Liver function studies	Normal; mild rise in aminotransferase levels	84450–84460
CMV antibody titer	Elevated	86644–86645
Culture of secretions	Virus isolated	87999
Radiographs of chest	Diffuse interstitial pneumonia	71010

Immunosuppressed Children

Test	Results Indicating Disorder	CPT Code
Complete blood count	Neutropenia, atypical lymphocytosis, thrombocytopenia	85007
Serum aminotranferase	Elevated	84450–84460
Radiographs of chest	Interstitial pneumonia	71010
Culture of secretions	Virus isolated	87999

Differential diagnosis:

Infants

Toxoplasmosis is more likely to be associated with hydrocephalus, microphthalmia, and chorioretinitis.

Hepatitis B produces elevated aspartate transaminase (AST) greater than 800 U/L.

Lymphocytic choriomeningitis virus is confirmed by serologic studies.

Children and Adolescents

Infectious mononucleosis produces pharyngitis and lymphadenopathy and is caused by Epstein-Barr virus (EBV).

Immunosuppressed Children

Bacterial and fungal infections are in the differential.

Radiation pneumonitis is in the differential.

Treatment: For retinitis, give ganciclovir, 5 mg/kg intravenously twice daily for 14 to 21 days, or foscarnet, 60 mg/kg intravenously every 8 hours for 14 to 21 days (not recommended in children because drug is deposited in bone, teeth, and cartilage and causes renal impairment).

Follow-up: For infants with congenital infection, observe growth and development closely.

Sequelae: Mortality rate in infants with congenital infection is 30%. Infection in newborns may result in delayed development and hearing loss (5–15% of asymptomatic infants born with the virus); during the perinatal period, severe pneumonia may result from the infection. In immunosuppressed children, the possible retinitis may result in blindness.

Prevention/prophylaxis: Screening of blood and milk donors for the presence of CMV.

Referral: Refer patient to a pediatrician for admission to the hospital for intravenous therapy.

Education: Teach parents to practice proper hand-washing techniques and not to allow sharing of eating utensils. Emphasize the importance of CMV screening of donors of blood, milk, and organs for transplant.

DIPHTHERIA

SIGNAL SYMPTOMS ▶ red pharynx with gray membrane in tonsillar areas, fever

| Diphtheria | ICD-9CM: 032.1 |

Description: Diphtheria is an acute infection of the upper respiratory tract or the skin with an incubation period of 1 to 6 days. Laryngeal diphtheria is characterized by the formation of a gray membrane over the pharynx, causing respiratory difficulties, cervical lymphadenopathy, and edema of the neck ("bull neck").

 Clinical Pearl: Diphtheria is a reportable disease.

Etiology: The causative agent is the toxin-forming *Corynebacterium diphtheriae,* a gram-positive, club-shaped rod.

Occurrence: Five or fewer cases are reported each year.

Age: All ages.

Ethnicity: Not significant.

Gender: Occurs equally in males and females.

Contributing factors: Nonimmunized children and adults; the presence of carriers within the community.

Signs and symptoms: The parent gives a history of a mild sore throat, moderate fever, and malaise that abruptly progresses to severe prostration. The child is usually taken to the clinic at this time.

Physical examination reveals an acutely ill child with a rapid pulse not related to the fever and a pharyngeal grayish membrane surrounded by an area of erythema and edema. The cervical lymph nodes are swollen, resulting in an associated swelling of the neck. There is respiratory stridor.

Diagnostic tests:

Test	Results Indicating Disorder	CPT Code
Nasal smears from nose and throat on Löffler's and tellurite agar (require 16–48 hr)	Identification of organism	87999
Complete blood count	Evidence of hemolytic anemia and thrombocytopenia with rapid destruction of RBCs; WBCs usually normal	85007

Differential diagnosis:

Streptococcal pharyngitis is differentiated by the absence of a pharyngeal grayish membrane.

Infectious mononucleosis produces lymphedema and hepatosplenomegaly.

Laryngeal obstruction may be a result of epiglottitis; observe for characteristic posture and "drooling." In cases of suspected epiglottitis, do not examine the pharynx.

Treatment: Within the first 48 hours, administer diphtheria antitoxin. Administer penicillin G, 150,000 mg/kg per day intravenously for 10 days. If patient is penicillin-allergic, administer erythromycin, 40 mg/kg per day orally in three to four divided doses for 10 days. Admit to the hospital, and isolate for 1 to 7 days; usual hospital stay is 10 to 14 days. Three consecutive negative throat cultures, beginning 24 hours after completion of antibiotic regimen, are required before lifting isolation.

Restrict carriers to the home. Administer erythromycin, 40 mg/kg per day orally in three or four divided doses for 10 days; penicillin V, 50 mg/kg per day; or benzathine penicillin G, 600,000 to 1,200,000 U intramuscularly (IM). Three consecutive negative throat cultures, beginning 24 hours after completion of antibiotic regimen, are required before lifting isolation. For immunized household contacts, observe for signs of illness.

Follow-up: Weekly follow-up after hospitalization for cardiac and neurologic evaluations.

Sequelae: Myocarditis occurs 2 to 40 days after the onset of the illness; characterized by a rapid, thready pulse, ST-T wave changes, arrhythmias, hepatomegaly, and fluid retention. Polyneuritis occurs during the first or second week after onset. The nerves involving the palate and the pharynx, then the optic nerve, and later the peripheral motor nerves are affected. Bronchopneumonia is often fatal.

Prevention/prophylaxis: Routine childhood immunizations.

Referral: Refer patient for hospitalization.

Education: Instruct parents in the importance of immunizations.

HUMAN HERPESVIRUS 6

SIGNAL SYMPTOMS▶ rose-pink macular rash, discrete, preceded by high fever

Human herpesvirus 6 (HHV-6)   ICD-9 CM: 057.0

Description: HHV-6 infection, formerly called *roseola infantum* or *exanthem subitum*, is a viral illness characterized by a high fever lasting 3 to 7 days. The fever is followed by an erythematous, discrete, rose-pink macular or maculopapular rash, which lasts 6 hours to 3 days. (Fig. 13–3). The virus has been associated with multiple sclerosis. The virus may become reactivated in an immunocompromised child.

Etiology: Infection caused by HHV-6. Virus is excreted in blood during the first 5 days of infection and subsequently in saliva and stool but rarely in urine.

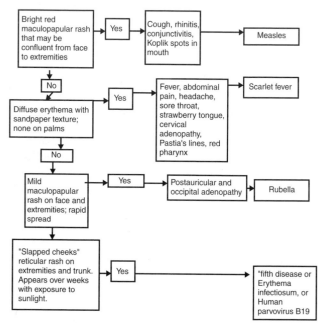

Figure 13–3. Determining the cause of a red rash.

Occurrence: Common; no seasonal variation.

Age: Occurs in children 3 months to 4 years old; 90% of cases occur in children younger than 2 years.

Ethnicity: Not significant.

Gender: Occurs equally in males and females.

Contributing factors: Exposure to the virus; immunosuppression. Increased risk factors may include poverty and multiple siblings.

Signs and symptoms: Child had a high fever for several days and now has a red rash reported to start initially on the trunk. May have a history of vomiting and mild diarrhea. Physical examination reveals the presence of a small, discrete, rose-pink macular or maculopapular rash.

Diagnostic tests: None.

Differential diagnosis:

Measles has accompanying coryza, runny nose, cough, conjunctivitis, and Koplik spots present. The rash usually starts on the face.

Rubella has incubation period of 14 to 21 days, with prodromal respiratory symptoms and postauricular and occipital nodes. The maculopapular rash begins on the face.

Scarlet fever has usual age of onset of 2 to 10 years; the rash is erythematous and diffuse and has a sandpaper texture. Scarlet tongue and Pastia's sign are noted; there is no rash on the face.

Erythema infectiosum is characterized by the "slapped cheeks" appearance and by the distribution and lacy pattern of the rash.

Treatment: Treatment is supportive. Give acetaminophen, as needed, for fever control; increase fluid intake.

Follow-up: None.

Sequelae: Approximately 10% of children experience febrile seizures. Reactivation of the virus occurs only in immunosuppressed patients. In rare cases, encephalitis can occur.

Prevention/prophylaxis: None.

Referral: None.

Education: Teach parents the importance of adequate fluid intake and methods of fever control.

HUMAN IMMUNODEFICIENCY VIRUS AND ACQUIRED IMMUNODEFICIENCY SYNDROME

SIGNAL SYMPTOMS known exposure of an infant to maternal HIV; recurrent feeding, weight gain, or immune system problems

Acquired immunodeficiency syndrome (AIDS)	ICD-9 CM: 042
HIV illness	ICD-9 CM: 042
HIV infection	ICD-9 CM: 08
HIV-2 infection	ICD-9 CM: 079.53

Description: HIV infection, with AIDS being the end of its clinical course, causes the slow demise of the body's immune system, affecting the renal, cardiac, integumentary, respiratory, neurologic, and gastrointestinal systems. When the body's immune system is unable to thwart any form of infection, AIDS results. AIDS is fatal in nearly all cases. There are a few long-term survivors, but their ultimate outcome is still uncertain.

Etiology: AIDS is caused by HIV-1 and less commonly by HIV-2. It is an RNA cytopathic retrovirus.

Occurrence: Childhood AIDS is the ninth leading cause of death in children aged 1 to 4 years and seventh in adolescents and adults aged 15 to 24. Childhood AIDS constitutes 2% of all reported cases of AIDS in the United States. Approximately 8% to 10% of infants HIV-positive at birth remain positive and die of AIDS when mother and infant have received appropriate prophylaxis.

Age: Infancy and adolescence are the most common age groups.

Ethnicity: Not significant.

Gender: Occurs equally in males and females.

Contributing factors: Transplacental transmission of HIV, contact with body fluids of HIV-positive persons, unprotected sexual activity with multiple partners, transfusions of contaminated blood, and sharing of needles among persons with needle-dependent drug addiction.

Signs and symptoms: The infant may be brought to the clinic because of feeding problems, recurrent diarrhea, persistent or recurrent diaper rashes or generalized rashes, or respiratory problems. Older children may present with fever, myalgia, sore throat, lymphadenopathy, or rash. Clinical manifestations of HIV infection include generalized lymphadenopathy, hepatomegaly, splenomegaly, oral candidiasis, parotitis, and cardiomyopathy. There may also be developmental delay, failure to thrive, and pneumonia (most serious cases caused by *Pneumocystis carinii*). Chronic parotid swelling is common in children with AIDS. Kaposi's sarcoma and B-cell lymphoma are rare in children with AIDS.

Diagnostic tests:

Test	Results Indicating Disorder	CPT Code
Western blot	Positive	86689
Polymerase chain reaction	Positive	83898
CD4 helper T suppressor cell	Decreased	86360
Erythrocyte sedimentation rate	Increased	85651
Hemoglobin and hematocrit	Decreased	83051
Immune complex assay	Increased	86332
Hepatic function panel	Increased	80076
Complete blood count	Lymphocytosis, leukopenia, neutropenia, thrombocytopenia	85031
Lactate dehydrogenase	Elevated	83615

Differential diagnosis:

Failure to thrive is differentiated by evaluating for feeding problems related to poor parenting skills or other physical causes.

For central nervous system disorders, atrophy and calcification in the basal ganglion and the frontal lobe may be shown on imaging studies in patients with brain infections.

Anemias are differentiated by low leukocyte count and elevated erythrocyte sedimentation rate.

For systemic candidiasis, evaluate for diabetes.

For pneumonia, observe for evidence of atypical findings on chest x-ray. Lymphoid interstitial pneumonitis produces diffuse interstitial reticulonodular infiltrates, often with hilar adenopathy.

Treatment: Treatment of presenting systemic manifestation. The predominant drug used for treatment of AIDS is zidovudine (AZT), 2 mg/kg per dose four times daily for the first 6 weeks of life. After 1 month of age, trimethoprim-sulfamethoxazole (Bactrim) is added. In older children, treatment regimens must follow guidelines for antiviral treatment and recommendations for starting regimens (Table 13–3).

Preferred initial treatment involves any of the following combinations:

Table 13–3   Guidelines for Initiating Antiretroviral Therapy

Clinical Category	CD4 cell count	Plasma HIV RNA	Recommendations
Symptomatic	Any value	Any value	Treat
Asymptomatic AIDS	Any value	Any value	Treat
Asymptomatic	CD4 200–350 cells/mm^3	Any value	Treatment usually offered with viral loads of <20,000 cells/mL owing to lower probability of AIDS-defining diagnosis within 3 years
Asymptomatic	CD4 >350 cells/mm^3	>30,000 (bDNAO) or >55,000 (RT-PCR)	Still some controversy whether to initiate treatment because these levels are at viral threshold. When doubt exists, monitor CD4 cell count*

* CD4 counts <350 and with any viral load count should be treated. CD4 counts of 350 to 500 but viral loads >5000 should be treated. If the viral load is <5000, it is up to the protocol at the particular clinic. With CD4 counts >500 and viral loads <5000, treatment is deferred, and values are monitored. If viral loads are 5000 to 30,000, treatment may be considered but is not required. Treatment should be started with viral loads >30,000,
Source: DHHS Guidelines. Contact: www.hivatis.org. August 22, 2001.

- Two nucleosides and a protease inhibitor (PI)
- Two nucleosides and two PIs
- Two nucleosides and a nucleoside analogue reverse transcriptase inhibitor (NNRTI)

Because the regimens are constantly evolving and new drugs are becoming available, the nurse practitioner should consult the HIV website or an HIV center for current recommendations for efficacious treatment. The above-listed regimen can serve as a guideline for the nurse practitioner. The following are the most commonly used drugs for antiviral therapy for children.

Amprenavir (Agenerase) (PI). This agent is not recommended in children younger than 4 years old. For children 4 to 12 or 13 to 16 but weighing less than 50 kg, use oral solution 22.5 mg/kg twice daily or 17 mg/kg three times daily with a maximum dose of 2.8 g per day. For children 13 to 16 and weighing greater than 50 kg, give 1.4 g twice daily.

Lamivudine (Epivir) (NNRTI), solution 10 mg/1 mL. For children 3 months to 16 years, give 4 mg/kg twice daily with maximum dose of 150 mg twice daily.

Hivid (NNRTI). For children older than 6 months and weighing 7 to 14 kg, give 12 mg/3 mg per kg; for children weighing 15 to 40 kg, give 10 mg/2.5 mg per kg. For children weighing more than 40 kg, maximum dose is 400 mg/100 mg twice daily.

Zidovudine (Retrovir) (NNRTI) syrup 50/5. For children 6 weeks to 12 years, give 160 mg/m^2 every 8 hours with a maximum dose of 200 mg.

Efavirenz (Sustiva) (NNRTI) 50-, 100-, and 200-mg capsules. Pretreat children with antihistamines. For children older than 3 years, give 200 mg daily; for children weighing 15 to 25 kg, give 150 mg daily; for children weighing 20 to 25 kg, give 300 mg daily; for children weighing 25 to 32.5 kg, give 350 mg daily; for children weighing 32.5 to 40 kg, give 400 mg daily; and for children weighing more than 40 kg, give 600 mg daily. (Avoid high-fat meals when taking this drug.)

Nelfinavir (Viracept) (PI). For children 2 to 13 years, give 20 to 30 mg/kg three times daily with a maximum dose of 750 mg three times daily; for children older than 13, give 1.25 mg twice daily with a maximum dose of 750 mg twice daily.

Nevirapine (Viramune) (NNRTI). This agent is not recommended for children younger than 2 months. For children 2 months to 8 years, give 4 mg/kg per day for 14 days if no rash, then increase to 7 mg/kg twice daily. For children 8 years, initially give 4 mg/kg per day and if no rash increase to twice daily.

Stavudine (Zerit) (NNRTI) liquid 1 mg/mL. For children weighing less than 30 kg, initially give 1 mg/kg every 12 hours. For children weighing more than 30 kg, give 40 mg every 12 hours. Withdraw drug immediately if peripheral neuropathy occurs.

Acyclovir (Zovirax) (nucleoside analogue) 200 mg/5 mL. Give 2 mg/kg per dose four times daily for 6 weeks. Then consult for increases in dosage.

Note: Other drugs may be used and in different combinations; it is in the best interest of the child to consult an established HIV center.

Follow-up: Follow-up for "well-baby" care should be done at routine intervals. All usual immunizations should be given with the exception of oral polio vaccine. Measles-mumps-rubella vaccine should be given at 12 months if there is no severe immunosuppression. Influenza vaccine should be given every year after age 6 months with the pneumococcus vaccine administered every 3 years after age 2 years. At present, varicella vaccine is not indicated because of insufficient data, but most health care providers administer Varivax if no serious immunosuppression is noted. Coordinate activities with an AIDS health care treatment center.

Sequelae: Ultimately death occurs. In children with perinatal infections, survival ranges from 2.5 months to 10 years. In persons infected later—through blood transfusions, unprotected sex, or the sharing of needles—incubation is longer, and the survival period is longer.

Prevention/prophylaxis: Use of a latex condom, especially one with nonoxynol 9, is important in breaking the chain of the spread of disease. Avoidance of exchange of any and all bodily fluids helps to decrease the risk of HIV infection. Needle-dependent drug addicts should not share needles. An AIDS vaccine is not available at this time.

Referral: Refer HIV-positive patients and children with a presumptive diagnosis of AIDS to an AIDS treatment facility for treatment.

Education: Provide education for patients, their families, and the community related to resources and treatment options. Educate parents about the overall disease process and survival rates. Caution parents to report all health changes to the health care provider immediately. This should be done because often opportunistic infections can worsen the prognosis when left untreated. Make counseling available to the child and the parents.

HUMAN PARVOVIRUS B19 (ERYTHEMA INFECTIOSUM)

SIGNAL SYMPTOMS▶ maculopapular lesions on face ("slapped cheek"), trunk, buttocks, and extremities; lacy pattern

Human parvovirus B19	ICD-9 CM: 057.0

Description: Infection with human parvovirus B19, commonly called *fifth disease,* is a mild, contagious, erythematous illness characterized by mild flu-like symptoms that diminish in about 3 days, followed in 7 to 10 days by a characteristic rash that is mildly pruritic. The rash fades but may be exacerbated by sunlight (e.g., warm baths) or stress. The rash is considered to be an immune response to the virus. The child is contagious until the eruption of the rash. Spread occurs by respiratory droplets.

Etiology: The causative agent is human parvovirus B19, not the canine variety.

Occurrence: Common, usually in winter or spring outbreaks.

Age: Usually occurs in school-age children, ages 5 to 15 years.

Ethnicity: Not significant.

Gender: Occurs equally in males and females.

Contributing factors: Contact with the respiratory droplets (via coughing) of an infected person.

Signs and symptoms: The child presents with a red rash that the parent states started on the face and spread to the trunk, buttocks, and extremities. There may be a recollection of contact with an infected person. There may be a history of a mild flu-like illness (low-grade fever, malaise, sore throat, coryza) 7 to 10 days before the eruption of the rash (50%). The parent, depending on the timing of the visit, may report that the rash had faded and has now reappeared.

Examination of the skin reveals maculopapular lesions on the face ("slapped cheek"), trunk, buttocks, and extremities, especially the thighs. The palms, soles, and circumoral area are rash-free. The confluent lesions with central clearing give the characteristically lacy appearance. The rash may feel warm.

Diagnostic tests:

Test	Results Indicating Disorder	CPT Code
Complete blood count	Mild leukopenia followed by leukocytosis and lymphocytosis	85007
Serum IgM	Elevated	82657
Serum IgG	Elevated	86001

Viral cultures are of no clinical use.

Differential diagnosis:

Measles is differentiated by prodromal symptoms.

Rubella is differentiated by lymphadenopathy.

Scarlet fever has pharyngitis and other systemic symptoms.

Treatment:

Nonpharmacologic

Comfort measures include cool baths. Avoid sunlight and heat exposure, scratching, and warm baths.

Pharmacologic

If itching is acute, may give an age-appropriate antipruritic.

Follow-up: Usually none.

Sequelae: Children with chronic hemolytic anemia are at risk for the development of aplastic crisis. In immunosuppressed children, a pancytopenia may develop. If the adolescent patient is pregnant, the fetus is at increased risk for hydrops fetalis. Older adolescents may have a reactive arthritis for 2 to 4 weeks after the rash.

Prevention/prophylaxis: None. By the time these children are examined, they are usually no longer contagious.

Referral: Refer child to a pediatrician in cases of suspected complications.

Education: Instruct parent and child about prolonged exposure to sunlight and other factors that may exacerbate the reappearance of the rash.

INFECTIOUS MONONUCLEOSIS

SIGNAL SYMPTOMS red pharynx with petechiae on palate and uvula

Infectious mononucleosis	ICD-9 CM: 075

Description: Infectious mononucleosis, known as the "kissing disease," is an acute, self-limiting, communicable disease caused by EBV. It is transmitted through nasal or oropharyngeal secretions. The incubation period is 30 to 50 days; recovery usually takes 3 to 6 weeks, and recurrence is rare. In most cases, the disease is mild, but some fatalities have been noted when severe liver damage occurs or in otherwise immunocompromised individuals.

Etiology: Contact with EBV.

Occurrence: Common.

Age: Occurs primarily in adolescents.

Ethnicity: Not significant.

Gender: Occurs equally in males and females.

Contributing factors: Contact with the saliva of playmates and family members; contact with symptomatic carriers.

Signs and symptoms: Young children may have no symptoms or a mild, nonspecific febrile episode; older children complain of sore throat, malaise, anorexia, and swollen glands. Parents may not be able to identify the contact source.

Physical findings include enlarged, firm, mildly tender lymph nodes, particularly the posterior and anterior cervical nodes. On palpation, there may be an enlarged spleen (50% of cases) and an enlarged liver (30% of cases), which are frequently tender. Swelling of the eyelids is frequently observed, as are petechiae on the soft palate. A macular, scarlatiniform, or urticarial rash may be present.

Diagnostic tests:

Test	Results Indicating Disorder	CPT Code
Complete blood count	Leukopenia early, lymphocytosis. Changes may not be noted until third week of illness	85057
Monospot test	Positive if titer is significant. 50% positive in first weeks, 90% positive by fourth week. Usually negative in children <5 years old	86308
Heterophil antibodies	90% older children positive, <50% positive in children <5 years old. Does not appear until after second week of illness. May continue to be positive for 1 year	86308– 86310
Bilirubin	Slightly elevated	82247
AST	Elevated; 4 × normal value	84450
Anti-EBV antibodies	Detection of IgM antibody to the viral capsid antigen or the rise of IgG antibody after several weeks; detection of IgG–viral capsid antigen antibody with absence of Epstein-Barr nuclear antigen late in the illness	86663– 86665

 Clinical Pearl: If child is not allergic to penicillin, give penicillin or ampicillin, 250 mg single dose, and wait for the eruption of the characteristic rash.

Differential diagnosis:

Lymphadenopathy has more generalized adenopathy.

In pharyngitis/streptococcal infection, there is no splenomegaly; neutrophilic leukocytosis is present.

In hepatitis, there is no splenomegaly; liver function studies are grossly abnormal.

Rubella has atypical lymphocytosis, but pharyngitis is unremarkable; there is no marked adenopathy and splenomegaly, and the illness has a shorter duration.

Adenoviruses have conjunctivitis, mild adenopathy, upper respiratory symptoms (cough), and fewer atypical lymphocytes.

Leukemia is differentiated by peripheral blood smear morphology.

Treatment:

Nonpharmacologic

Symptomatic treatment is as follows:

- Increased fluid intake
- Fever control with use of acetaminophen
- Increased rest with children exhibiting fatigue
- Exclusion from school or attendance on a part-time basis
- Exclusion from sports activities until danger of liver involvement is past
- Exclusion from sports in cases of splenomegaly for 6 to 8 weeks

Pharmacologic

For pharyngitis symptoms, administer penicillin V, 250 mg four times a day for 10 days.

Follow-up: Follow-up at 2-week intervals for evaluation of splenomegaly and further hematologic and antibody evaluations.

Sequelae: Hepatitis, splenic rupture, and encephalitis are uncommon complications. For children with immunosuppression, induced either by genetics or chemotherapy, progressive EBV infections may develop.

Prevention/prophylaxis: No kissing of known contacts or use of utensils that foster the transfer of infective agents through saliva.

Referral: Refer patients with liver, spleen, neurologic, or hematologic involvement to pediatrician or internist.

Education: Instruct parents in the importance of limiting activity of children with hepatic or splenic involvement. Instruct parents in the proper handling and cleaning of utensils used by the infected child.

LYME DISEASE

SIGNAL SYMPTOMS ▶ an erythema migrans rash: a round or oval lesion with central clearing

| Lyme disease | ICD-9 CM: 088.81 |

Description: Lyme disease is a tick-borne illness caused by the spirochete *Borrelia burgdorferi*. The characteristic rash may appear within 3 to 30 days of the bite and usually fades within 3 to 4 weeks.

Clinical Pearl: This is a reportable disease.

Etiology: *B. burgdorferi,* a spirochete that lives in the midgut of nymphal and adult deer ticks (*Ixodes dammini,* East and Midwest; *Ixodes pacificus,* West), is passed to humans by bites from infected ticks.

Occurrence: High occurrences in summer and early fall. In the United States, the highest incidence rates are in the Northeast and Mid-Atlantic states; lower rates occur in the North Central, Pacific, and Southeast, with the lowest incidence rates in the Great Plains and Mountain states. Lyme disease also occurs in horses, cattle, dogs, and cats. In 2000, Colorado, Georgia, Hawaii, Montana, New Mexico, and South Dakota reported no cases.

Age: Seen usually in children, age 2 years and older, particularly 5- to 9-year-olds. Cases of gestational Lyme disease have been reported.

Ethnicity: Not significant.

Gender: Slightly more prevalent in males.

Contributing factors: Outdoor activity in an endemic area.

Signs and symptoms: Client has a history of a tick bite.

There are three stages with different clinical manifestations that may overlap.

Stage 1: Skin rash (erythema chronicum migrans) usually appears 3 to 30 days after the bite and gradually expands to form a large, plaque-like, erythematous, nonscaly, annular lesion that may be 20 cm. The central portion of the lesion may be clear, erythematous, and indurated. Lesions are often hot and may burn, prickle, or itch. Lesions occur most commonly in warm, moist areas, such as the popliteal spaces, groin, armpits, and under the breast; lesions are not found in mucosal areas. In less than 10% of patients, smaller secondary annular lesions appear in a few days as a result of dissemination of the spirochete. Duration of an average untreated initial lesion is 3 weeks; it often has a bluish hue and may recur for 1 year or more. Other symptoms are fever, fatigue, headaches, myalgias, malaise, and arthralgias. Flu-like symptoms include fever, malaise, neck pain, and no respiratory or gastrointestinal symptoms.

Stage 2: Occurs 1 week or months after the initial bite. Self-limiting cardiac symptoms are most common in males and last 3 days to 6 weeks. In untreated cases, neurologic complications include meningitis, encephalitis, and cranial neuritis (15–31%). The seventh cranial nerve is the one most frequently involved. Other nerves may be involved, and symptoms may be migratory.

Stage 3: Arthritis begins 4 weeks after the skin lesion. Large joints (most commonly the knees) are affected. Attacks are intermittent, may last for days or weeks, and may recur over 1 year. Arthritis may result in destruction of the joint. Fever may be high.

Diagnostic tests: Diagnosis relies on clinical presentation and a careful history, especially of travel to an endemic area and outdoor activities. The following results confirm the diagnosis.

Test	Results Indicating Disorder	CPT Code
C-reactive protein	Positive	86140
Erythrocyte sedimentation rate	Elevated	85651
ELISA	Antibodies not present until 3–6 weeks after bite; IgM titers positive at values <1:160; IgG titers positive at values <1:320	87449
Spinal fluid (in cases of possible meningitis)	Elevated protein and pleocytosis	87040
Rheumatoid factor	Negative by latex agglutination	86430
Western blot test	Positive	86689

Blood cultures rarely identify the agent.

Differential diagnosis:

Stage 1 rash may be confused with cellulitis, erythema multiforme, erythema marginatum rheumaticum, fungal infections, or eczema. The syndrome may be confused with viral influenza.

Stage 2 may be confused with Bell's palsy, viral meningitis, lead poisoning, or rheumatic fever.

Stage 3 may be confused with arthritis.

Treatment: The earlier effective treatment is initiated, the better the prognosis (Table 13–4).

Follow-up: Monitor treatment and progression of illness, being watchful for complications.

Table 13–4   Treatment of Lyme Disease

Recommended Drug	Dosages for Adults	Dosages for Children
Oral Amoxicillin	500 mg tid	50 mg/kg per day divided in three doses, not to exceed 500 mg per dose
Doxycycline	100 mg bid (not recommended for pregnant or lactating women)	1–2 mg/kg bid, not to exceed 100 mg per dose (not recommended for children <8 years old)
Alternative: Cefuroxime axetil	500 mg bid	30 mg/kg per day bid, not to exceed 500 mg per dose
Parenteral Ceftriaxone	2 g once a day	75–200 mg/kg per day divided into three or four doses, not to exceed 6 g per day
Alternative: Penicillin G	18–24 million U per day divided into doses given q4h	200,000–400,000 U/kg per day divided into doses given q4h, not to exceed 18–24 million U per day

Sequelae: Inadequate treatment may result in cardiac complications, arthritis, and neuropathies.

Prevention/prophylaxis: The following precautions should be taken.

In wooded areas, wear light-colored clothing and tall socks, and tuck pants into boots.

Scan the body for ticks often because ticks may take 24 hours to begin feeding.

Use repellents containing diethyltoluamide (DEET) or permethrin or citronella.

 Clinical Pearl: Do not use products with concentrations of DEET greater than 10%; be careful of children because of systemic absorption. Permethrin should not be applied to a child's skin.

Keep any suspicious ticks labeled with site at which they were obtained and body site.

If symptoms occur, the tick may be checked by the Centers for Disease Control for the presence of the spirochete.

Referral: Consult and collaborate with a physician for confirmation of the diagnosis and plan of care. Report case to state epidemiologist.

Education: Teach parents and community about the tick, the cycle of the organism, and methods for prevention, such as wearing proper clothing and using repellents. Teach parents and children how to remove ticks properly.

When removing a tick, do not squeeze the body of the tick.

Grasp the body of the tick close to the skin with tweezers.

Gently pull straight out without twisting motion. If you use fingers to remove the tick, wear gloves or protect fingers with a tissue and wash hands thoroughly afterward.

MEASLES

SIGNAL SYMPTOMS ▶ red-brown discrete macular rash with blanching with pressure, prodromal Koplik spots on upper buccal mucosa

| Measles | ICD-9 CM: 056.9 |

Description: Measles (rubeola) is an acute, highly contagious viral illness with an incubation period of 8 to 12 days. The disease can be transmitted from the first or second day before to the fifth day after the eruption of the rash.

 Clinical Pearl: This is a reportable disease.

Etiology: *Morbillivirus,* a genus in the Paramyxoviridae family.

Occurrence: Occurs more frequently in the winter and spring.

Age: Primarily infants and children.

Ethnicity: Not significant.

Gender: Occurs equally in males and females.

Contributing factors: Some research has suggested that measles contracted from the opposite sex and transmission intensity (e.g., home exposure versus outside-home exposure) result in a more severe case. Infants of mothers born after 1963 are more susceptible to measles than are infants born to older mothers.

Signs and symptoms: The child may present to the clinic with a history of exposure to measles in the past 9 to 14 days and a rash. The child had a fever, conjunctivitis, and cough before the rash appeared. The rash consists of discrete, brownish red macules progressing to papular or morbilliform. The rash is blotchy or confluent: The skin between the lesions is normal. Examination of the oral cavity reveals white lesions on the buccal mucosa from before the rash appeared and lasting 12 to 24 hours after the rash's appearance (Koplik spots). The rash began behind the ears and sides of neck, progressing to the trunk and extremities.

Diagnostic tests: None.

Differential diagnosis:

   The incubation period of rubella is 14 to 21 days, with prodromal respiratory symptoms and postauricular and occipital nodes. The maculopapular rash begins on the face.

   The usual age for scarlet fever is 2 to 10 years. The rash is erythematous and diffuse and has a sandpaper texture; scarlet tongue and Pastia's sign are noted, and there is no rash on the face.

   Erythema infectiosum is differentiated by the "slapped cheeks" appearance and the distribution and characteristically lacy pattern of the rash.

Treatment: Symptomatic for fever control with use of acetaminophen.

Follow-up: Usually none.

Sequelae: Otitis media, bronchopneumonia, croup, and diarrhea often occur as a result of the measles. Encephalitis, which occurs in 1 in 1000 cases, can result in severe, permanent brain damage. Death can occur in 3 in 1000 cases.

Prevention/prophylaxis: Immunization at 15 months is recommended, with a second immunization between ages 4 and 6. The dose is 0.5 mL, administered subcutaneously.

Referral: Usually none.

Education: Instruct parents in the importance of immunizations. Instruct pregnant adolescents about the risks of fetal exposure to measles.

MUMPS

Mumps	ICD-9 CM: 072.9

Description: Mumps, characterized by swelling of the parotid gland, is a systemic, acutely contagious disease transmitted by nasopharyngeal secretions. The communicable period is 1 day before until 3 days after parotid swelling. The incubation period is 16 to 18 days (range 12–25 days). To reduce transmission, children should be excluded from school until 9 days after parotid gland swelling.

 Clinical Pearl: This is a reportable disease.

Etiology: The etiologic agent is *Paramyxovirus*.

Occurrence: Mumps is more common in late winter and spring. Since the use of mumps vaccine, the incidence has been greatly reduced.

Age: Peak age group is 10 to 14 years.

Ethnicity: Not significant.

Gender: Occurs equally in males and females.

Contributing factors: Contact with *Paramyxovirus*.

Signs and symptoms: The child complains of tenderness and pain in the jaw; may have had trouble swallowing. Parents have often done the "pickle test," stimulating the parotid and causing increased pain. Often there is no history of immunization (Fig. 13–4).

Enlargement of the parotid gland, usually bilaterally, is a significant sign. Approximately 30% of patients have no apparent swelling of the glands, however. Severe tenderness and pain often accompany swelling. On examination, the ear is displaced upward and outward, with obliteration of the angle of the jaw. Stensen's duct orifice is red and swollen, and yellow exudate may be expressed.

Diagnostic tests:

Test	Results Indicating Disorder	CPT Code
ELISA	Indication of infection:	87449
Hemagglutination	not usually done	86000
Tissue culture of urine, spinal fluid, and throat washings for complement fixation	Confirms infection or vaccination: not usually done	87220
WBC count	Leukocyte counts usually normal	85048

Differential diagnosis:

In cervical adenopathy, the ear usually does not protrude.
Cat-scratch fever usually does not involve the parotid gland.

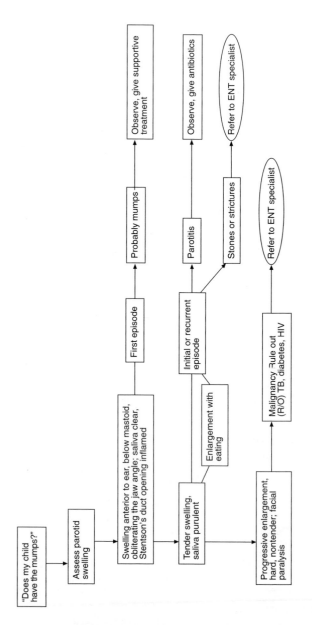

Figure 13–4. Evaluation of parotid swelling. (ENT, ear, nose, and throat; HIV, human immunodeficiency virus; R/O, rule out; TB, tuberculosis.)

In pharyngitis/streptococcal infection, leukocytosis is present, and the parotid gland is not usually involved.

In parotitis, the exudate from Stensen's duct is pustular; leukocytosis and neutrophilia are noted.

Tooth infection is determined by examination of the oral cavity.

Enteroviral meningitis has elevated serum amylase.

In pancreatitis, serum amylase may be elevated. Obtain lipase and amylase isoenzymes to evaluate pancreatic function; transient pancreatitis may be evident by the presence of abdominal pain.

Treatment: Treatment is symptomatic. Fluid should be increased; usually soft foods are tolerated better until the swelling begins to decrease.

Follow-up: Usually none.

Sequelae: Meningeal signs have been reported, with encephalitis occurring in 1 in 6000 cases. Unilateral orchitis is common when the infection occurs after puberty, but this rarely results in sterility and resolves in 1 to 2 weeks. Nerve deafness, which may be transient, causing the inability to distinguish high tones, may occur. Facial paralysis is a rare complication.

Prevention/prophylaxis: Mumps vaccine, 0.5 mL subcutaneously at age 12–15 months and repeated at age 4 to 6. Mumps vaccine cannot be administered to immunocompromised children except for HIV-positive children. Children receiving immunosuppressive therapy should not be immunized, but children with HIV should be immunized.

Referral: None, unless meningeal signs appear.

Education: None.

PERTUSSIS

SIGNAL SYMPTOMS ▶ cough with inspiratory whoop

Pertussis	ICD-9 CM: 033.9

Description: Pertussis (whooping cough) is an acute, highly contagious respiratory illness with an incubation period of 6 to 20 days. There are three stages.

Catarrhal stage (1–2 weeks): Rhinorrhea, conjunctival infection, lacrimation, mild cough, and low-grade fever are present. Infants tend to have profuse nasal discharge.

Paroxysmal stage (≥2–4 weeks): This is more severe, with a forceful, repetitive cough during which a characteristic "whoop" is produced as a result of increased respiratory effort. There is facial redness or cyanosis, bulging eyes, salivation, and distention of neck veins during the coughing episode. Post-tussive emesis often occurs. Exhaustion resulting from paroxysmal coughing spells is a common complaint.

Convalescent stage (1–2 weeks): Paroxysmal coughing and vomiting decrease. Leukocytosis ($>20,000$–$50,000$) is characteristic.

 Clinical Pearl: This is a reportable disease.

Etiology: The causative agent is *Bordetella pertussis*. A similar disease, parapertussis, is caused by *Bordetella parapertussis*. The specific cause is the released toxin that causes lymphocytosis and other symptoms.

Occurrence: Not common now because of childhood immunizations.

Age: Most common in children younger than 1 year and young adults.

Ethnicity: Not significant.

Gender: Occurs more frequently in females.

Contributing factors: Unrecognized symptomatic family members.

Signs and symptoms: Parents describe the characteristic whoop of, and the exhaustion after, the coughing spells; vomiting may occur after a coughing episode. There is an associated low-grade fever. The patient has no history of immunization.

On physical examination, the coughing episodes are observed to be accompanied by cyanosis and sweating. The coughing is severe, having the characteristically loud inspiration (whoop) after 10 to 30 coughs. The child is listless and exhausted. Mild respiratory symptoms, such as rhinitis and sneezing, may be present.

Diagnostic tests:

Test	Results Indicating Disorder	CPT Code
WBC count (catarrhal stage)	20,000–30,000 with 70–80% lymphocytes	85408
Nasopharyngeal swabs for culture using chocolate agar or Bordet-Gengou agar containing an antimicrobial agent	Positive for *B. pertussis*	87220
Radiographs of chest	Thickened bronchi, sometimes a "shaggy" heart border indicative of bronchopneumonia, patchy atelectasis	71010
Serum agglutinins	Positive late in illness, no diagnostic value	86156–86157

Differential diagnosis:

Bronchitis has no characteristic cough or marked elevation in WBC count.

Cough in pneumonia is not as severe, and WBC counts are not as elevated.

With aspiration of foreign body, chest x-ray usually reveals the foreign body; there is no characteristic cough or marked elevation in WBC count.

Parapertussis is a milder illness and usually is found in Europe.

Treatment:

Nonpharmacologic

Increase hydration, and give frequent, small feedings. Avoid respiratory irritants.

Pharmacologic

Administer erythromycin, 40 to 50 mg/kg per day in four divided doses for 14 days. If patient is allergic to erythromycin, give ampicillin, 100 mg/kg in four divided doses. Albuterol dosage (tachycardia is a common side effect, and aerosol methods may improve a paroxysmal episode) for ages 2 to 5 years is 0.1 mg/kg orally three times daily (not to exceed 2 mg three times daily); for ages 6 to 11 years, give albuterol, 2 mg/kg orally three or four times daily. Cough suppressants are not useful in decreasing paroxysmal coughing episodes.

Follow-up: Weekly during the most severe part of the illness, then as needed.

Sequelae: Pneumonia is the most common complication of pertussis. Atelectasis, aspiration pneumonia, subconjunctival hemorrhage, umbilical or inguinal hernia, and rarely intracranial hemorrhage can occur. Death occurs in 10 in 1000 cases.

Prevention/prophylaxis: Immunization is the most important method of prevention. Pertussis vaccine, given in combination with diphtheria and tetanus (DPT), is administered at 2, 4, 6, and 15 months of age. In newborns whose mothers have pertussis, erythromycin can be given (50 mg/kg per day) for 14 days.

Family and hospital contacts should be treated with erythromycin prophylactically.

Referral: None, unless complications develop.

Education: Emphasize the importance of immunizations.

ROCKY MOUNTAIN SPOTTED FEVER

SIGNAL SYMPTOMS▶   red or hemorrhagic maculopapular rash on wrist and ankles, fever

Rocky mountain spotted fever	ICD-9 CM: 083.9

Description: Rocky Mountain spotted fever is a tick-borne illness characterized by fever and a rash. There is an incubation period of 2 to 8 days. The offending tick is the dog tick in the East, the Lone Star tick in the Southwest, and the wood tick in the West.

 Clinical Pearl: This is a reportable disease.

Etiology: *Rickettsia rickettsii* is the causative organism. The organism multiplies within the endothelial lining and smooth muscle cells of blood vessels, causing generalized vasculitis.

Occurrence: Has been reported in every state except Maine; states with the most cases are North Carolina and Oklahoma. It is a seasonal illness that usually occurs from April to September.

Age: All ages, but particularly children age 5 to 9 years.

Ethnicity: Not significant.

Gender: Occurs equally in males and females.

Contributing factors: Rural, wooded areas most often in the spring and summer. Tick must be attached for at least 4 hours.

Signs and symptoms: History reveals outdoor activities and a history of a tick bite. The patient presents with a high fever of abrupt onset, myalgia, and a headache that is severe and persistent. Vomiting and diarrhea occur 2 to 6 days after fever. A rose-red macular or maculopapular rash appears on palms, soles, and extremities; becomes petechial and spreads centrally; blanches on pressure; and is exacerbated by warmth in 95% of cases. Conjunctivitis, splenomegaly, muscle tenderness, edema, and meningism may also occur.

Diagnostic tests:

Test	Results Indicating Disorder	CPT Code
WBC count	Normal or slightly decreased with a shift to the left during the first week, leukocytosis reported in the second week	85048
RBC count	Platelets are depressed	85585
Urinalysis	Hematuria present	81000
Complement fixation titers for Rocky Mountain spotted fever	May increase after 14 days of illness	86000
Fibrinogen	Depressed, disseminated intravascular coagulation	85384–85385
Creatinine	Increased	825665
Liver function studies	Elevated aspartate transaminase, alanine transaminase; depressed bilirubin, total protein, and albumin	84450–84460
Weil-Felix	*Proteus* Ox-19 and Ox-2 single titer of >1:160 (fourfold increase)	100.00
Immunofluorescent biopsy of skin	Identification of organism	86255

Differential diagnosis: Differential diagnosis includes a large variety of illnesses ranging from measles to collagen diseases. The epidemiologic data of the season, the history of a tick bite, and the type of rash should facilitate making the diagnosis.

Treatment:

Nonpharmacologic

Remove tick by gentle upward traction with forceps to avoid contaminating self or patient with material from the crushed tick.

Pharmacologic

Administer antibiotic therapy.

> For children weighing less than 45 kg, give doxycycline, 4.4 mg/kg per day in two divided doses orally or intravenously.
>
> For children and nonpregnant women, give doxycycline, 100 mg twice daily orally or intravenously. Administer until there are clinical signs of improvement, usually within 24 to 72 hours.

To restore circulation, consider fluid management with replacement if needed. Presence of noncardiogenic pulmonary edema may require mechanical ventilation with positive end-expiratory pressure to correct hypoxemia.

In cases of intravascular coagulation and hemorrhage, replacement of platelets and clotting factors is necessary.

Follow-up: Weekly follow-ups to evaluate disease status and efficacy of therapy.

Sequelae: Complications and death may occur from severe vasculitis in brain, heart, and lung. The mortality rate is estimated at 5% to 7%.

Prevention/prophylaxis: Give patient and family the following instructions.

> Remove tick early.
>
> In wooded areas, wear light-colored clothing and long socks, and tuck pants into boots.
>
> Scan body for ticks often.
>
> Use repellents, but be careful with children because of the risk of systemic absorption.
>
> Keep any suspicious ticks labeled with site at which they were obtained and body site.

Referral: Refer patient for hospitalization.

Education: Teach parents the importance of wearing protective clothing and using insect repellents. Teach parents and children the proper technique for tick removal.

RUBELLA

SIGNAL SYMPTOMS ▶ macular rash, faint and evanescent; abrupt fever; tender postauricular nodes

Rubella	ICD-9 CM: 056.9

Description: Rubella (German or 3-day measles) is an acute, viral infection with an incubation period of 14 to 21 days that usually presents as a mild illness. Communicable period is 2 days before to 7 days after the appearance of the rash. The characteristic rash begins on the face and lasts 3 days or less. Asymptomatic illness occurs in 25% to 50% of cases.

Clinical Pearl: This is a reportable disease.

Etiology: *Rubivirus,* family Togaviridae, is the causative agent.

Occurrence: The peak incidence is in early spring or late winter. Incidence has decreased because of the increase in immunized children.

Age: Any pediatric age group.

Ethnicity: Not significant.

Gender: Occurs equally in males and females.

Contributing factors: Exposure to infected children; nonimmunized status. Fetuses exposed to rubella at 1 to 4 months' gestation have an increased risk of congenital rubella.

Signs and symptoms: The child presents with the complaint of a "red rash" that started on the face; the child is usually afebrile. There may have been nonspecific respiratory symptoms before the onset of the rash (prodromal phase). Adolescents and adults (usually women) may complain of transient polyarthralgia and polyarthritis, but this is less common in young children.

There is a fine, pink, discrete, macular rash that becomes punctate or scarlatiniform on the second day, with fine desquamation as the rash fades. Postauricular and occipital nodes may be noted early, progressing to generalized lymphadenopathy.

Diagnostic tests:

Test	Results Indicating Disorder	CPT Code
Complete blood count	Leukopenia, low platelet count	85007

Congenital Rubella

Test	Results Indicating Disorder	CPT Code
Complete blood count	Low platelet count; hemolytic anemia with pleiocytosis	85007
Liver function studies	Abnormal	80076
IgM rubella antibody titer	Elevated; total serum IgM level elevated	86709
IgG	Depressed	86001
IgA	Depressed	86332

Pregnant Women

Test	Results Indicating Disorder	CPT Code
Antibody studies	A fourfold rise in antibody titer obtained 1–2 weeks apart is diagnostic; the fetus is considered at risk, particularly in the first trimester	86762

Differential diagnosis:

Measles is differentiated by accompanying coryza, runny nose, cough, conjunctivitis, and Koplik spots present.

The usual age at onset for scarlet fever is 2 to 10 years. The rash is erythematous and diffuse and has a sandpaper texture. Scarlet tongue and Pastia's sign are present. There is no rash on the face.

Erythema infectiosum is differentiated by the "slapped cheeks" appearance and the distribution and characteristically lacy pattern of the rash.

Contact dermatitis has a rash not characteristic of rubella.

Lymphadenopathy usually has more nodes involved.

Treatment: Nonpharmacologic treatment is symptomatic.

Follow-up: None, unless the patient is pregnant or has any other evidence of complications.

Sequelae: Encephalitis and thrombocytopenia are rare complications. Congenital rubella usually is associated with anomalies that involve the cardiac, ophthalmic, auditory, and neurologic systems.

Prevention/prophylaxis: Immunization is the most effective method of control. If a pregnant woman is exposed, a blood specimen is obtained to measure the rubella titer as soon as possible. If negative, a second specimen is obtained 3 to 4 weeks later; if positive, infection is assumed to have occurred, and the risk to the fetus increases. Although immunization should ensure against fetal exposure, it is wise to do the titers.

Referral: None.

Education: Teach the importance of immunizations.

SCARLET FEVER

SIGNAL SYMPTOMS ▶ brilliant red edematous pharynx with gray or white exudate or membrane on pharynx

Scarlet fever	ICD-9 CM: 034.1

Description: Scarlet fever is an acute, infectious bacterial infection involving the respiratory system, skin, soft tissue, and blood. There is a characteristic rash that begins within 12 to 48 hours of onset of symptoms and a scarlet-colored tongue preceded by the complaint of a severe sore throat. The incubation period is 24 to 48 hours.

Careful treatment is necessary to reduce the risk of cardiac and renal complications.

Etiology: Infection with Group A β-hemolytic streptococcus.

Occurrence: Fairly common.

Age: Any pediatric age group.

Ethnicity: Not significant.

Gender: Occurs equally in males and females.

Contributing factors: Exposure to the bacteria.

Signs and symptoms: The child presents with a history of acute onset of fever (>103–104°F) accompanied by chills, vomiting, headache, and sore throat. The characteristic rash may or may not be present, depending on how long the parent waited before seeking medical services.

Physical examination reveals a hyperemic, edematous pharynx covered with a gray-white exudate; the pharynx is inflamed. The tongue is white with projections of red, edematous papillae (early sign), progressing to a scarlet-colored tongue with prominent red papillae ("strawberry tongue"). The rash is red, punctate, or finely papular and blanches when touched; the rash begins in the axillae, groin, and neck but becomes generalized except on the face within 24 hours. Circumoral pallor and Pastia's sign are noted. The skin desquamates as illness resolves.

Diagnostic tests:

Test	Results Indicating Disorder	CPT Code
Throat culture	Positive	86308
Quick streptococcal test	Positive	86203–84606

Differential diagnosis:

> The incubation period for rubella is 14 to 21 days; the patient has prodromal respiratory symptoms and postauricular and occipital nodes. The maculopapular rash begins on the face.

> Erythema infectiosum is differentiated by the "slapped cheeks" appearance and the distribution and characteristically lacy pattern of the rash.

> Measles has accompanying coryza, runny nose, cough, conjunctivitis, and Koplik spots present.

> Infectious mononucleosis has positive EBV titers and generalized lymphadenopathy.

> In enterovirus, usually the WBC count is normal; often the rash is more prominent on the soles and palms.

> Roseola is usually seen in children younger than age 2 years; the patient has upper respiratory symptoms and abrupt onset of fever, followed by the rash.

Treatment: The treatment of choice is penicillin. Give long-acting benzathine penicillin G, 600,000 U intramuscularly for children weighing less than 60 lb, 1.2 million U intramuscularly for children weighing more than 60 lb. If patient is allergic to penicillin, administer erythromycin, 40 mg/kg per day for 14 days.

Follow-up: Repeat throat culture in 1 week.

Sequelae: When the infection is severe, bacteremia, pneumonia, meningitis, deep soft tissue infections, or streptococcal toxic shock syndrome may result. Inadequately treated infections can result in rheumatic fever, cardiac involvement, and renal problems.

Prevention/prophylaxis: Throat cultures should be done for all who are in close contact with infected persons. Prophylactic penicillin should be administered, 400,000 U per dose four times daily for 10 days or 600,000 U intramuscularly (single dose), or erythromycin, 40 mg/kg per day for 14 days.

Referral: None.

Education: Instruct parents and children not to use eating or drinking utensils after the infected person. Stress the importance of completing the treatment regimen.

VARICELLA

SIGNAL SYMPTOMS red small papules on trunk or face, fever

Varicella	ICD-9 CM: 052.9

Description: Varicella (chickenpox) is a viral, highly contagious, acute disease with an incubation period of 14 to 21 days. The communicable period is 1 day before eruption of vesicles until 6 days after the last lesion appears or when all crusts have formed.

Etiology: Infection with varicella-zoster virus, a member of the herpesvirus group.

Occurrence: More common in spring and winter.

Age: All pediatric age groups.

Ethnicity: Not significant.

Gender: Occurs equally in males and females.

Contributing factors: Contact with infected children; common in day care centers and schools.

Signs and symptoms: The child presents with a history of exposure to other infected children, usually mild fever, and the presence of the characteristic pruritic rash, which usually begins on the scalp. Physical examination of the skin reveals macules or papules: small, red, elevated, teardrop-shaped vesicles, with an erythematous ring 1/4 to 1/2 inch in diameter. The rash occurs in "crops"; that is, all stages are present as new lesions appear.

Diagnostic tests:

Test	Results Indicating Disorder	CPT Code
Tzanck smear	Positive	87207
Immunofluorescent staining of vesicular lesions	Positive	87999

Differential diagnosis:

> Impetigo bullosa is characterized by fewer lesions, no typical vesicles, and response to antibiotic agents.
>
> Coxsackievirus has fewer lesions and less crusting.
>
> Insect bites have no typical vesicles.

Treatment:

Nonpharmacologic

Treatment is symptomatic for fever and itching. Cool oatmeal baths (Aveeno) are often soothing.

Pharmacologic

 Clinical Pearl: Avoid administering aspirin because of the association between the use of aspirin and the development of Reye's syndrome.

For itching, prescribe diphenhydramine (Benadryl), 1.25 mg/kg (4–6 mg/kg per day), every 6 hours, or hydroxyzine (Atarax), 0.5 mg/kg (10 mg) every 6 hours per day.

Some research has recommended administration of acyclovir, 80 mg/kg per day in four divided doses, for children aged 3 to 24 months to reduce symptoms, interrupt vesicle formation, and accelerate the healing process. Acyclovir must be administered within the first 24 hours after the onset of the illness. Some research has suggested that the use of ibuprofen may be associated with the later development of streptococcal infections.

Follow-up: Usually none.

Sequelae: Bacterial superinfection of lesions can occur. *Streptococcus pyogenes* is the bacteria most often associated with varicella complications. Encephalitis, pancreatitis, hepatitis, or pneumonia can develop in immunocompromised children. Older persons who acquire chickenpox are at risk for pneumonia.

When the infection is reactivated from a latent form after the primary infection, it is called *herpes zoster,* also known as *shingles*.

Prevention/prophylaxis: Isolation of infected children from other children can prevent the spread of the disease. Varicella vaccine, given at 15 months, produces immunity. It is recommended that varicella vaccine (live attenuated vaccine) be administered to healthy persons older than 1 year of age who are varicella-susceptible within 3 days of exposure. Pregnant women, persons who are allergic to vaccine components, and persons who are immunocompromised should be given varicella-zoster immune globulin to prevent or modify the disease.

Referral: None for well children. Refer infected immunosuppressed children and neonates, in whom varicella is a life-threatening illness, to a pediatrician or infectious disease specialist.

Education: Teach the importance of hygienic measures, such as keeping the nails short, to reduce the risk of superinfections.

REFERENCES

Anemia, Iron Deficiency

DeLoughery, T: Anemia: an approach to diagnosis. Hematol Oncol Clin 1, January 1999.

Reid, D: Iron deficiency anemia linked with cystic fibrosis disese severity. Chest 121:48, 2001.

Anemia, Sickle Cell

Dix, H: New advances in the treatment of sickle cell disease: Focus on perioperative significance. AANA J 69:281, 2001.

Marwah, S., et al: Reduced vitamin E antioxidant capacity in sickle cell disease is related to transfusion status but not to sickle crisis. Am J Hematol 69:144, 2002.

Prasad, A: Zinc deficiency in patients with sickle cell disease. Am J Clin Nutr 75:181, 2002.

Zemel, B, et al: Effect of zinc supplementation on growth and body composition in children with sickle cell disease. Am J Clin Nutr 75:300, 2002.

Cat-Scratch Fever

Armengol, C, and Hendley, J: Cat-scratch disease encephalopathy: A cause of status epilepticus in school-aged children. J Pediatr 134:635, 1999.

Lex, J: Catscratch disease. EMed J 2, Aug 9, 2001.

Loutit, J: Contemporary management of cat-scratch disease. Clin Advis Nurse Pract 4:30, 2001.

Walter, R, and Eppes, S: Cat scratch disease presenting with peripheral facial nerve paralysis. Pediatrics 101:e13, 1998.

Cytomegalovirus

Nadelman, C, and Newcomer, V: Herpes simplex virus infections. Postgrad Med 107:189, 2000.

Oshiro, B: Cytomegalovirus infection in pregnancy. Contemporary OB/GYN Nov 1, 1999.

Wright, R, et al: Congenital lymphocytic choriomeningitis virus syndrome: A disease that mimics congenital toxoplasmosis or cytomegalovirus infection. Pediatrics 100:e9, 1997.

Diphtheria

Singh, M, and Saba, P: Diphtheria. eMed September 27, 2001.

Human Herpesvirus 6

Akhyani, N, et al: Tissue distribution and variant characterization of human herpesvirus (HHV)-6: Increased prevalence of HHV-6A in patients with multiple sclerosis. J Infect Dis 182:1321, 2000.

Caserta, M, et al: Human herpesvirus 6. Clin Infect Dis 33:829, 2001.

Lanphear, B, et al: Risk factors for the early acquisition of human herpesvirus 6 and human herpesvirus 7 infections in children. Pediatr Infect Dis J 17:792, 1998.

Suga, S, et al: Prospective study of persistence and excretion of human herpesvirus-6 in patients with exanthem subitum and their parents. Pediatrics 102:900, 1998.

Human Immunodeficiency Virus Infection and Acquired Immunodeficiency Syndrome

American Academy of Pediatrics, Committee on Pediatric AIDS and Committee on

Adolescents and Human Immunodeficiency Virus Infection: The role of the pediatrician in prevention and intervention. Pediatrics 107:188, 2001.

American Academy of Pediatrics, Committee on Pediatric AIDS: Human immunodeficiency virus/acquired immunodeficiency syndrome education in schools. Pediatrics 101:933, 1999.

American Academy of Pediatrics, Committee on Sports Medicine and Fitness: Human immunodeficiency virus and other blood borne viral pathogens in the athletic setting. Pediatrics 104:1400, 1999.

American Academy on Pediatrics, Committee on Pediatric AIDS and Committee on Infectious Diseases: Issues related to human immunodeficiency virus transmission in schools, child care, medical setting, the home and community. Pediatrics 104:318, 1999.

Bartlett, J, and Gallant, J: 2001–2002 Medical Management of HIV Infection. Johns Hopkins University, Division of Infectious Diseases, Baltimore, MD, 2001

Cappanelli, E, et al: Pharmacokinetics and tolerance of zidovudine in preterm infants. J Pediatr 142:1, 2003.

Futterman, D, et al: HIV and AIDS in adolescents. Pediatr Clin North Am 47:171, 2000.

Keller, M: Immunizations rarely associated with significant increase in HIV plasma RNA in children in combination with retrovirals, Pediatric Infection Disease Journal, 7(26), 2000.

Luber, A: To ABT or not ABT—a reevaluation of pharmacokinetics in HIV clinical patients. Medscape HIV/AIDS J 6:1, 2000.

Luzuriagna, K, and Sullivan, L: Prevention and treatment of pediatric HIV infection. JAMA 280:17, 1998.

Neilson, K: Pediatric HIV infection. HIV Clin Manage 12:1, 1999.

Tevas, P: Early initiation of antiretroviral therapy: The case for caution. Medscape HIV/AIDS eJournal 8:1, 2002.

Human Parvovirus B19 (Erythema Infectiosum)

Koch, W, et al: Serologic and virologic evidence for frequent intrauterine transmission of human parvovirus B19 with a primary maternal infection during pregnancy. Pediatr Infect J 17:489, 1999.

Sabella, C, and Goldfarb, J: Parvovirus B19 infections. Am Fam Physician 60:1455, 1999.

Taked, S, et al: Renal involvement induced by human parvovirus b19 infection. Nephron 89:280, 2001.

Infectious Mononucleosis

Godshall, S, and Kirchner, J: Infectious mononucleosis: Complexities of a common syndrome. Postgrad Med 107:175, 2000.

Newcom, K: Infectious mononucleosis: A clinical review. Advance NP 9:37, 2001.

Lyme Disease

American Academy of Pediatrics, Committee on Infectious Diseases: Prevention of Lyme disease (RE9942). Pediatrics 105:142, 2000.

Aucott, J, et al: Lyme disease: The debate continue. Patient Care Nurse Pract 4:38, 2001.

Dennis, D, et al: Now you can prevent Lyme disease. Patient Care Nurse Pract 2:20, 1999.

Gammons, M, and Salem, G: Tick removal. Am Fam Physician 66:643, 2002.

Gerver, M, and Shapiro, ED: Late Lyme disease: Clearing up confusion. Contemp Pediatr 18:46, 2001.

Klempner, MS, et al: Intralaboratory reliability of serologic and urine testing for Lyme diseae. Am J Med 110:217, 2001.

Rothermel, H, et al: Optic neuropathy in children with Lyme disease. Pediatrics 108:477, 2001.

Wormser, G, et al: Guidelines from the Infectious Disease Society of America: Practice guidelines for the treatment of Lyme disease. Clin Infect Dis 31:1, 2000.

Measles

Aaby, P: Assumptions and contradictions in measles and measles immunization research: Is measles good for something? Soc Sci Med 41:673, 1995.

Centers for Disease Control and Prevention: Epidemiology of measles—United States, 1998. MMWR Morb Mortal Wkly Rep 48:749, 1999.

Papania, M, et al: Increased susceptibility to measles in infants in the United States. Pediatrics 104:e59, 1999.

Mumps

Adelman, W, and Joffe, A: The adolescent with a painful scrotum. Contemp Pediatr 3:111, 2000.

Pertussis

Grant, C, and McKay, EJ: Pertussis encephalopathy with high cerebrospinal fluid antibody titers to pertussis toxin and filamentous hemagglutinin. Pediatrics 102:986, 1998.

Smith, C, and Taylor, D. Quieting the '100-day' cough: A primer on pertussis. Adv NP Oct:60, 2000.

Rocky Mountain Spotted Fever

Gammons, M, and Salem, G: Tick removal. Am Fam Physician 66:643, 2002.

Gayle, A, and Ringdahl, E: Tick-borne diseases. Am Fam Physician 64:461, 2001.

Ghali, F, et al: Location, location, location. Contemp Pediatr Aug 1998.

McKinnon, H, and Howard, T: Evaluating the febrile patient with a rash. Am Fam Physician 62:804, 2000.

Thorner, A, et al: Rocky Mountain spotted fever. Clin Infect Dis 27:1353, 1998.

Rubella

Centers for Disease Control: Rubella and congenital rubella syndrome—United States, January 1, 1991–7 May, 1994. MMWR Morb Mortal Wkly Rep 43:391, 1994.

Varicella

Laskey, A, et al: Endocarditis attributable to group A β-hemolytic streptococcus after uncomplicated varicella in a vaccinated child. Pediatrics 106:e40, 2000.

Lesko, S, et al: Invasive group A streptococcal infection and nonsteroidal anti-inflammatory drug use among children with primary varicella. Pediatrics 107:1108, 2001.

Schmitt, H, et al: *S. pyogenes* a frequent cause of complications in children with varicella. Pediatrics 108:e79, 2001.

Slack, C, et al: Post-varicella epiglottitis and necrotizing fasciitis. Pediatrics 105:e13, 2000.

Zerr, D, et al: A case-control study of necrotizing fasciitis during primary varicella. Pediatrics 103:783, 1999.

Chapter 14

PSYCHOSOCIAL PROBLEMS

ANOREXIA

SIGNAL SYMPTOMS ▶ lack of appetite for food

| Anorexia | ICD-9 CM: 307.1 |

Description: Anorexia is a serious eating disorder characterized by failure to maintain an adequate weight appropriate for age and height. May be categorized as mild (15% below ideal body weight [IBW]), moderate, (20% below IBW), or severe (30% IBW). Anorexia is due to a pervasive fear of becoming fat or gaining weight despite current underweight status and to a significant distortion of perceived body size or body shape (Fig. 14–1).

Etiology: Unknown, but there seems to be a familial pattern.

Occurrence: Occurs in 1% of teenagers.

Age: Age distribution shows a bimodal distribution of onset at 12 to 14 years and at 17 to 18 years.

Ethnicity: Not significant.

Gender: The female-to-male ratio is 20:1; 90% to 95% of anorectic patients are female.

Contributing factors: Major transitions, such as entering high school or college or marrying; "finicky" eating in childhood; and perfectionist behavior seem to be factors. Of girls age 9 to 12, 75% diet three to five times in a year, setting the pattern for disordered eating. Teenage vegetarians may be at greater risk for developing eating disorders.

Signs and symptoms: The caregiver complains that the child "plays with her food and is losing weight." The child contradicts the caregiver about her food intake but is concerned that she is "too fat." During the history, the girl should be asked what she considers the perfect weight, whether she is on a diet, what she does to maintain her weight (anorectic girls have a history of excessive exercise), and what she thinks of her current weight. It is helpful to obtain a weight history to determine the

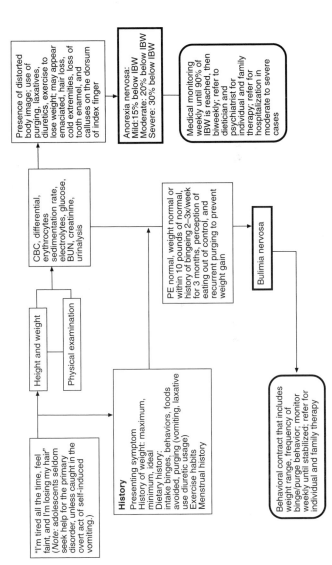

Figure 14–1. Evaluation of eating disorders. (BUN, blood urea nitrogen; CBC, complete blood count; IBW, ideal body weight; PE, physical examination.)

child's growth pattern. Postmenarchal females should be asked about the frequency of periods and amount of the flow. Past diet history should be noted. Amenorrhea (non–pregnancy related) of at least three consecutive cycles can occur secondary to anorexia. The Eating Attitudes Test and the Eating Disorder Inventory are useful assessment tools.

The physical examination may be normal. Loss of subcutaneous fat may not be evident until the patient disrobes. Bradycardia or hypotension may be present. There may be dry skin, cold extremities, limpness and loss of sheen of the hair, prominent ribs, and a scaphoid abdomen. Growth charts are abnormal in prepubertal and pubertal children with signs of anorexia nervosa of 6 months' duration or longer. Projected heights should be calculated as well as the ideal weight.

Diagnostic tests:

Test	Results Indicating Disorder	CPT Codes
Complete blood count	Assess nutritional status	85007
Erythrocyte sedimentation rate	Excludes inflammatory bowel disease or collagen vascular disease	85651
Serum electrolyte	Hypochloremic alkalosis and hypocalcemia owing to vomiting	80551
Urinalysis	Concentrated in early stages, not in late stages	81000
Serum total protein and albumin	Usually normal	82040 84160–84165

Differential diagnosis:

With cancer, diabetes mellitus, hyperthyroidism, or chronic renal disease, there is weight loss but no fear of obesity or disturbance of body image.

Depression may present with loss of appetite and weight loss.

Treatment:

Nonpharmacologic

Treatment is multidisciplinary, involving a primary care provider, mental health professional, and dietitian. The first goal is for the patient to increase caloric intake to gain weight. The dietitian plans a diet sufficient for weight gain. If there are no severe metabolic disturbances, the patient can be treated on an outpatient basis, with weekly visits to members of the treatment team. Mental health counseling includes not only the patient, but also the entire family.

Contracting has been found to be a useful strategy. The contract should include long-term weight goals, rate of weight gain (1/2 to 1 lb per week), amount of allowable exercise, frequency of visits, and the minimum weight that requires hospitalization (25–30% of IBW). Other criteria for hospitalization include a pulse rate in the 40s, low blood pressure, low blood glucose (<60 mg/dL), dehydration, electrocardiogram (ECG) abnormalities, and food refusal.

Pharmacologic

A daily multivitamin and mineral supplement should be given. To minimize osteoporosis risk, give calcium, 1200 mg, and vitamin D, 400 IU; if indicated, prescribe a phosphorus supplement to prevent serum hypophosphatemia.

Follow-up: Height, weight, and subcutaneous fat are measured weekly; chest and abdominal examinations are also done weekly.

Sequelae: Complications, which are many, involve all body systems. Among the complications are amenorrhea or irregular menses, decreased triiodothyronine (T_3) and increased reverse triiodothyronine (rT_3), (thyroxine [T_4] and thyroid-stimulating hormone [TSH] levels are normal), dehydration, osteoporosis, bradycardia, congestive heart failure, dental erosion (if anorexia is accompanied by vomiting), pancreatitis, constipation, hematuria, leukopenia, anemia, and stunted growth. The mortality rate is 10%, with 2% to 5% committing suicide.

Prevention/prophylaxis: Reduce the messages children get about the "perfect" weight. Assist girls in forming a positive self-image.

Referral: Consult with or refer patient to a primary care physician for definitive diagnosis and admission to the hospital, if necessary. Refer patient to a mental health counselor for family therapy, to a dietitian for appropriate meal planning, and to a support group.

Education: Instruct patient and family about the illness. Provide factual knowledge, not myths. Teach patient about eating and appropriate eating patterns; many have lost sight of what constitutes a normal eating pattern. Alert parents to the possibility of the child's use of web-based proanorectic sites.

ANXIETY

SIGNAL SYMPTOMS▶ fears not appropriate for age and developmental level

Anxiety	ICD-9 CM: 300.0

Description: Anxiety is a vague, uneasy feeling whose source is unknown or nonspecific. Normal developmental anxiety is categorized as follows:

- Stranger anxiety (5 months to $1\frac{1}{2}$ years, with a peak at 6–12 months)
- Separation anxiety (7 months to 4 years, with a peak at 18–36 months)
- Anxiety from or even phobia of the dark and "monsters" (3–6 years)

"Appropriate" anxiety is a feeling that occurs when anticipating a painful or frightening experience, when avoiding the memory of such an experience, and in instances of child abuse. There are three major anxiety disorders:

- Anxiety states
- Phobic anxiety
- Post-traumatic stress disorder

Anxiety is different from fear: Fear is a response to a known, external, real threat.

Etiology: Unknown. Possible disruption of parent-infant relationship and a history of a stressful event, situational change, or chronic illness.

Occurrence: Occurs in 10% of school-age children and adolescents.

Age: Any age. Age-normal fears or anxieties can develop into anxiety disorders.

Ethnicity: Not significant.

Gender: Occurs equally in males and females.

Contributing factors: Environmental factors, such as emotional overstimulation, family discord or violence, and harsh disciplinary methods.

Signs and symptoms: The child may present with a history of increased dependence on home and parents, avoidance of social interaction outside the family, avoidance of anxiety-producing stimuli, decreased school performance, increased self-doubt and irritability, and ritualistic behaviors (e.g., washing, counting). Caregivers may have observed increased fear and worries, uneasiness and apprehension, and frightening themes in play and fantasy. They may also have noted decreased concentration, hyperactivity, dizziness and lightheadedness, shortness of breath, panic, and sleep disturbances. The child may also complain of heart palpitations, nausea and vomiting, fatigue, and headaches or stomachaches.

Physical findings may be negative. If the child is seen during an episode, findings may reveal shortness of breath, flushing, sweating, dry mouth, or tachycardia. Effective interviewing to elicit a detailed history is important, as is behavioral observation of an episode if possible. Whole person drawings may elicit information regarding self, relationships, and fears. Adolescents can complete the Hamilton Anxiety Rating Scale as an adjunct to diagnosis.

Diagnostic tests: None. To rule out organic/physiologic causes, the following can be performed.

Test	Results Indicating Disorder	CPT Codes
Drug screen	Evidence of toxic substances	80100
Thyroid panel	Hypothyroidism or hyperthyroidism	84481/84482
Blood glucose	Hypoglycemia	82947
Complete blood count	Anemia	85007
ECG	Presence of arrhythmias or mitral valve prolapse	93042

Differential diagnosis:

Drug history differentiates abuse of illicit substances, medications, alcohol, and recreational substances (caffeine, chocolate).

Hyperthyroidism is differentiated by T_4 and T_3 elevation and TSH suppression.

Anemia is differentiated by hemoglobin levels less than 11 g/dL.

Hypoglycemia is differentiated by fasting blood glucose levels less than 60 mg/dL.

Hypoxemia is differentiated by partial pressure of oxygen (PO_2) decreased in pulmonary disease, hypoventilation, anemia, and carbon monoxide poisoning (PO_2 normal in anxiety).

ECG shows abnormalities and differentiates cardiopathy, such as arrhythmia, high-output state, and mitral valve prolapse.

Treatment:

Nonpharmacologic

Cognitive-behavioral therapy is used with the development of coping skills. Psychotherapy is recommended for the child and the family. Establish an open, trusting relationship with the child. Promote well-being by prescribing a balanced diet and exercise.

Pharmacologic

TRICYCLIC ANTIDEPRESSANTS

Give imipramine, 3 to 5 mg/kg per day in two divided doses. Start dosage at 1 mg/kg per day and increase to no more than 3 mg/kg per day every 4 to 5 days, as tolerated. Clinical effectiveness may not be seen until 4 to 6 weeks after initiation of treatment.

Tricyclic antidepressants seem to have more cardiotoxic effects in children than in adults. Observe for heart rates greater than130 beats/min, blood pressure 130/85 mm Hg, and changes in the ECG. Anticholinergic responses are also seen with the use of tricyclic antidepressants.

SELECTIVE SEROTONIN REUPTAKE INHIBITORS

The following selective serotonin reuptake inhibitors (SSRIs) are recommended.

Fluoxetine: In children younger than 12 years old, start at 5 to 10 mg per day with a maintenance dose of 10 to 30 mg; in adolescents, begin with 10 mg per day and maintain at 20 to 40 mg per day.

Sertraline: In children younger than 12 years, start at 25 mg per day and maintain at 100 to 150 mg per day; in adolescents, begin with 25 to 50 mg per day and maintain at 150 to 200 mg per day.

Fluvoxamine: In children younger than 12 years, start at 25 mg per day and maintain at 100 to 200 mg per day; in adolescents, begin with 25 to 50 mg per day and maintain at 150 to 300 mg per day.

ANTIANXIETY AGENT

Buspirone is specifically an antianxiety agent. Begin with 5 mg per day with weekly titrations upward to 20 to 30 mg per day in divided doses (0.2–0.6 mg/kg per day).

Follow-up: At each dosage increase, then every 3 to 4 months, obtain height, weight, pulse, blood pressure, and ECG readings.

Sequelae: Long-term effects of childhood anxiety problems are unknown.

Prevention/prophylaxis: Anticipatory guidance for parents to help them deal with their child's normal fears in an appropriate manner.

Referral: Consult or collaborate with a psychiatrist for definitive diagnosis and pharmacologic intervention when anxieties exceed developmental norms.

Education: Educate parents about normal childhood development. Instruct parents in the dosage, purpose, and side effects of antianxiety medications.

ATTENTION-DEFICIT/
HYPERACTIVITY DISORDER

SIGNAL SYMPTOMS▶ persistent pattern of inattention, hyperactivity, and impulsivity

Attention-deficit disorder	ICD-9 CM: 314
Attention-deficit/hyperactivity disorder	ICD-9 CM: 314.01

Description: ADHD is a multifaceted, chronic disorder in which the child exhibits difficulty sustaining attention, controlling impulses, and inhibiting activity level to meet the demands of a given situation. It is a neurologically based problem involving an interference in the brain's ability to procure, store, process, and produce information. Approximately 50% of the behaviors persist into adulthood. The disorder has two forms: (1) impulsivity and hyperactivity and (2) inattention, disorganization, and difficulty completing tasks (Fig. 14–2).

Etiology: There seems to be a pattern of hereditary transmission. It has also been suggested that ADHD may be related to birth complications or to a disease of or trauma to the central nervous system. Research has not supported a relationship to food additives. Current theories suggest an imbalance of neurotransmitters, such as dopamine, in the premotor cortex and superior frontal cortex (chromosomes 5 and 11), or the genes that regulate norepinephrine.

Occurrence: Occurs in an estimated 9% to 12% of school-age children.

Age: Occurs in children (usually <7 years old); may persist into adolescence and adulthood.

Ethnicity: Not significant.

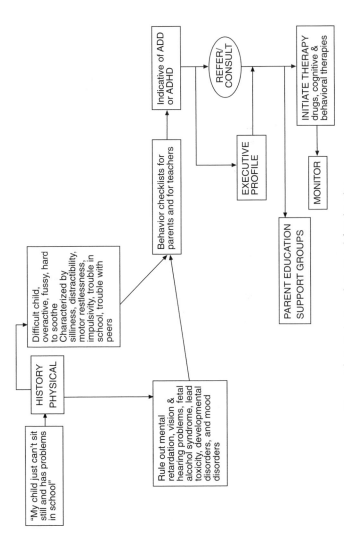

Figure 14–2. Evaluation of attention-deficit disorder.

Gender: Hyperactivity is more prevalent in males (3:1); attention deficit with inattention occurs in males and females.

Contributing factors: Chaotic households; possibly a family history of similar behavior. Maternal smoking during pregnancy may increase risk.

Signs and symptoms: The child is brought to the clinic because of behavior, noted either in the home or in the classroom, consisting of disruption, lack of attention, or daydreaming. Physical findings are negative. Data related to birth and developmental history should be gathered, gross and fine motor skills assessed, and a family and home assessment conducted. An in-depth assessment of the behavior requires interviews with the parents, child, and teachers. Impulsive and disruptive behaviors are seen to a greater degree and frequency than what is considered appropriate for developmental age. These behaviors are reported to have been present for at least 6 months, and they are evident in two or more settings, such as home and school (Table 14–1). These children often have comorbid conditions, such as depression, sleep disorders, anxiety, and disruptive behavior disorders.

Table 14–1   Diagnostic Criteria for Attention-Deficit/Hyperactivity Disorder

A. Either 1. or 2.:
  1. Six (or more) of the following symptoms of **inattention** have persisted for at least 6 months to a degree that is maladaptive and inconsistent with developmental level:
    Inattention
    a. Often fails to give close attention to details or makes careless mistakes in schoolwork, work, or other activities
    b. Often has difficulty sustaining attention in tasks or play activities
    c. Often does not seem to listen when spoken to directly
    d. Often does not follow through on instructions and fails to finish schoolwork, chores, or duties in the workplace (not due to oppositional behavior or failure to understand instructions)
    e. Often has difficulty organizing tasks and activities
    f. Often avoids, dislikes, or is reluctant to engage in tasks that require sustained mental effort (such as schoolwork or homework)
    g. Often loses things necessary for tasks or activities (e.g., toys, school assignments, pencils, books, or tools)
    h. Is often easily distracted by extraneous stimuli
    i. Is often forgetful in daily activities
  2. Six (or more) of the following symptoms of **hyperactivity/impulsivity** have persisted for at least 6 months to a degree that is maladaptive and inconsistent with developmental level:
    Hyperactivity
    a. Often fidgets with hands or feet or squirms in seat
    b. Often leaves seat in classroom or in other situations in which remaining seated is expected
    c. Often runs about or climbs excessively in situations in which it is inappropriate (in adolescents or adults, may be limited to subjective feelings of restlessness)
    d. Often has difficulty playing or engaging quietly in leisure activities
    e. Is often "on the go" or often acts as if "driven by a motor"
    f. Often talks excessively
    Impulsivity
    g. Often blurts out answers before questions have been completed
    h. Often has difficulty awaiting turn
    i. Often interrupts or intrudes on others (e.g., butts into conversations or games)

Table 14–1 Diagnostic Criteria for Attention-Deficit/Hyperactivity Disorder

B. Some hyperactive-impulsive or inattentive symptoms that caused impairment were present before age 7 years

C. Some impairment from the symptoms is present in two or more settings (e.g., at school [or work] and at home)

D. There must be clear evidence of clinically significant impairment in social, academic, or occupational functioning

E. The symptoms do not occur exclusively during the course of a Pervasive Developmental Disorder, Schizophrenia, or other Psychotic Disorder and are not better accounted for by another mental disorder (e.g., Mood Disorder, Anxiety Disorder, Dissociative Disorder, or a Personality Disorder)

Code based on type:
314.01 Attention-Deficit/Hyperactivity Disorder, Combined Type: If both Criteria A1 and A2 are met for the past 6 months
314.00 Attention-Deficit/Hyperactivity Disorder, Predominantly Inattentive Type. If criterion A1 is met but Criterion A2 is not met for the past 6 months
314.01 Attention-Deficit/Hyperactivity Disorder, Predominantly Hyperactive-Impulsive Type: If Criterion A2 is met but Criterion A1 is not met for the past 6 months
Coding note: For individuals (especially adolescents and adults) who currently have symptoms that no longer meet full criteria, "In Partial Remission" should be specified

Source: Reprinted with permission from the Diagnostic and Statistical Manual of Mental Disorders, ed 4. Copyright 1994, American Psychiatric Association.

Diagnostic tests:

Test	Results Indicating Disorder	CPT Code
Thyroid panel	Rule out hypothyroidism/hyperthyroidism	84881/84482
EEG	Rule out seizure disorder	95816
Serum lead	Rule out lead toxicity	83665

EEG, electroencephalogram.

Computed tomography (CT), magnetic resonance imaging (MRI), and EEG are of no diagnostic use.

Psychological testing is done to rule out mental retardation and to test cerebral function.

The Conners, ACTeRs, or Schnelle test, or the Nursing Evaluation for Attention-Deficit Disorders, is given. Behavior rating scales are disclosed to the parents and teachers.

Vision and hearing screening tests are performed to check for deficits; the child qualifies for interventions under Public Law 94-142 if deficits are found.

Early studies using Altopane imaging for the diagnosis of ADHD showed that in adults there was a 70% increase in the dopamine transporter density, whereas in Parkinson's disease, the uptake was decreased. In 2001, the Food and Drug Administration approved trials to study the use of Altopane to diagnose ADHD.

Differential diagnosis:

Children with hearing deficits may have hyperactivity.

Poor parenting skills may result in a child with impulsive behaviors.

Besides having vocal tics, patients with Tourette's syndrome also have motor tics. The disorder may be exacerbated by the stimulant medications used for ADHD.

Mental retardation is usually not seen in cases of ADHD.

Fetal alcohol syndrome is differentiated by family history and facies.

Lead toxicity is differentiated on the basis of laboratory data.

Sleep disturbances (retiring late, arising early) may mimic ADHD.

Absence seizures (history of daydreaming or staring spells) should be ruled out by EEG.

Hypothyroidism is differentiated on the basis of laboratory data.

Treatment:

Behavioral Management

Parents should be given the following strategies.

Reduce environmental stimuli.

Focus on the child's positive traits, increasing his or her self-esteem.

Keep things as organized as possible, give the child responsibilities (e.g., list of chores), and reward progress (e.g., with gold stars).

Be specific, make directions simple, and make eye contact with the child.

Use the "time out" method of discipline; a kitchen timer can be useful as a means of increasing the child's sense of time.

Adolescents may benefit from making daily lists of what they want to accomplish; keeping an appointment book or planning calendar; keeping a notepad handy to write down ideas or items they want to remember; breaking down projects into smaller tasks that are more manageable; and posting schedules, plans, or errands. When they achieve their goals, they should reward themselves.

Pharmacologic

STIMULANTS

Methylphenidate (Ritalin), 0.2 to 0.5 mg/kg per dose. Usual dosing is before school and at noon; depending on behavior, a third dose may be given in the late afternoon (approximately 4 PM). Dosage should be titrated upward weekly, to 5 to 60 mg per day, by the primary care provider. Peak action is within 2 hours, and the effects dissipate within 6 hours. Children usually have weekends and summers off therapy. A sustained-release formulation (Ritalin-SR), 20 mg, is taken once daily. Ritalin LA, 20 mg, is given once daily in the morning. Ritalin is contraindicated in children with a history (personal or familial) of motor tics or Tourette's syndrome,or if family members have untreated substance abuse disorders.

Metadate CD is an extended-release capsule for once-daily use (10-

and 20-mg tablets). This agent is not recommended for children younger than age 6.

Adderal is an amphetamine mixture, 5 to 30 mg per day or 5 to 15 mg twice daily. Adderal XR is given once daily. Do not give in the evening.

Concerta, 18 to 54 mg daily. Swallow whole in the morning; do not chew, crush, or divide.

Dextroamphetamines are similar to methylphenidate in therapeutic onset and duration of action. Usual dosage is 2.5 to 10 mg per dose before school and at noon. The action of sustained-release capsules (Spansules) may last 8 hours. Not recommended for children younger than age 3.

Focalin, 2.5 mg, is given twice daily.

ANTIDEPRESSANTS

Bupropion (Wellbutrin), 50 to 100 mg three times daily. Wellbutrin SR, 100 to 150 mg twice daily.

Desipramine (Norpramin), 1 to 2 mg/kg per day in two divided doses. This drug is contraindicated in children with a family history of cardiac disease or who have a known seizure disorder.

α-ADRENERGIC AGONISTS

Clonidine, in conjunction with methylphenidate, is initiated at 0.05 mg at bedtime. Dose is increased after 3 to 5 days by giving an additional 0.05 mg in the morning. Dosage can be increased by 0.05 mg alternating morning, noon, and evening until the total daily dose is 0.3 mg in three divided doses (3 to 5 mm/kg per dose). By adding clonidine to the treatment regimen, the dosage of methylphenidate may often be decreased by 30% to 50%. Clonidine is contraindicated in patients with known renal or cardiovascular disease.

 Clinical Pearl: A baseline ECG should be obtained before therapy is started.

Pemoline tablets (Cylert), 37.5 mg per day single dose. Not recommended as a first-line agent because of liver toxicity.

NONSTIMULANT

Atomoxetine (Strattera), 0.5 mg/kg per day. The dosage can be increased to 100 mg per day.

Follow-up: Monitor patient every 2 weeks until dosage is stable. Monitor for side effects, such as decreased appetite, headache, stomachache, and insomnia. Medications are contraindicated in children with hypertension. Monitor growth and development. Regularly monitor behavior, school achievement, and response to medication. Monitor hepatic function every 6 months.

Sequelae: Without interventions, these children experience increasing problems in school, increasing their feelings of failure and worthlessness. Of juvenile crime, 50% to 70% is estimated to have been perpetrated by children with ADHD and conduct disorders; of these children, 50% to 60% continue to have symptoms into adulthood, experiencing problems with work and personal relationships.

Prevention/prophylaxis: None.

Referral: Refer patient to a Children's Developmental Center or a mental health center. Refer parents and older children to a support group if possible.

Education: Instruct parents and teachers that the disorder may be inherited and may persist into adulthood, but that treatment is available. Refer parents to support groups. Instruct parents about the dosage, purpose, and side effects of the medications. Ensure that parents understand the importance of a complete evaluation before a definitive diagnosis. Some parents demand a diagnosis of ADHD and treatment to obtain the related financial benefits.

AUTISTIC SPECTRUM DISORDER

SIGNAL SYMPTOMS▶ child has difficulty relating to others with problems in language development and other behavioral manifestations

Autistic spectrum disorder	
Autistic disorder	ICD-9 CM: 299.0
Pervasive developmental disorder (PDD)	ICD-9 CM: 299.8
Rett's syndrome	ICD-9 CM: 330.8
Asperger's syndrome	ICD-9 CM: 299.0

Description: *Autistic spectrum disorder* is the current term for a group of disorders including autistic disorder; PDD, not otherwise specified; Rett's syndrome; and Asperger's disorder—all of which manifest a common deficit in the ability to relate to others.

Autistic disorder: A developmental disorder characterized by the loss of the ability to communicate, the loss of previously accomplished developmental milestones, and a sense of the child living in his or her own world. This is the third most common developmental disorder. Autism is a complex developmental problem usually observed and diagnosed between 12 and 36 months of age. Autism interferes with the normal development of the brain and specifically affects the areas of social interaction and communication skills. Often characterized by repetitive behavior such as hand flapping, rocking, and head banging, children have difficulty with verbal and nonverbal communication, social interaction skills, and engaging in leisure or play activities. They often form unusual attachments to objects and people and resist any changes in their routines and environment.

PDD, not otherwise specified: A developmental disorder characterized by impairment of the quality of social interaction and communications; impairment does not meet the full criteria for autistic disorder.

Rett's syndrome: A neurodegenerative disorder that primarily affects females, who present with microcephaly, stereotypical hand movements (hand wringing), social withdrawal, and loss of communication skill.

Asperger's syndrome: A less severe developmental disorder of autistic-like children with normal intelligence. They have delays in speech and language, have abnormal interactions with peers, and tend to be concrete, rote thinkers. Many are able to control their behavior and are considered socially acceptable. There is repetitive speech, coordination difficulty, obsessive rituals and routines, and difficulty relating to people.

Etiology: Unknown; a suggested cause is central nervous system dysfunction or an abnormality occurring at the time of fetal brain development. Possible involvement of *GABRB3* gene on chromosome 15q.

Occurrence:

Disorder	Age	Ethnicity	Gender	Occurrence
Autistic disorder	Probably present at birth; onset best seen between the ages of 12 and 36 mo	Ethnicity is not significant	Male-to-female ratio is about 4:1	1:500 individuals
PDD, not otherwise specified	First year of life		More common in boys (4:1)	Occurs in 10–12 per 10,000 children
Rett's syndrome	5–48 mo		Occurs primarily in girls	
Asperger's syndrome	Early childhood		Occurs in boys and girls	

Contributing factors:

Autistic disorder: There seems to be increased incidence in children with perinatal problems such as rubella, phenylketonuria, encephalitis, and fragile X syndrome. One quarter of families with an autistic child have family members with language-related problems.

PDD: Extended time of exposure and reexposure while undergoing treatment for plumbism has been suggested as a contributing factor in PDD. There may be a sibling with PDD.

Signs and symptoms:

History

Autistic disorder: Parents of children who were previously developmentally appropriate report that the child is no longer able to communicate needs through verbal or nonverbal means, resists being touched and cuddled, has lost most facial expressions, resists eye-to-eye contact, lacks spontaneous make-believe play ability, and is more isolated than previously. These deficits can be summarized as delays or abnormal functioning in at least one of the following three areas: (1) communication, (2) symbolic or imaginative play, or (3) social interaction.

 Clinical Pearl: Parents are often noted to say that the child seems to be "in a world of their own, unaware of their surroundings anymore."

PDD, not otherwise specified: The parent may report a different cry during the child's infancy, feeding problems, colic and sleep problems; in older children, families report aggressive, violent, or out-of-control behaviors, tantrums, or problems with speech.

Rett's syndrome: Development of multiple defects after a period of normal functioning. Between 5 and 48 months of age, head growth decelerates, and there is loss of hand skills, speech, and eating disturbances. Impairment of gait or trunk movements is noted. There may be a history of periodic apnea during wakefulness, intermittent hyperventilation, breath-holding spells, peripheral vasomotor disturbances, or seizures. Studies have shown a prolonged QT interval.

Asperger's syndrome: Motor skills are delayed or motor clumsiness is noted. There is no delay in speech, language, cognitive development, or self-help skills.

Physical Examination

Physical findings are not remarkable. The developmental assessment reveals delays in meeting milestones, particularly in language and social skills. In Rett's syndrome, the lack of head growth is evident, and there is impairment of gait and trunk movements. There may be loss of teeth owing to bruxism.

Diagnostic tests: No diagnostic tests can be done in the laboratory. A detailed history from the parent or caregiver is important as to when behavioral changes were noted and what those were. These children should be referred to a developmental center where specific psychological evaluation can be done (1) to determine if they are autistic and (2) to assess their degree of impairment and help to develop a plan of care that will optimize their life. Vision and hearing screening should be normal. In older children and adolescents, use of diagnostic tools such as the Autism Behavior Checklist and the Autism Diagnostic Interview is suggested.

Differential diagnosis:

With vision and hearing problems, language development is often
delayed, but developmentally delayed children usually are
interested in interpersonal interaction.

With mental retardation, 70% have an IQ of less than 70.

Metabolic disorders are diagnosed by laboratory evaluations.

Fragile X syndrome is a genetic condition diagnosed by
chromosomal studies.

Williams syndrome is a rare disorder; children are "elf-like" in
appearance with many symptoms common to autism.
Developmental specialists and pediatric neurologists best
differentiate this syndrome.

Landau-Kleffner syndrome has losses in speech, which usually occur
between 3 and 7 years of age. An EEG can determine the presence
of this disorder.

Treatment:

Nonpharmacologic

Because of the variability and severity of symptoms as expressed, any
treatment considered should be planned for the specific individual.
These children may receive occupational therapy, physical therapy,
speech therapy, behavioral and social skills training, and educational
tutoring. Consistency among the caregivers regarding expectations, rules,
and behavioral management is important.

Autistic disorder: The most widely accepted programs include the
Lovaas Program, Applied Behavioral Analysis (ABA), Discrete Trial
Training, Picture Exchange Communication System (PECS),
Auditory Integration Therapy (AIT), and TEACCH program. All of
these programs depend on highly motivated and dedicated teachers
and parents who provide a structured program modified for each
child.

Pharmacologic

AUTISTIC DISORDER

Haloperidol, 0.5 to 4 mg per day, to modify disruptive, hyperactive,
and aggressive behavior.

Fenfluramine may be helpful in children with elevated serotonin.

Naltrexone may help control self-injurious behavior.

Respiradol, 0.5 mg up to 5 mg once a day, may be used and has
been shown to decrease certain characteristic repetitive behaviors.

Use of stimulants may make the symptoms more severe, but these
agents can be used in some cases for improvement of attention
behaviors.

Medications for sleep difficulty include chloral hydrate (Noctec) and
diphenhydramine (Benadryl). Mirtazapine (Remeron), for sleep
disorders, has value in resetting the sleep cycle.

Drugs found to have no validity in altering or improving autism include secretin, intravenous immunoglobulin therapy, and transfer factor.

PERVASIVE DEVELOPMENTAL DISORDER,

NOT OTHERWISE SPECIFIED

Clinical trials are ongoing for the use of risperidone (optimal dosage range 0.75 to 1.5 mg daily, in divided doses) for fidgetiness.
Methylphenidate may be used if ADHD coexists.
Fluoxetine (Prozac), an SSRI, may be used to reduce rituals or compulsions.

Follow-up: Continuous follow-up by primary care providers, educational consultants, psychologists, and physical and occupational therapists is necessary in some form for the rest of the autistic child's life.
Sequelae:
Autistic disorder: Continued and worsening inability to function in the world, complete a successful educational program, form meaningful relationships, or live independently. Seizure disorders may eventually be seen in approximately 25% of autistic children; one in six may become gainfully employed as adults; one in six are able to function in structured environments. The best prognosis is in children of normal intelligence and in children who have symbolic language skills by age 5 years.
Prevention/prophylaxis: Appropriate prenatal care for the mother.
Referral: As soon as a child is suspected to have autism, he or she should be referred to a comprehensive diagnostic and treatment center.
Education: Parents should be instructed regarding the wide spectrum of disabilities that may be seen accompanying this disorder. Families should be referred to a support group and receive assistance in seeking the most highly qualified health care providers, educational programs, psychologists, and other treatment team members so that the earliest possible treatment can be instituted. Parents should also be told that there is great variation in the severity of this disorder and that with good care a child can achieve and be successful.

The child's rights with regard to educational opportunities should be presented to the parents and assistance given to them with the child's Individual Education Plan and any other resources they need to access the optimal health care plan for their child.

BREATH HOLDING

SIGNAL SYMPTOMS▶   voluntary or involuntary stoppage of breath

Breath holding	ICD-9 CM: 786.9/312.81 (older child)

Description: Breath holding is a paroxysmal, spontaneous, reflexive event occurring during expiration in healthy children that resolves in time. Breath holding is categorized as cyanotic, in which the child is provoked (anger, frustration, disciplinary measures), cries, becomes noiseless, becomes cyanotic, becomes limp, and may lose consciousness, and pallid, in which breath holding is usually in response to fear or injury; the cry is less, and the child turns pale. Rarely is seizure activity seen after loss of consciousness.

Etiology: Involuntary breath holding and loss of consciousness caused by cerebral anoxia. There is a family history is 25% of cases. It has been suggested the genetic pattern is an autosomal dominant trait with reduced penetrance.

Occurrence: Occurs in 5% of children younger than age 6 years; 60% have cyanotic spells, 20% have pallid spells, and 20% have both.

Age: Occurs in children age 6 months to 6 years.

Ethnicity: Not significant.

Gender: Occurs equally in males and females.

Contributing factors: Trigger events that upset or frustrate the child. May be associated with pica and iron-deficiency anemia. Mothers with negative perceptions of the child and child behavior as well as altered perceptions as a competent parent.

Signs and symptoms: The child presents with a history of breath-holding spells. Physical examination is negative.

Diagnostic tests: None. If frequency increases, test for the following.

Test	Results Indicating Disorder	CPT Code
EEG	Rule out seizure disorders	95816
Complete blood count	Rule out anemia	85007

Differential diagnosis:

> With epilepsy, the EEG results are abnormal, and there is usually no precipitating event.
>
> Sleep apnea is differentiated by the history, which reveals that episodes occur while child is asleep.
>
> Rett's syndrome is a neurodegenerative disorder that affects females, who present with microcephaly, stereotypical hand movements, social withdrawal, and loss of communication skills that are related to a psychological disorder.
>
> Vasovagal syncope rarely occurs before the age of 12 years.

Treatment:

Nonpharmacologic

Parents should do the following:

> Monitor the event, but treat it in a matter-of-fact manner because it is impossible to protect the child from all upsetting events.

Help the child to control his or her responses to upsetting events.
Prevent self-injurious behavior.

As in temper tantrums, the child's demands that precipitated the "spell" should not be granted. In the case of syncope, the parent should place the child in the lateral supine position to protect the head and prevent aspiration. Parents should maintain a patent airway, but not do cardiopulmonary resuscitation unless true respiratory arrest has occurred.

Pharmacologic

In pallid breath-holding spells with significant bradycardia, the implantation of a pacemaker has been found to be effective.

Follow-up: None.

Sequelae: There may be a link between the pallid type and syncopal episodes in adulthood.

Prevention/prophylaxis: For pallid spells accompanied by bradycardia or asystole, atropine, 0.01 mg/kg per dose, has been used to prevent spells. Help the young child to learn more appropriate measures to deal with the frustrations of growing up.

Referral: Refer to a neurologist if there is increased frequency or any question as to diagnosis.

Education: Educate parents in techniques to assist the child in dealing with frustrations. Be supportive to parents, and reassure them that their child will outgrow this behavior.

BULIMIA

SIGNAL SYMPTOMS ▶ excessive appetite

Bulimia	ICD-9 CM: 783.6

Description: Bulimia nervosa is a serious eating disorder of two types: purge and exercise. Bulimia is characterized by the following:

- Recurrent episodes of secretive binge eating (two times per week for 3 months) followed by self-induced vomiting (90%) and the use of laxatives (50–75%) or diuretics (10–34%) to compensate for the eating
- Excessive exercise and concern about weight or body shape
- Lack of control over the eating
- Use of restrictive diets
- Other impulsive behaviors

Binge eating is defined as rapid consumption of large amounts of food (5000–20,000 calories of high-carbohydrate food at a time)

Etiology: Unknown, although there seems to be a familial link.

Occurrence: Occurs in 2% to 15% of teenagers and 15% to 30% of college-age girls.

Age: Primarily occurs in older adolescents.

Ethnicity: Primarily in white females.

Gender: Females account for 90% of the bulimic population; 10% are males. History may reveal gender differences: Males tend to be concerned with sexual identity and maintaining body shape and muscle tone; females are concerned with perception of body image.

Contributing factors: Low self-esteem and personalities characterized by overachievement and perfectionism seem to be implicated. Bulimic females frequently have a history of being obese. Additionally, 60% of female bulimia patients have been sexually abused. Bulimia in males and females may be a form of self-medication for depression, anxiety, and loneliness. Coaches who encourage dehydration before weigh-ins and before games or matches may play a role in the subsequent binge eating among players.

Signs and symptoms: The child is brought to the clinic usually because the caregiver has noticed the self-induced vomiting after meals. Bulimia may be suspected during the history taking for an initial complaint of depression. Ask the following questions:

What does the child consider the perfect weight?

Is the child on a diet?

What does the child do to maintain her weight? (These is usually a history of excessive exercise.)

What does the child think of her current weight?

It is helpful to obtain a weight history to determine the patient's growth pattern. Postmenarcheal females should be asked about the frequency of periods and the amount of blood flow. Inquire about past diet behavior. The Eating Attitudes Test and the Eating Disorder Inventory are useful assessment tools.

Physical findings may include weight that is normal or slightly above normal; salivary gland enlargement; esophagitis; callus formation on knuckles of first and second fingers from inducing vomiting; and erosion of dental enamel on posterior surface of the front teeth from constant contact with stomach acid (see Fig. 14–1).

Comorbid conditions include affective disorders, obsessive-compulsive disorder, substance abuse, and events related to risk-taking behaviors, such as kleptomania and sexual promiscuity.

Diagnostic tests:

Test	Results Indicating Disorder	CPT Codes
Complete blood count	Assess nutritional status	85007
Erythrocyte sedimentation rate	Exclude inflammatory bowel disease or collagen vascular disease	85651
Electrolyte studies	Hypochloremic alkalosis Hypocalcemia owing to vomiting Metabolic acidosis owing to laxative use	80051
Urinalysis	Concentration levels	81000
Serum total protein and albumin	Usually normal	82040 84160–84165

Differential diagnosis: Disorders that cause vomiting are many; bulimia is unique in that the patient focuses on body image or fears of obesity.

Treatment:

Nonpharmacologic

A multidisciplinary team, including a primary care physician, mental health counselor, and dietitian, should be formed. Contracting has been found to be a useful strategy. The contract should include long-term weight goals, rate of weight gain or loss, amount of allowable exercise, strategies to reduce the number of bingeing and vomiting episodes, and the frequency of visits to health care professionals.

Pharmacologic

Imipramine, initiated at 30 to 40 mg and increased to 150 to 300 mg daily or until a satisfactory response is achieved, has had some success. Give at night to improve therapeutic levels. Do not give to persons with cardiac dysfunction.

Fluoxetine, 20 mg per day, is given, up to 60 mg per day for children 16 years old and older.

 Clinical Pearl: Bupropion is contraindicated in purging patients because of increased risk of seizures.

Follow-up: Weekly visits with the health care team to evaluate progress.

Sequelae: Gastric dilation, esophageal tears, diarrhea, dental decay, cardiac abnormalities, and irregular menses are medical complications. Approximately 5% commit suicide, and 80% are clinically depressed.

Prevention/prophylaxis: Reduce the messages children get as to the "perfect" weight. Assist girls in forming a positive self-image. Educate teachers and coaches not to encourage poor habits such as fasting/bingeing cycles in children.

Referral: Consult with or refer patient to a primary care physician for definitive diagnosis and admission to the hospital if necessary. Refer patient and family to a mental health counselor for family therapy. Refer patient to a dietitian for appropriate meal planning. Refer patient and parents to support groups.

Education: Instruct patient and family about the illness. Provide factual knowledge, not myths. Teach patient about eating and appropriate eating patterns; many have lost sight of what constitutes a normal eating pattern.

DEPRESSION

SIGNAL SYMPTOMS▶   alteration in mood

Depression	ICD-9 CM: 311

Description: Depression is an intense, persistent state of unhappiness often related to a recent event that lasts for days or often weeks and interferes with the ability to experience pleasure or to be productive.

Etiology: There may be a genetic predisposition, as noted by occurrence secondary to depression in the mother; there may also be a familial tendency toward negative interpretations of life events, such as developmental situations (entering adolescence, going away to college) or chronic illness.

Occurrence: Occurs in 1% to 3% of preadolescent children and 3% to 6% of adolescents. Incidence is higher in children with a family history of depression.

Age: Any age.

Ethnicity: Not significant.

Gender: Probably occurs equally in males and females younger than age 14 years; after age 14, more females affected.

Contributing factors: Rejection by peers, failure to achieve expectations, parent-child conflicts (may be "trigger" factors), history of abuse, and a poor home environment.

Signs and symptoms: The child may present with any of the clinical manifestations listed in Table 14–2.

Adolescents often have difficulty talking about their sadness; rather, they exhibit acting-out behaviors, particularly toward the parents.

Physical findings may be negative. Somatic symptoms must be investigated because they are often signs and symptoms of other organic disorders (Fig. 14–3).

Table 14–2 Clinical Manifestations of Depression in Children and Adolescents

Symptom	Clinical Manifestations
Dysphoric mood	Tearfulness; sad, downturned expression; unhappiness; slumped posture; quick temper; irritability; anger
Anhedonia	Loss of interest and enthusiasm in play, socializing, school, and usual activities; boredom; loss of pleasure
Fatigability	Lethargy and tiredness; no play after school
Morbid ideation	Self-deprecating thoughts, statements; thoughts of disaster, abandonment, death, suicide, or hopelessness
Somatic symptoms	Changes in sleep or appetite patterns; difficulty in concentrating; bodily complaints, particularly headache and stomachache

Source: Clark, RB: Psychosocial aspects of pediatrics and psychiatric disorders. In Hay, W, et al (eds): Current Pediatric Diagnosis and Treatment. Appleton & Lange, Stamford, CT, 1994, p. 170, with permission.

Diagnostic tests: None. Behavioral checklists, such as the Short Screening Scales for Anxiety and Depression (Goldman et al, 1988), may be helpful for an initial assessment. Testing for diagnostic differentials includes the following.

Test	Results Indicating Disorder	CPT Code
Complete blood count	Hemoglobin <11g/dL indicates anemia	85007
Thyroid panel	Low T_3 and T_4 and elevated TSH indicate hypothyroidism	84481–84482
Epstein-Barr antibody titer	Elevated in chronic fatigue syndrome	86663
Drug screen	Evidence of substance abuse	80100
Blood glucose levels	<60 mg/dL indicates hypoglycemia; >160 mg/dL indicates hyperglycemia	82947

Perform a general medical examination along with weight and blood pressure measurements before initiating treatment with SSRIs and other types of medications.

Differential diagnosis:

Chronic fatigue syndrome is differentiated by low-grade fever, enlarged lymph nodes, sore throat, and an elevated Epstein-Barr antibody titer.

Hypothyroidism is differentiated by clinical laboratory findings and by clinical features such as dry skin and dry, brittle hair.

Concomitant chronic illness, such as diabetes, hypoglycemia, anemia, or epilepsy, may contribute to depression.

Substance abuse is differentiated by a drug screen. Children often use or abuse chemicals to change the way they feel and as another

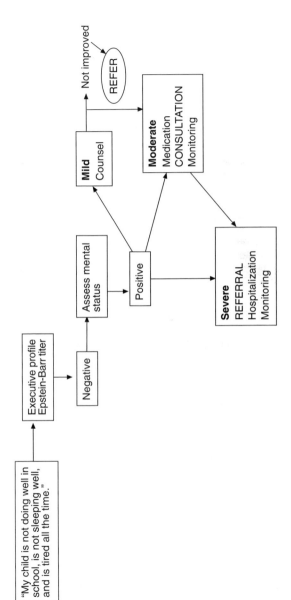

Figure 14–3. Evaluation of depression.

way of "acting out," not realizing that a secondary effect is depression.

Treatment:

Nonpharmacologic

Behavioral therapy involves individual psychotherapy for the child, particularly cognitive therapy; family therapy is indicated to teach parents how to meet the child's emotional needs more effectively.

Pharmacologic

Imipramine (tricyclic antidepressant): Starting dose is 1 mg/kg per day; increase by 0.25 mg every 4 to 5 days to 3 mg/kg per day. Contraindicated in cases of known cardiac disease, seizure disorder, or electrolyte abnormalities or a family history of cardiomyopathy.

 Clinical Pearl: Before starting treatment with tricyclic antidepressants, screen for cardiac problems, seizure disorder, and liver profiles. Monitor cardiovascular function by ECG with each dosage increase greater than 3 mg/kg per day.

Patients taking tricyclic antidepressants may experience anticholinergic effects, headaches, and sleep disorders. Interactions occur with antidepressants and stimulants: Plasma levels of antidepressants are lower in combination with barbiturates and cigarette smoking; plasma levels are increased in combination with phenothiazines, methylphenidate, and oral contraceptives.

SSRI: Usually once-daily dosing, in the morning, is sufficient. There are no known contraindications. Side effects may be increased psychomotor activity, headache, insomnia, and gastrointestinal distress. May interact with other antidepressants, leading to higher than expected blood levels.

Fluoxetine: Initially, 5 to 10 mg per day; increase by 5 to 10 mg every 2 weeks, as tolerated, to a maximum dose of 40 mg per day.

Sertraline: Therapeutic dose to 50 to 150 mg per day.

Paroxetine: Therapeutic dose to 10 to 40 mg per day.

Bupropion (other category): Dosage range is 150 to 375 mg per day in divided doses. In adolescents, maximum dosage should be less than 450 mg per day. Bupropion is contraindicated in seizure disorder. Few anticholinergic or cardiotoxic effects. Adverse effects include headache, increased psychomotor activity, anorexia, insomnia, and induction of seizures with doses greater than 450 mg per day.

Follow-up: Weekly follow-up until stabilized on medication, then every 3 to 4 months. For patients on tricyclics, follow-up every 3 to 4 months, taking height, weight, pulse, and blood pressure measurements and performing an ECG. For patients on SSRIs and other medications, follow-up with a medical examination, including weight and blood pressure measurements, every 3 months.

Sequelae: Depressed children have school problems because depression interferes with memory and concentration, leading to failure and low self-esteem. Of children with an initial episode occurring between ages 8 and 13, 75% have a recurrence later in life.

Prevention/prophylaxis: Active listening to the child and awareness of "nuances" of behavior with appropriate interventions.

Referral: Consult/collaborate with a primary care physician or psychiatrist before forming a definitive diagnosis and initiating pharmacologic interventions. The child may require hospitalization for severe depression.

Education: Be supportive to parents as they learn to listen to their children and learn to meet the child's emotional needs more effectively. Instruct parents about the dosage, purpose, and side effects of medications.

EMOTIONAL ABUSE

SIGNAL SYMPTOMS▶ mistreatment through verbal or nonverbal expressions

Emotional abuse	ICD-9 CM: 995.82

Description: The repeated pattern of rejecting, isolating, verbally terrorizing, ignoring, corrupting, verbally assaulting, and overpressuring a child to the extent they believe they are worthless, flawed, unloved, unwanted, endangered, or only of value in meeting another's needs. These behaviors may be categorized as follows.

Mild emotional abuse: There is no malicious intent and no immediate danger of harm to child.

Moderate emotional abuse: There are elements of malicious intent or danger of emotional harm, but not both.

Severe emotional abuse: There are elements of malicious intent and the infliction of emotional harm on the child.

Etiology: Child's failure to meet expectations of parents, teachers, and peers.

Occurrence: Accounts for approximately 7% of reported child abuse. The abuse may occur at home, day care, school, or during team sports.

Age: All pediatric age groups.

Ethnicity: Not significant.

Gender: Occurs equally in males and females.

Contributing factors: Excessive expectations for age by parents, teachers, and significant others.

Signs and symptoms: The child may present with a history of sleep disorders, somatic symptoms (stomachaches, headaches), or avoidance behaviors (refusal to go to school, running away). Physical findings reveal a negative examination related to the somatic complaints. Observations of the child reveal a child with loss of self-esteem and hypervigilant behaviors.

Diagnostic tests: None except those in relation to the somatic complaints.

Differential diagnosis: Evaluate the somatic complaints.

Treatment: Child and family therapy.

Follow-up: Monitor child's progress in relation to somatic complaints.

Sequelae: May result in a chronic condition of low self-esteem or substance use and abuse.

Prevention/prophylaxis: Parent effectiveness training.

Referral: Only 20 states have mechanisms in place to deal with reports of emotional abuse. Usually not referred to child protective services unless the abuse is severe. Refer the child to mental health counseling, and refer the family to family therapy.

Education: Involve parents in parent effectiveness training. Educate parents in appropriate behaviors.

FAILURE TO THRIVE

SIGNAL SYMPTOMS▶   inadequate weight gain

Failure to thrive (FTT)	ICD-9 CM: 783.41

Description: FTT refers to young children with inadequate weight gain, usually below the third percentile on a standard growth chart, and weight less than 80% of the median weight for height for age and gender.

Etiology: The causes of FTT can be categorized as either nonorganic or organic.

Nonorganic causes relate to maternal factors, such as poor mother-child bonding; poor feeding techniques, including the child's excessive consumption of fruit juice; nutritional beliefs of the mother; errors in formula preparation; and child neglect.

Organic causes relate to a variety of chronic or serious childhood conditions, such as chromosomal disorders, fetal alcohol syndrome, immunodeficiency diseases, tumors, intestinal obstruction, renal failure, cystic fibrosis, celiac disease, and central nervous system pathology.

Occurrence: FTT accounts for 3% to 5% of admissions to teaching hospitals: 44% have environmental causes, 37% have organic causes, and 19% have no known cause.

Age: Any age, dependent on underlying cause.

Ethnicity: Not significant.

Gender: Occurs equally in males and females.

Contributing factors: Family dysfunction, maternal depression, and postpartum depression have been implicated in nonorganic FTT. It is more common in children living below the poverty level.

Signs and symptoms: The child may have a history of poor feeding, vomiting, or diarrhea. The child may have a diagnosis of an organic illness. Findings reveal inadequate weight gain and weight changes that are below norms for age/weight percentile on standard charts. Standardized charts are particularly useful when serial weights are not available. The child is observed to have frozen watchfulness, minimal smiling, decreased vocalization, resistance to being held, and self-stimulating rhythmic behaviors (Fig. 14–4).

Diagnostic tests:

Obtain a diet history that includes how the formula is prepared.

Observe parent-child interaction; watch the child being fed.

Investigate possibilities of environmental deprivation.

Test	Results Indicating Disorder	CPT Code
Complete blood count	Assessment of anemias or possible infection	82947
Urinalysis	Rule out infections	81000
Thyroid panel	Decreased T_4 and elevated TSH indicate hypothroidism	84482/ 84481
Serum electrolytes	Rule out metabolic disorders	80051
Erythrocyte sedimentation rate	Elevated in infectious processes	85651
If gastrointestinal symptoms: stool culture and guaiac	Rule out blood loss	87045 82270
Serum albumin, alkaline phosphatase, calcium, and phosphorus	Assessment of protein status and biochemical rickets (severe malnutrition)	84160– 84165 84075 82310 84100
Bone age	If normal, rules out systemic chronic disease or hormonal abnormality	76020

Differential diagnosis: To identify specific causes of organic FTT.

Central nervous system pathology or neuromuscular disease should be suspected if the child presents with the inability to suck or swallow.

If child presents with chronic diarrhea, cystic fibrosis, or celiac disease, suspect a maldigestion or malabsorption problem.

Poor nutrient use is observed with renal failure and inborn errors of metabolism.

Tumors, inborn errors of metabolism, and intestinal obstruction can cause vomiting.

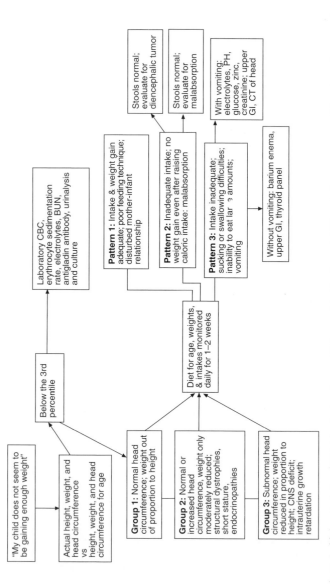

Figure 14—4. Evaluation of failure to thrive. (BUN, blood urea nitrogen; CBC, complete blood count; CNS, central nervous system; CT, computed tomography; GI, gastrointestinal.)

Regurgitation is seen in gastroesophageal reflux or rumination syndrome.

Suspect an elevated metabolic rate in cases of thyrotoxicosis, chronic disease such as heart failure, inflammatory lesions, immunodeficiency diseases, and burns.

Patients with chromosomal disorders and fetal alcohol syndrome all have reduced growth potential.

Treatment: Increase caloric intake to 150 kcal/kg per day. Number of calories per ounces of formula may be increased by adding less water (13 oz formula concentrate mixed with 10 oz water = 24 kcal/oz high-calorie formula) or by the addition of carbohydrates. Record amount of feedings, and obtain before-breakfast weights daily. Involve parents in the interventions, particularly in planning an organized program of early infant stimulation. Treat the underlying organic cause if one is found. Older children may benefit from increased milk products, margarine, oil, and peanut butter.

For infants and toddlers who do not gain weight by oral feedings, supplement the diet by tube feedings.

Follow-up: Regular monitoring of growth and development during the first 2 years of life. Initially, see child weekly for evaluation of weight gain; as weight gain stabilizes, follow-up at 1- to 3-month intervals.

Sequelae: Children hospitalized for FTT exhibit mental retardation (15–67%), school learning problems (37–67%), and behavioral disturbances (28–48%) by 3 to 11 years of age.

Prevention/prophylaxis: Emphasis in the prenatal period on infant nutrition, including formula preparation and parent-child interaction, assists in preventing nonorganic FTT.

Referral: If outpatient treatment fails, malnutrition is severe, or other circumstances put the child at risk, refer child for hospitalization.

Education: Educate parents and caregivers in proper feeding techniques and daily requirements for adequate nutrition. Educate parents in parenting techniques to promote bonding.

MUNCHAUSEN SYNDROME BY PROXY

SIGNAL SYMPTOMS ▶ factitious production of symptoms in children for emotional gain for others

Munchausen syndrome by proxy   ICD-9 CM: 301.51

Description: Munchausen syndrome by proxy is a form of child abuse characterized by a parent, usually the mother (98%), who induces signs and symptoms of illness in a child.

Etiology: Three types of parents are prone to be perpetrators:

Help seekers report illness in the child to convey distress in their personal lives.

Active inducers give the appearance of being perfect parents, resist treatment, and try to hide their psychological problems.

Doctor addicts, because of their obsession with the child's health, become paranoid regarding the treatment team; these parents tend to change doctors and hospitals often.

Occurrence: Unknown. These children have a 9% mortality rate.

Age: Occurs mainly from infancy to age 2, rarely in children older than 6.

Ethnicity: Not significant.

Gender: Occurs equally in males and females.

Contributing factors: Often occurs in a nuclear family in which both parents live together, but the father is typically not involved in child rearing and the mother is devoted to the child.

Signs and symptoms: Diarrhea, neurologic impairment, seizures, and vomiting are common presenting symptoms. A careful history reveals an unexplained persistent or recurrent illness whose signs and symptoms do not correlate with the history or appearance of the child. There is evidence of the child's failure to respond to standard medical treatment, repeated hospitalizations, and parents' demand for vigorous medical evaluation. The child's separation from the mother results in the absence of reported signs and symptoms.

Possible indicators of Munchausen syndrome by proxy include a mother who has had previous medical or nursing experience. The mother is calm, socializes with the staff, and appears not too concerned about child's illness. A history may reveal that the mother had an illness similar to that of the child. She is overprotective, not leaving the child alone; there are repeated requests for evaluation and care of the child. The physical examination focuses on the presenting complaint. Other children may have died from similar conditions.

Diagnostic tests:

Video surveillance of parent-child interaction. Permission from the judicial system is required before videotaping.

Removal of parent from the room to see whether illness abates (evidenced by absence of gastrointestinal complaints or apneic episodes).

Differential diagnosis: Because of confusing findings, the differential diagnosis is focused on validating the presenting complaint. Close observation of parent-child interaction may require hospitalization in suspect cases.

Treatment: Confront the parent and advise her to undergo counseling. Treatment for the child may involve removal of the child from the home by protective services.

Follow-up: Follow-up for remission of symptoms.

Sequelae: Depending on the degree of abuse and time until diagnosis, sequelae range from no long-term symptoms to death.

Prevention/prophylaxis: Appropriate parenting skills.

Referral: Refer child to protective services. Refer parent and child to mental health services for counseling/psychotherapy.

Education: Educate the parent in parenting skills.

PHYSICAL ABUSE

SIGNAL SYMPTOMS mistreatment using physical means

Physical abuse	ICD-9 CM: 995.54

Description: Physical abuse is a deliberate assault on a child using excessive force or hitting with a closed fist or other instrument.

Etiology: May be triggered by behaviors in the child, such as persistent crying, toileting accidents, spilling, and disobedience.

Occurrence: Occurs in 1% to 2% of children in the United States; accounts for 2000 deaths per year.

Age: Occurs in all pediatric age groups, but primarily in children younger than age 6 years (one third of cases occur in infants <1 year old, and half occur in children age 1 to 6).

Ethnicity: Not significant.

Gender: Occurs equally in males and females.

Contributing factors: Increased parental stress (<10% of parents have psychotic or criminal personalities) and parental substance abuse are among the factors implicated in physical abuse of children and domestic violence in the home.

Signs and symptoms: The child presents with a vague history of injuries. Indicators of abuse include a discrepant history (i.e., inconsistent with the injury) and a delay in seeking medical care. A pattern of increased severity of injury is seen if no intervention occurs. The child has a history of multiple hospitalizations or multiple caretakers for injuries. The child may also have a history of behaviors that trigger the assaults.

Perform a careful, complete physical examination including height and weight. Record place, size, shape, and color of any bruises or burns. Bruising in cases of abuse is usually confined to the buttocks or lower back. Observe for distinctive patterns of bruising that suggest use of a belt, cords, pinches, and choke holds. Some burns, such as those from irons, cigarettes, or submersion into scalding water, have a distinctive pattern. Perform a funduscopic examination of the eye to look for retinal hemorrhages (particularly helpful in diagnosing shaken baby syndrome). Examine the eardrums, oral cavity, and genitalia for evidence of trauma. Evaluate the musculoskeletal system for tenderness and range of motion. Obtain color photographs of injuries, taking care to label with name, location, date, and time. Signs and symptoms of acute abdomen (e.g., rupture of the liver, spleen, intestines) may be the result of striking or squeezing the abdomen.

Diagnostic tests:

Test	Results Indicating Disorder	CPT Code
Radiographs of skull, thorax, spine, and long bones in children <5 if abuse is suspected	Periosteal tears in shaken baby syndrome Coexistence of new and old injuries indicates long-term presence of abuse	70250 72270 73592 73090 73092
CT scan or MRI if shaken baby syndrome is suspected	Presence of subdural hemorrhages	70470
If bruising: prothrombin time	Depressed: acquired deficiency in clot formation	85210
Partial thromboplastin time	Depressed: acquired deficiency in clot formation	85730

Investigate the family situation: Look for a caregiver who is stressed, has a history of abuse during childhood, has unrealistic expectations for the child, and is socially isolated.

Differential diagnosis:

Differentiate accidental injuries (accidental bruising is most common over the forehead, bony prominences, and anterior tibia).

Dermatologic conditions such as impetigo and contact dermatitis may be confused with healing cigarette burns.

Differentiate injuries resulting from unrestrained motor vehicle accidents.

Treatment: Inform the parents that the clinic is required to report the suspected abuse. Develop a multidisciplinary plan along with child protective services.

Treat the specific injury.

Follow-up: Follow-up as indicated for the presenting injury. Follow-up as part of the multidisciplinary team, providing services for the child and family.

Sequelae: Child is at risk for permanent injury or death.

Prevention/prophylaxis: Identification and education of high-risk parents in proper parenting skills. Support groups such as Parents Anonymous.

Referral: Consult with child protection authorities to initiate a multidisciplinary investigation. Report suspected abuse to local authorities.

 Clinical Pearl: Nurse practitioners are mandated reporters.

Hospitalize the child while investigation continues to determine the safety of the home environment.

Education: Teach proper parenting skills. Educate parents, caregivers, and babysitters regarding the hazards of shaking infants and the need to support the head at all times.

SCHIZOPHRENIA

SIGNAL SYMPTOMS▶ disordered thinking, affect, socializing, action, language, or perception

Schizophrenia	ICD-9 CM: 299.9

Description: Schizophrenia is any group of psychotic disorders characterized by withdrawal from reality and illogical thought patterns, such as delusions and hallucinations. In adolescents, it is a chronic disorder.

Etiology: Unknown. Genetic patterns, defects of the frontal lobe, and dopamine imbalance have been suggested as causative factors.

Occurrence: Rare. Estimated incidence is 1 to 2 in 10,000 children younger than 15 years old.

Age: Onset occurs in children age 5 to 15.

Ethnicity: Not significant.

Gender: Occurs equally in males and females.

Contributing factors: Dysfunctional family relationships and a family history of schizophrenia may be contributing factors.

Signs and symptoms: The child is brought to the clinic because of somatic complaints or behavioral problems. Findings include rambling or illogical speech patterns, bizarre thought content, and hallucinations or delusions. Physical findings are normal.

Diagnostic tests:

Test	Results Indicating Disorder	CPT Code
Drug screen	Presence of illicit substances	80100
Ceruloplasmin levels	Normal values are 23–43 mg/dL: elevated in Wilson's disease	82390
EEG	Assess for brain tumors	95816
MRI		70551–70553

 Clinical Pearl: Before initiating antipsychotic pharmacotherapy, obtain a baseline complete blood count, liver function tests, and ECG if patient has a history of cardiac disease or arrhythmias.

Differential diagnosis:

Differentiate normal growth and development. Children younger than age 8 normally have a vivid fantasy life; however, rambling speech and bizarre thought content are differentiating characteristics.

In adolescents, learning disabilities may mimic schizophrenia.

Mania in adolescents is characterized by increased activity, energy, and irritability.

In Wilson's disease, there may be psychiatric symptoms as a result of hepatic degeneration.

Treatment: The goal of treatment is to ease psychotic symptoms, reduce risk of relapse, teach skills, and support parents.

Nonpharmacologic

Institute behavioral therapy. Train child in appropriate life, social, and cognitive skills through a structured day treatment center.

Pharmacologic

Haloperidol: Begin dose at 0.5 to 1 mg per day, increasing by 0.5 mg every 3 to 5 days until there are clinical effects or side effects, up to a maximum of 4 mg per day. Dosage is usually twice a day. Available in tablets, intramuscular formulation, intravenous formulation, concentrate, and decanoate. Effects may take 2 to 3 weeks to become fully apparent. Before initiating drug regimen, examine for abnormal movements, then watch for cognitive slowing and one or more extrapyramidal symptoms.
Contraindicated in patients with poorly controlled seizures, cardiac arrhythmias, agranulocytosis, previous neuroleptic malignant syndrome, and tardive dyskinesia.

Risperidone: Start at 0.25 mg per day and increase up to 6 mg per day. Available in tablets and liquid.

Clozapine: 12.25 mg one to two times, then increase to 450 mg per day as maximum dose. This drug is under investigation for children who do not respond to typical neuroleptics. Starting dose is 6.25 mg with weekly increases of 6.25 mg as needed.

Olanzapine: 5 to 10 mg daily in children and adolescents with weekly increases by 2.5- or 5-mg increments to a target dose of 20 mg per day.

Extrapyramidal symptoms are a side effect of antipsychotic drugs. Family members should be advised of the possibility.

 Clinical Pearl: When recognizing dystonic reactions, parents should administer 25 to 50 mg of diphenhydramine, discontinue the antipsychotic drug, and contact the physician or emergency department.

Follow-up: Monitor progress, in collaboration with the attending psychiatrist, every 3 months for signs of tardive dyskinesia.

Sequelae: Schizophrenia is a chronic disorder with remissions and exacerbations that affect school and work performance as well as social interactions and relationships.

Prevention/prophylaxis: None.

Referral: Consult with and refer patient to a psychiatrist.

Education: Provide support for family, emphasizing the provision of a calm environment and the importance of clear communication. Instruct parents about dosage, purpose, and side effects of medications. Instruct parents to have diphenhydramine on hand for the treatment of dystonic reactions to an antipsychotic drug.

SELF-INJURIOUS BEHAVIOR

SIGNAL SYMPTOMS▶   injuries to the body produced by self

| Self-injurious behavior | ICD-9 CM: 300.9 |

Description: Self-injurious behaviors range from mild piercing of ears to more severe suicidal behaviors.

Suicide is a self-injurious behavior that functions as a maladaptive attempt actively to solve a problem. Possibly 70% of children have experienced a loss, a failure, or an arrest before attempting suicide. Before attempts, children may appear depressed and irritable, may withdraw from social activities, and show a loss of interest in usual activities. The incidence of suicide in adolescents and young adults tripled between 1952 and 1992.

Self-mutilation is the participation in the deliberate destruction of body tissue without suicidal intent; it is considered a form of self-directed violence. Body art, tattoos and insertion of body jewelry in tongue, navel, eyebrow, nipple, or genitalia, is a form of self-mutilation.

Etiology:

Suicide: Sadness, despair, and depression account for 50% of suicides; anger accounts for 20% of impulsive suicides; and substance abuse accounts for 20%. The remaining 10% are due to unknown causes. Firearms, hanging, carbon monoxide poisoning, and deliberate drug overdose are the most common methods in successful suicides. Panic attacks have been attributed to suicide ideation and attempts in adolescents.

Self-mutilation: This is a biologically driven behavior, a response to psychological and environmental stressors. Adolescents have described motivation as "for shock value," a rite of passage, and a sign of commitment.

Occurrence:

Suicide: Second leading cause of death in 15- to 24-year olds. Attempts outnumber success 100:1. In children younger than 14, for completed attempts, the rate is 0.7 in 100,000; for adolescents age 15 to 19, the rate is 11.3 per 10,000; there are 50 to 100 attempts for every success. The most common means of suicide is ingestion of pills.

Self-mutilation: Underreported, but some studies have found 750 cases per 100,000 in the general population of adolescents and adults. Self-mutilation is becoming more common; it seems to parallel the increase in child abuse. Self-mutilation is common in children who are mentally retarded.

Age:

Suicide: May occur in preschool children, but it is more common in adolescents.

Self-mutilation: Usually begins in adolescence but with mental retardation may begin at any age.

Ethnicity:

Suicide: Highest suicide rate is in white adolescent males. Native Americans and Alaskan Natives have a high rate of suicides. Hispanic youth have a higher rate of suicide attempts than whites or blacks.

Self-mutilation: Not known.

Gender:

Suicide: Prepubertal males and adolescent females are the most likely to attempt or succeed. Females outnumber males in attempts, but males are more successful in completing the act.

Self-mutilation: Occurs in males and females.

Contributing factors:

Suicide: Alcohol or drug abuse; psychosis; poor impulse control; parental conflict; previous attempts; family history of suicide; experiences that lead to guilt, shame, or humiliation; situations in which the child feels trapped, helpless, and hopeless; suicides among circle of friends; adoption. Close family connectedness is seen as a protector for adolescent suicide.

Self-mutilation: Organic conditions, such as Lesch-Nyhan disease and Tourette's syndrome; severely retarded patients, particularly if they are institutionalized; overwhelming stress; pathologic childhood experiences such as sexual and physical abuse. May be associated with substance abuse, bulimia, or anorexia.

Signs and symptoms:

History

Suicide: There may be a history of past or present suicide threats or gestures; reports of giving away personal possessions; or a written statement in which life is described as futile.

Self-mutilation: Multiple episodes of nonlethal self-injury, usually with a razor blade, but any sharp object may be used. The forearm (opposite the handedness) is the foremost site, but any part of the body is subject to the self-cutting. Criteria for diagnosis have been suggested by Fovazza and Rosenthal (1993): (1) preoccupation with physically harming self, (2) recurring failure to control impulse to do bodily harm (repetitive addictive acts), (3) feelings of tension that increase before the act, (4) feelings of gratification or relief during and after the act, (5) the act not associated with suicidal intent or in response to hallucinations or delusions.

Physical Examination

Suicide: The child may appear depressed. Other physical findings are not significant. Questions to be asked during the interview for assessment of suicide risk should include: How have you been feeling (inside and outside) (feelings of hopelessness, helplessness, wanting to give up)? Have you been feeling "down" or discouraged (how often, how long, and how severe)? Do these feelings interfere with your life (school, home, eating, sleeping)? Have you ever thought of suicide? Have you ever made a plan (include means)? Is there someone to whom you can go for help? Inquire about any loss or a suicide attempt or success among the child's circle of friends.

Self-mutilation: Findings range from tattoos or the insertion of body jewelry at various body sites to persistent scratches or cuts or lesions as a result of "picking" at the skin.

 Clinical Pearl: Inform the appropriate persons when you deem child is at high risk for suicide; hospitalize, with immediate referral to a mental health professional.

Diagnostic tests: None.

Differential diagnosis:

Self-mutilation: Rule out organic disorders whose behaviors include self-injury. Typically, Tourette's syndrome manifests in head banging; in Lesch-Nyhan disease, the manifestation is finger biting; mental retardation may take the form of scratching, biting self, and head banging. Rule out psychiatric disorders. Common manifestations in obsessive-compulsive behavior are hair pulling and skin picking; in schizophrenia, the form taken is usually in response to "voices." Assess for anxiety, depression, stressors, and family history of trauma. Explore with the patient other forms of addictive behavior, such as substance abuse.

Treatment:

Suicide: Consider any threat or attempt serious, and do not leave child alone. Meet and discuss the situation with the parent and the child. Listen to the child and the parents as they describe their feelings and perceptions. Individual counseling for suicide threats and attempts is often appropriate. Admit the child to the hospital immediately if you determine the potential for suicide is high, the child is in severe depression and intoxication, and in situations in which concern for the child's safety is paramount.

Self-mutilation: Behavioral interventions should include improving communication skills, raising self-esteem, identifying a support group, and finding persons the patient can turn to for individual support. In cases of infection related to body piercing or tattoos, systemic antibiotics are given.

Follow-up: Monitor any medication with which an underlying depression or other behavior is being treated.

Sequelae:

Suicide: Actual death, either intended or accidental. Aborted or incomplete suicide attempts may result in permanent injury.

Self-mutilation: Infection at site of tattoos or body piercings. Difficulty in removing the body jewelry in emergency situations. Allergies related to the dyes used in application of tattoos and the metal in the jewelry. Keloid formation at site of tattoos.

Prevention/prophylaxis:

Suicide: Treatment for depression. Active life skill education for children identified as high risk.

Self-mutilation: Prevention of complications through proper skin care. Advise patients never to self-pierce. Advise for vaccination against hepatitis B, and obtain tetanus immunization before piercing.

Referral:

Suicide: Refer child and parents to a mental health professional immediately.

Education: Reassure parents and child that the problems are understood. Educate parents and general public in the signs and symptoms of at-risk behaviors. Educate the child regarding the risk factors of self-mutilation, such as infection, possible allergic reactions, and blood-borne diseases. Inform the child particularly with body piercing the site may take 1 year to heal.

SEXUAL ABUSE

SIGNAL SYMPTOMS ▶ mistreatment through sexual activity

Sexual abuse	ICD-9 CM: 995.53

Description: Sexual abuse is the engaging of a child in sexual activities that are not understood by the child (i.e., the child cannot give informed consent) and that violate sexual taboos. Activities include exhibitionism; fondling; child pornography; and oral, anal, and genital contact. The categories of sexual abuse may or may not include the following:

- *Incest*—sexual abuse by a close relative that includes sexual intercourse
- *Molestation*—sexual abuse by a stranger that may or may not include penetration
- *Rape*—forced genital contact
- *Sexual assault*—violent or nonviolent manual, oral, or genital contact

Etiology: Pedophilia or a family structure that considers incest normal.

Occurrence: There are 250,000 reported cases per year; severe or chronic cases of child abuse are found in 1% to 3% of children. Most offenders are male; adolescents constitute 20% of offenders. Of boys younger than 18, 31% have been sexually molested.

Age: All pediatric age groups.

Ethnicity: Not significant.

Gender: Most victims are female.

Contributing factors: Fear of perpetrator, low self-esteem, and ignorance of what is acceptable touching behavior by family members or strangers.

Signs and symptoms: The child may be brought to the clinic because the parent suspects the child has been or is currently being sexually abused; the parent may report a sexualized play in a developmentally immature child, or the child has related events that are compatible with the diagnosis, such as "He plays with my bottom, and sticks his finger in there." Boys may exhibit inappropriate sexual behavior, suicidal ideation, and concentration deficits. If a boy is younger than the age of sexual activity and has a gonorrheal infection, suspect abuse.

The parent may report behavioral changes, such as sleep disturbances, nightmares, or night terrors; appetite disturbances (e.g., anorexia, bulimia); nocturnal enuresis; neurotic or conduct disorders; withdrawal, guilt, or depression; temper tantrums, aggressive behavior, suicidal ideation, or threats of running away; hysterical or conversion reactions; or excessive masturbation.

The school may have referred the child to the clinic because of inappropriate classroom behaviors.

Older children may be brought to the clinic because of substance abuse, suspected promiscuity, prostitution, or sexual abuse of other children by the victim.

Medical conditions or complaints that might lead one to suspect sexual abuse are recurrent abdominal pain; genital, urethral, or anal trauma; sexually transmitted diseases; recurrent urinary tract infections; enuresis or encopresis; or pregnancy.

Referrals may also be made to the clinic by protective services or law enforcement, usually as a result of a complaint by a parent.

Any history taking—whether it is a discussion with the child to investigate a definite complaint or a direct discussion because of what is suspected—should be done in a compassionate, nonjudgmental manner, with consideration for the age and developmental level of the child. Issues to be discussed are who the perpetrator is or was, the relationship to the victim, the duration of the abusive situation, and what was done to the child. Neither the nurse practitioner nor the person accompanying the child should prompt the child by posing leading or suggestive questions. Use of a doll with body parts and a child's drawings of self and family may facilitate the history taking.

Physical findings may be negative or nonspecific for abuse. Possible indicators of sexual abuse include bruises to the hard or soft palate, grasp marks, and the presence of a foreign body in the vagina or rectum. Perform a vaginal examination in the young child; the knee-chest position is a good position for viewing. In the older child, use the lithotomy position. Findings that are consistent with sexual abuse are disruptions of hymenal tissue (e.g., clefts or notches, absence of hymen, scars), anal scars, or skin tags outside the midline. The anus may be dilated 15 to 20 mm, and there is absence of stool in the ampulla. Children who have been previously abused may have labial adhesions, edema of the perineal tissues, and perianal fissures. In prepubertal boys, maintenance of a penile erection during the examination may be seen.

Diagnostic tests: The laboratory evaluation of the sexually abused child must include the collection of specimens that will be acceptable as forensic evidence. Obtain the following.

Test	Results Indicating Disorder	CPT Code
Wet mount of vaginal, oral, and rectal specimens	Presence of motile sperm	87210
Aspirate of cervical mucus	Presence of motile sperm	89330
Rectal, throat, vaginal/ endocervical cultures	Positive for *Neisseria gonorrhoeae*	87070
Throat, vulvovaginal, urethral, and rectal cultures	Presence of *Chlamydia*	87070
Blood for VDRL and HIV If chancre present, dark-field examination	Positive for syphilis Positive for *Treponema pallidum*	86592 87164
Culture of vaginal discharge	Presence of *Trichomonas vaginalis*	87070
Vaginal secretions (wet mount)	Presence of bacterial vaginosis Presence of *T. vaginalis*	87210
Vaginal culture	Positive for herpes simplex virus	87252
Biopsy of herpetic lesion (if present)	Positive for human papillomavirus	87252
If child is postmenarchal: blood or urine for pregnancy test	Positive for pregnancy	84702 81025

VDRL, Venereal Disease Research Laboratory; HIV, human immunodeficiency virus.

If possible, blood for hepatitis B and HIV from the perpetrator and blood for HIV from child at time of abuse and 3, 6, and 12 months later should be tested.

Specimens for Police Report, if Indicated

If there was a struggle, obtain fingernail scrapings for blood or fabric. Collect loose hairs or threads of fabric from the body or clothing. Collect air-dried specimens from the vagina, cervix, rectum, and mouth for testing for sperm antibodies, blood, and acid phosphatase. Inspect the body and clothing for fluorescence of sperm using Wood's lamp.

Differential diagnosis: Related to somatic complaints that may have brought the child to the clinic.

Normal Sex Play versus Sexual Abuse

Normal sex play occurs among children of the same developmental and cognitive levels. The children may play "house" or "doctor," touching their own or each other's genitals. The children have agreed to this infrequent activity. They feel guilty about their play, which is a normal response, and no physical injury results.

Suspect child abuse if there is an age gap in a relationship between a younger child and an older child (or young adult): If the younger child is younger than 13, a 5-year age difference is suspicious; if the younger child is older than 13, a 10-year age difference is suspicious. (*Note:* If the younger child has cognitive impairment, the age differences may be less.) In these cases, there is coercion by force or emotional pressure to complete the act, and the activity is not consistent with the developmental levels of the participants. The victim has a negative response, such as anger or fear. There is documented evidence of a physical injury as a result of the activity. Strongly suspect sexual abuse in a prepubertal child who has been diagnosed with gonorrhea.

Treatment:

Nonpharmacologic

The child and family need extensive counseling from a mental health professional.

Pharmacologic

Infections to be treated include the following:

Sexually transmitted diseases, confirmed (see Chapter 9)

Recurrent urinary infections (see Chapter 8)

Nonspecific vaginitis (see Chapter 9)

Risk of pregnancy: Oral contraceptives are options for emergency contraception, including an estrogen/progestin such as norgestrel and ethinyl estradiol (Orval), 2 tablets at the time of examination and 2 tablets 12 hours later (may prevent pregnancy within 72 hours of sexual intercourse), or Lo/Ovral, Levlen, or Levora, 4 tablets; or progestin only, such as levonorgestrel, 1 0.75-mg tablet followed by 1 tablet 12 hours later, or Ovrette, 20 tablets (1.5 mg norgestrel) followed by 20 tablets 12 hours later.

Prophylactic antibiotics are given if the parent requests them, a sexually transmitted disease is suspected, follow-up of child is uncertain, or the assault on the adolescent occurred within 72 hours.

Ceftriaxone, 125 mg intramuscularly single dose, for gonorrhea or incubating syphilis

Erythromycin, 50 mg/kg per day for 7 days divided into four doses, maximum 500 mg four times daily ($>$8 years old); or azithromycin, 1 g orally single dose; or doxycycline, 100 mg orally twice daily for 7 days ($<$8 years old and adolescents), for chlamydia

Give hepatitis B immunoglobulin, 0.5 mL intramuscularly, for hepatitis B.

Follow-up: Patient should return in 10 days for evaluation of therapeutic response in cases of infection. Obtain a serologic test for syphilis in 6 weeks.

Sequelae: Children who have a history of sexual abuse are at risk for becoming perpetrators. Some also develop low self-esteem or eating disorders, attempt or commit suicide, or engage in shoplifting or prostitution.

Prevention/prophylaxis: Effective parental education in appropriate parenting skills. Teaching children about what constitutes inappropriate touching behavior by another person.

Referral: Referral/report to child protective services for follow-up of family. The police should also be notified. May wish to refer patient to a pediatrician specializing in sexual abuse cases for initial workup and court appearance as the expert witness. Document completely and accurately all findings using drawings to describe any unusual findings.

The child may need to be admitted to the hospital for treatment of injuries and for personal safety. Refer the offender for treatment of psychological problems.

Education: Teach children what constitutes—and how to protect themselves against—inappropriate touching behavior from others. Teach parent effectiveness training. Educate the community regarding the prevalence of this problem and the ultimate outcomes.

SLEEP DISORDERS

SIGNAL SYMPTOMS▶   disruption in sleeping patterns

Primary sleep disorders (parasomnias)	ICD-9 CM 780.59
Secondary sleep disorders (dyssomnias)	NEC 780.56; nonorganic 307.47
Night terrors	ICD-9 CM: 307.46

Sleepwalking	ICD-9 CM: 307.45
Narcolepsy	ICD-9 CM: 347
Obstructive sleep apnea	ICD-9 CM: 780.57
Nightmares	ICD-9 CM: 307.47
Night awakenings	ICD-9 CM: 780.50
Disorders of initiating and maintaining sleep	ICD-9 CM: 780.50
Delayed sleep phase syndrome	ICD-9 CM: 780.50

Description: Primary sleep disorders are episodic, usually with a family history, and are characterized by an abnormal polysomnography.

Night terrors occur during non–rapid eye movement (REM) sleep and within 2 hours of sleep; they are associated with sleepwalking, screaming, and other bizarre behavior. When awakened, the child is disoriented and incoherent and has no memory of the event the next day.

Sleepwalking occurs early in the sleep cycle and is characterized by the child walking purposelessly and sedately. Alernatively, although less common, the child may be agitated and rush from the bed. May have inappropriate speech or confused mumblings.

Narcolepsy, a chronic neurologic disorder, is characterized by irresistible sleeping episodes; may be associated with cataplexy and disturbed nocturnal sleep.

Obstructive sleep apnea is characterized by prolonged partial upper airway obstruction or complete obstruction that disrupts normal ventilation during sleep and normal sleep patterns.

Nocturnal enuresis is bed wetting (see Chapter 8).

Nightmares are vivid frightening dreams that occur during REM sleep, followed by awakening in the latter part of the night; the child is alert, can describe the images, and is sometimes able to recall and talk about them the following day.

Secondary sleep disorders are more commonly characterized by normal polysomnography and usually have a behavioral component.

Night awakenings describe an infant who awakens after sleep has been initiated and insists on parental reassurance before returning to sleep.

Disorders of initiating and maintaining sleep occur when an infant or toddler resists bedtime routine.

Delayed sleep phase syndrome describes a teenager who reports being wide awake during the late evening and unable to initiate sleep until 3 or 4 A.M. (see Fig. 1–1).

Etiology:

Obstructive sleep apnea is caused by mechanical or structural problems in the airway that cause cessation or reduction of airflow. The most common cause is enlarged tonsils and adenoids.

Narcolepsy is a chronic neurologic disorder.

An infant older than 4 months whose night awakenings persist is considered a "trained night crier."

Disorders of initiating and maintaining sleep may have their roots in developmental issues such as autonomy and separation.

Occurrence:

Obstructive sleep apnea: Occurs in 1% to 2% of children.

Nightmares: Occur in 25% to 50% of children in the susceptible age group.

Night terrors: Occurs in 3% of susceptible age group.

Sleepwalking: Occurs in 15% of children age 5 to 12 years.

Narcolepsy: Occurs in 0.04% of general population.

Delayed sleep phase syndrome: 7% of adolescents.

Night awakenings: 95% of newborns cry after awakening and require parental reassurance. By age 1 year, 60% to 70% have learned to self-soothe themselves and return to sleep.

Age:

Obstructive sleep apnea: all age groups.

Nightmares: Children 3 to 5 years.

Sleepwalking: Children 5 to 12 years.

Night terrors: Children 3 to 8 years and adolescents.

Night awakenings: Infants usually less than 1 year of age.

Disorders of initiating and maintaining sleep: toddler and school-age children.

Delayed sleep phase syndrome: Adolescents.

Ethnicity:

Obstructive sleep apnea: More prevalent in African-Americans.

Nightmares: Not significant.

Gender:

Obstructive sleep apnea: equally in males and females (1:1).

Nightmares: Occurs equally in males and females.

Contributing factors:

Obstructive sleep apnea: Family history of asthma or multiple family histories of sleep disorders, including sudden infant death syndrome, allergies, enlarged tonsils or adenoids, craniofacial anomalies, and neuromuscular disease and obesity.

Nightmares: Stressful or frightening daytime events or anxieties may trigger nightmares; more frequently seen in sexually abused children.

Night terrors/sleepwalking: Family history is common.

Night awakenings: Parental behaviors associated with soothing the colicky infant have been suggested as contributing to night awakening behavior.

Signs and symptoms:

Obstructive sleep apnea: The parents report that the child stops breathing while sleeping or the child snores and is a chronic mouth breather. Episodes may occur 30 times per hour. These children may have daytime sleepiness and bedtime resistance. Social functioning is related to poor school performance.

Nightmares: The child is brought to the clinic with the complaint of "having nightmares." Ask the parent about the frequency of the episodes and about what is occurring at home, including the programs the child is allowed to watch on television that might trigger the dreams. Physical findings are negative. The child is willing to talk about the dreams.

Narcolepsy: The child has daytime sleepiness with daily unwanted sleep episodes. These children are often considered lazy, or learning disabled.

Night awakenings: The infant awakens during night and insists on some form of parental reassurance before returning to sleep.

Disorders of initiating and maintaining sleep: The child finds numerous excuses for delaying usual sleep routine.

Diagnostic tests: Tests are for obstructive sleep apnea and narcolepsy.

Test	Results Indicating Disorder	CPT Code
Polysomnography (obstructive sleep apnea, narcolepsy)	Irregular sleep patterns	95806–95807
Nocturnal pulse oximetry	97% positive predictive value for obstructive sleep apnea	82805

Differential diagnosis: None.

Treatment:

Obstructive sleep apnea: Adenotonsillar hypertrophy treated with nasal fluticasone spray decreased the frequency of episodes.

Nightmares: Parental reassurance.

Narcolepsy: Behavioral interventions to establish a regular sleep-wake schedule; a 20-minute nap three times a day is helpful. Methylphenidate, no more than 30 mg per day, has been found to be effective.

Delayed sleep phase syndrome: Resetting the brain clock by changing sleep schedule, exposure to bright natural light in the morning, and reduction in exposure to evening light. Adherence to the new sleep schedule is imperative, even on weekends, for prevention of relapse.

Disorders of initiating and maintaining sleep: Consistent sleep routines administered in a calm, firm manner. The use of articles such as stuffed animals or favorite blankets may be helpful.

Follow-up:

Obstructive sleep apnea: Monitor for reduction in episodes if either pharmacologic or surgical interventions are initiated.

Nightmares: None, unless occurrence increases.

Narcolepsy: Monitor progress and medication.

Sequelae:

Obstructive sleep apnea: Failure to thrive, increased diastolic blood pressure, poor school performance, aggressive hostile behaviors, death.

Nightmares: None.

Narcolepsy: Recurring accidents related to daily unwanted sleep episodes.

Delayed sleep phase syndrome: School failure, truancy, or tardiness.

Prevention/prophylaxis:

Nightmares: Attempt to keep the amount of stress in the home to a minimum. Monitor and guide television viewing in the susceptible age group.

Referral:

Obstructive sleep apnea: Sleep study center.

Nightmares: In severe cases, refer the child for psychological help.

Narcolepsy: Refer to sleep study center.

Education:

Nightmares: Parents need to know that this condition is self-limiting and needs little treatment and that the child will outgrow the problem.

Sleepwalking: Parents need to be sure that the home is safe: gates on staircases, no bunk beds, and windows and door are locked.

SUBSTANCE ABUSE

SIGNAL SYMPTOMS ▶ mistreatment of self through use/misuse of habituating substances

Substance abuse ICD-9 CM: 305.

Description: Substance abuse is the use and misuse of habituating substances in a manner that deviates from social norms. Current drugs of choice are alcohol, marijuana, and cocaine. Illicit use of hallucinogens is increasing in the United States with the Internet as a source for information for obtaining and using the drugs. Substance abuse may be classified as follows.

Experimental: This is infrequent, episodic use of a variety of drugs with peers that causes no problems at home, school, or work.

Recreational: This is episodic use of tobacco, alcohol, or marijuana with peers with the intent to become accepted or feel at ease.

Circumstantial: This is repeated use of drugs as a coping mechanism because of a learned association between use and decreased feelings of stress or anxiety. Can lead to physical or psychological dependency.

Habitual: Substances and their use involve all areas of life; drug use is its own reward.

Compulsive: Physiologic addiction to the substance exists; the child is unable to stop using without intervention. This type of addiction requires a multifaceted approach to treatment with multiple personal changes. Children and adolescents can become addicted in 1 to 4 years compared with men, who may be social drinkers for 20 to 30 years before showing addictive behaviors.

Etiology: Failure to develop appropriate coping skills.

Occurrence: According to a 1999 study, 33% of 12th graders and 9% of 8th graders reported they had been drunk at least once in the past 30 days; 23% of 12th graders and 10% of 8th graders had smoked marijuana; 35% of 12th graders and 18% of 8th graders smoked cigarettes; and the percentage of adolescents who reported using hallucinogenic drugs, cocaine, crack, heroin, and other drugs increased. Many children with a substance abuse problem had a coexisting mental health problem, such as depression, conduct disorder, and anxiety.

Age: Adolescence primarily, but is occurring increasingly in younger age groups.

Ethnicity: Not significant.

Gender: Occurs equally in males and females. There is an increase in the use of diet pills in females and cocaine use in males.

Contributing factors: Age at first use is correlated with a higher probability of continued use and abuse; low self-esteem, poor coping mechanisms, peer pressure, and a family history of substance abuse have been implicated. Other risk factors identified are friends who drink, a history of physical or sexual abuse, previous report of running away, threats, impulsivity, and the need for instant gratification.

Signs and symptoms: An adolescent rarely comes to the clinic asking for help but presents with symptoms related to organ systems affected by substance use or abuse. An adolescent may have presented previously in an emergency department because of intoxication or overdose states and have been referred for follow-up (Fig. 14–5). The teenager is often in denial, as are the parents, so it is necessary to confront the family openly regarding the issue of drug use, when suspected. Use of alcohol and drugs is often considered by society normal experimentation for this age

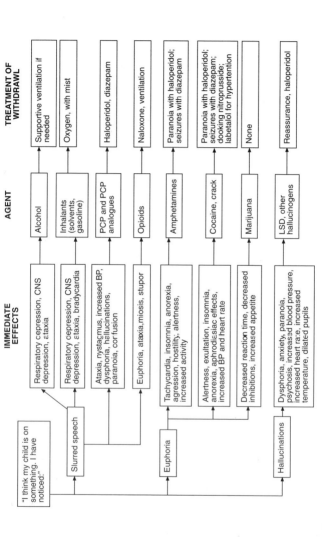

Figure 14-5. Differentiation of substances and treatment of withdrawal. (BP, blood pressure; CNS, central nervous system; LSD, lysergic acid diethylamide; PCP, phencyclidine hydrochloride.)

group. When taking the history of substance abuse, include questions related to types of drugs used, timing (e.g., daily, weekends), settings (e.g., alone, with friends), circumstances (e.g., to be accepted, to cope), and outcomes (e.g., problems with family, peers, school, law enforcement, work).

Few physical findings are associated with chronic use or abuse of substances in children. Alcohol use may cause gastritis and pancreatitis. Use of marijuana and tobacco is associated with bronchitis. Cocaine use may cause palpitations and chest pains. Serial observations that reveal changes in the adolescent's appearance and emotional tone may be the first clue that he or she is using or abusing substances (Fig. 14–6).

Diagnostic tests: The CAGE questionnaire is an easy screening tool for alcohol and substance abuse: "Have you ever felt you should *C*ut down on your drinking? Have people *A*nnoyed you by criticizing your drinking? Have you ever felt *G*uilty about your drinking? Do you ever have an *E*ye opener first thing in the morning?" Two or more positive responses indicate possible abuse. Drug screens are appropriate only when the patient presents with acute intoxication.

Differential diagnosis: A variety of complaints related to substance abuse may bring the child to the clinic (unless the child presents as a result of overdose or withdrawal). The complaints need to be evaluated and the child confronted as to the use of substances. The adolescent substance abuser is at risk for multiple problems. The normal risk-taking behavior of adolescents is enhanced by the addition of chemicals to the system (e.g., motor vehicle accidents owing to driving under the influence).

Treatment:

Mild (experimental): Anticipatory guidance as to future outcomes, education related to use and abuse, and exploration of drug-free alternatives.

Moderate (recreational): Participation in a drug-free support group and individual and family therapy. Continued relationship with patients as they participate in drug-free living.

Severe (circumstantial, habitual, or compulsive): Participation in a formalized treatment program separated from drugs and drug-using peer group. Continued relationship with patients as they participate in drug-free living.

Follow-up: Weekly visits until stabilized. Let patients know that you are there to support them in their new behaviors.

Sequelae: Medical consequences of substance use and abuse include blackouts, trauma and accidental injury, intoxication, and overdose. Examples of medical complications are tachycardia in cocaine users, gastritis related to alcohol use, cerebral ataxia from the inhalation of toluene, and extreme fatigue after amphetamine use.

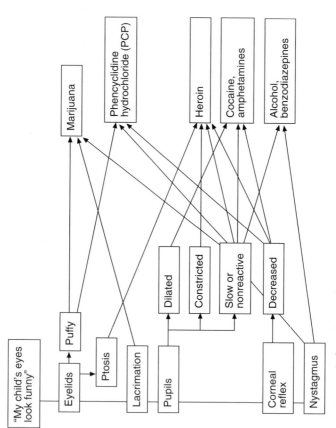

Figure 14–6. Evaluation of eyes to detect type of substance abuse.

Social consequences include conflicts with family, loss of friends, impulsive behavior (promiscuity, destruction of property, fighting), and automobile accidents. Disciplinary actions taken because of school problems, driving under the influence incidents, and thefts are also negative outcomes.

Prevention/prophylaxis: Collaborate with school officials to increase awareness of the dangers of drugs in children from kindergarten through 12th grade. Teach life skills programs for at-risk teenagers to increase their self-esteem and to enable them to learn appropriate coping mechanisms.

Referral: Refer patient for outpatient or inpatient treatment or to an alcohol and drug rehabilitation service that focuses on the needs of adolescents. Refer patient and family to a 12-step program (Alcoholics Anonymous, Narcotics Anonymous, Al-Anon). Refer patient and family to a mental health professional for individual and family therapy.

Education: Teach programs in schools to educate teenagers regarding the dangers and outcomes of substance abuse. Support parents as they work through their feelings of guilt and shame.

TEMPER TANTRUMS

SIGNAL SYMPTOMS ▶ excessive display of anger

Temper tantrums   ICD-9 CM: 312.1

Description: Temper tantrums are a common expression of anger and frustration at ages 12 months to 4 years, as children attempt to gain mastery over their environment.

Etiology: In some children, temper tantrums seem to be related to their temperament, whereas other children innately have a higher tolerance for frustration and ability to cope with difficult experiences.

Occurrence: Occur weekly in 50% to 80% of children younger than 4; in 5% to 20% of these cases, the tantrums are severe enough to be considered developmentally inappropriate.

Age: Occur primarily in children aged 1 to 4, but many occur in older age groups, such as in children who are immature for a particular age and have a developmental disorder.

Ethnicity: Not significant.

Gender: Occur equally in males and females.

Contributing factors: Frustrations brought about by environmental conditions (e.g., crowding), physical limitations (e.g., hearing loss, speech or language delay, hyperactivity), or side effects of medications. Some tantrums seem to be related to the child's temperament. Poor parenting skills may be a factor in that the child learns to use the tantrums as a means of gain (i.e., negative behavior is continually reinforced). Fatigue and increased irritability seem to contribute to these outbursts.

Signs and symptoms: The child presents with the following history when demands are not met: kicks, screams, throws self on floor, and may throw objects. Physical examination is negative. Obtain a history of the incidents, where they happen, "triggers," how many, how long, and the response of the parents. Obtain information related to family members who have problems dealing with anger (parents often are worried that the child is predestined to become like this person).

Diagnostic tests: None.

Differential diagnosis:

Precocious puberty and congenital adrenal hyperplasia is diagnosed by history (severe and persistent temper tantrums, masturbation, tall stature, and secondary sexual characteristics).

Treatment: Give parents guidelines for modifying their child's behavior, such as the following.

Construct an environment with a minimum of restrictions so that conflict is reduced and the need to say "no" is limited.

Use distraction when the child's frustration level increases.

Reward the child's positive responses.

Present the child with choices and options within a developmental framework to help him or her gain mastery over such situations.

If the child loses control and needs time to regain it, use the "time out" technique.

Do not use threats because they serve no purpose.

Do not allow the child to hurt self or others.

Do not give in to the child's demands.

Do not overreact to the episode, but set reasonable limits and provide direction for the child.

Follow-up: Well-child visits.

Sequelae: Increased lack of emotional control, anxiety, and depression.

Prevention/prophylaxis: Early identification of the angry child and reduction of risk factors, emphasis during health supervision visits on developmental issues and parent-child interactions.

Referral: None. If tantrums exceed what is appropriate for age and developmental level, however, refer child to a pediatric developmental specialist. If signs of adrenal hyperplasia are noted, refer to pediatric endocrinologist.

Education: Teach parents that temper tantrums are part of "normal" development, although they are unacceptable behavior. Teach parents effective behavior-modification techniques and parenting skills.

REFERENCES

Anorexia

American Psychiatric Association: Practice guidelines for the treatment of eating disorders (revisions). Am J Psychiatry 157(Suppl):1, 2000.

Cote, C: Dying to be thin: Recognition and management of eating disorders. ADVANCE NP 9:67, 2001.

Elliot, V: Doctors cry "how-to": Web sites for anorexia, bulimia. AMNews, August 12, 2002.

Gidwani, G, and Rome, E: Eating disorders: Identification and treatment in the adolescent patient. The Female Patient 24:15, 1999.

Panagiotopoulos, C, et al: Electrocardiographic findings in adolescents with eating disorders. Pediatrics 105:1100, 2000.

Patton, G, et al: Onset of adolescent eating disorders: Population based cohort study over 3 years. BMJ 318:765, 1999.

Pritts, S, and Susman, J: Diagnosis of eating disorders in primary care. Am Fam Physician 67:297, 311, 2003.

Seidenfeld, M, and Rickert, V: Impact of anorexia, bulimia and obesity on the gynecologic health of adolescents. Am Fam Physician 64:445, 2001.

Williams, R: Use of the Eating Attitudes Test and Eating Disorder Inventory in adolescents. J Adolesc Health Care 8:266, 1987.

Anxiety

Caroll, M, and Ryan-Wenger, N: School-age children's fears, anxiety, and human figure drawings. J Pediatr Health Care 13:24, 1999.

Walkup, J, et al: Fluvoxamine for the treatment of anxiety disorders in children and adolescents. N Engl J Med 344:1279, 2001.

Walsh, K: Welcome advances in treating youth anxiety disorders. Contemp Pediatr 9:66, 2002.

Williams, T, and Hodgman, C: Medication for the management of anxiety disorders in children and adolescents. Pediatr Ann 30:146, 2001.

Attention-Deficit/Hyperactivity Disorder

Adesman, A: New medications for treatment of children with attention-deficit/hyperactivity disorder: Review and commentary Pediatr Ann 31:514, 2002.

American Academy of Pediatrics, Committee on Quality Improvement and Subcommittee on Attention-Deficit /Hyperactivity Disorder: Clinical practice guideline: Diagnosis and evaluation of the child with attention-deficit/hyperactivity disorder. Pediatrics 105:1158, 2000.

American Psychiatric Association: Diagnostic and Statistical Manual of Mental Disorders, ed. 4. American Psychiatric Association, Washington, DC, 1994.

Brown, R, et al: Prevalence and assessment of attention-deficit/hyperactivity disorder in primary care settings. Pediatrics 107:e43, 2001.

Bush, B, et al: Correlates of ADHD among children in pediatric and psychiatric clinics. Psychiatr Serv 53:1103, 2002.

Flick, G: Controversies in ADHD: Fundamental questions being answered slowly, but scientifically. ADVANCE NP 10:34, 2002.

Glod, C: Attention deficit-hyperactivity disorder: An overview of assessment and treatment issues. ADVANCE NP 9:52, 2001.

Hannah, J: The role of schools in attention-deficit/hyperactivity disorder. Pediatr Ann 31:507, 2002.

Herrerias, C, et al: The child with ADHD: Using the AAP clinical practice guideline. Am Fam Physician 63:1803, 2001.

Hunt, R, et al: An update on assessment and treatment of complex attention-deficit hyperactivity disorder. Pediatr Ann 30:162, 2001.

Hunt, R, et al: An update on assessment and treatment of complex attention-deficit hyperactivity disorder. Pediatr Ann 30:162, 2001.

Leslie, L: The role of the primary care physician in attention-deficit/hyperactivity disorder. Pediatr Ann 31:475, 2002.

Michelson, D, et al: Atomoxetine in the treatment of children and adolescents with attention-deficit/hyperactivity disorder: A randomized, placebo-controlled, dose-response study. Pediatrics 108:e83, 2001.

Robin, A: Attention-deficit/hyperactivity disorder in adolescents. Pediatr Ann 31:485, 2002.

Ward, J: Finding answers: New radiopharmaceutical may settle ADHD treatment debate. ADVANCE NP 9:59, 2001.

Autistic Spectrum Disorder

American Psychiatric Association: Diagnostic and Statistical Manual of Mental Disorders, ed. 4. American Psychiatric Association, Washington, DC, 1994.

Berjerot, S, et al: Autistic traits in obsessive-compulsive disorder. J Psychiatry 55:169, 2001.

Bertrand, J, et al: Prevalance of autism in a United States population: The Brick Township, New Jersey, investigation. Pediatrics 108:1155, 2001.

Carpenter, M, et al: Understanding others' intentions in children with autism. J Autistic Dev Disord 6:589, 2001.

Cascio, R, and Kilmon, C: Pervasive developmental disorder, not otherwise specified: Primary care perspectives. Nurse Pract 22:11, 1997.

Dragich, J, et al: Rett syndrome: A surprising result of mutation in MECP2. Hum Mol Genet 9:2365, 2000.

Ellaway, C, et al: Prolonged QT interval in Rett syndrome. Arch Dis Child 80:470, 1999.

Estrada, B: MMR and autism: Suspect or superstition? Infect Med 18:183, 2001.

Hyman, S, and Levy, S: Autistic spectrum disorders: When traditional medicine is not enough. Contemp Pediatr 10:101, 2000.

Klauber, T: The significance of trauma and other factors in work with the parents of children with autism. J Child Psychother 33, 1999.

McDougle, C, et al: Risperidone treatment of children and adolescents with pervasive developmental disorders: A prospective open-label study. J Am Acad Child Adolesc Psychiatry 36:685, 1997.

Niklasson, L, et al: Chromosome 22q11 deletion syndrome (Catch 22): Neuropsychiatric and neuro psychological aspects. Dev Med Child Neurol 1:44, 2002.

Paricak-Vance, M, et al: Gene linked to autism. Am J Hum Genet 72, 2003.

Rosenwasser, B, and Axelrod, S: More contributions of applied behavioral analysis to education of people with autism. Behav Modif 26:2, 2002.

Ruffman, T, et al: Social understanding in autism: Eye gaze as a measure of core insights. J Child Psychol Psychiatry 8:1083, 2001.

Williams, P, et al: Eating habits of children with autism. Pediatr Nurs 26:259, 2000.

Breath Holding

Anderson, J, and Bluestone, D: Breath-holding spells: Scary but not serious. Contemp Pediatr January 1, 2000.

DiMario, F: Prospective study of children with cyanotic and pallid breath-holding spells. Pediatrics 107:265, 2001.

DiMario, F, and Sarfarazi, M: Family pedigree analysis of children with severe breath-holding spells. J Pediatr 130:647, 1997.

Kelly, A, et al: Breath-holding spells associated with significant bradycardia: Successful treatment with permanent pacemaker implantation. Pediatrics 108:698, 2001.

Mattie-Luksic, M, et al: Assessment of stress in mothers of children with severe breath-holding spells. Pediatrics 106:1, 2000.

Bulimia

American Academy of Pediatrics, Committee on Adolescents: Identifying and treating eating disorders. Pediatrics 111:204, 2003.

Buck, M: Using the atypical antipsychotic agents in children and adolescents. Pediatr Pharm 7, 2001.

Cote, C: Dying to be thin: Recognition and management of eating disorders. ADVANCE NP 9:67, 2001.

Field, A, et al: Relation of peer and media influences to the development of purging behaviors among preadolescent and adolescent girls. Arch Pediatr Adolesc Med 153:1184, 1999.

Foster, T, and Smith-Coggins, R: Bulimia. EMed J 2, Oct 31, 2001.

Gidwani, G, and Rome, E: Eating disorders: Identification and treatment in the adolescent patient. The Female Patient 24:15, 1999.

Seidenfeld, M, and Rickert, V: Impact of anorexia, bulimia and obesity on the gynecologic health of adolescents. Am Fam Physician 64:445, 2001.

Williams, R: Use of the Eating Attitudes Test and Eating Disorder Inventory in adolescents. J Adolesc Health Care 8:266, 1987.

Depression

Castigllia, P: Depression in children. J Pediatr Health Care 14:73, 2000.

McConnell, H: Does bullying cause emotional problems: A prospective study of young teenagers. BMJ 3232:480, 2001.

Melnyk, B, and Moldenhauer, Z: Current approaches to depression in children and adolescents. ADVANCE NP 24, 1999.

Newer antidepressants provide hope for effective drug treatment of depression in children and adolescents. Drug Ther Perspect 16:12, 2000.

Shoaf, T, et al: Childhood depression: Diagnosis and treatment strategies in general pediatrics. Pediatr Ann 30:130, 2001.

Son, S, and Kirchner, J: Depression in children and adolescents. Am Fam Physician: 62:2297, 2000.

Wade, T, et al: Emergence of gender differences in depression during adolescence: National panel result from three countries. J Am Acad Child Adolesc Psychiatry 41:190, 2002.

Emotional Abuse

Harmarman, S: Evaluating and reporting emotional abuse in children: Parent-based, action-focused aids in clinical decision-making. J Am Acad Child Adolesc Psychiatry July 2000.

Hamarman, S, and Bernet, W: Evaluating and reporting emotional abuse in children. J Am Acad Child Adolesc Psychiatry 39:928, 2000.

Nelms, B: Emotional abuse: Helping prevent the problem. J Pediatr Health Care 15:103, 2001.

Peterson, LW, et al: The use of children's drawings in the evaluation and treatment of child sexual, emotional, and physical abuse. Arch Fam Med 4:445, 1995.

Failure to Thrive

Blackman, J: Children who refuse food. Contemp Pediatr 5:200, 1998.

Careaga, M, and Kerner, J: A gastroenterologist's approach to failure to thrive. Pediatr Ann 29:558, 2000.

Munchausen Syndrome by Proxy

Hall, DE, et al: Evaluation of covert video surveillance in the diagnosis of Munchausen syndrome by proxy: Lessons from 41 cases. Pediatrics 105:1305, 2000.

Paulk, D: Munchausen syndrome by proxy: Tall tales and real hurts. Clin Rev 11:51, 2001.

Physical Abuse

American Academy of Pediatrics, Committee on Child Abuse and Neglect: Distinguishing sudden infant death syndrome from child abuse fatalities (RE0036). Pediatrics 107:437, 2001.

American Academy of Pediatrics, Committee on Child Abuse and Neglect: Distinguishing sudden infant death syndrome from child abuse fatalities (RE0036): Addendum. Pediatrics 108:812, 2001.

American Academy of Pediatrics, Committee on Child Abuse and Neglect: Shaken baby syndrome: Rotational cranial injuries—technical report (T0039). Pediatrics 108:206, 2001.

American Academy of Pediatrics, Committee on Child Abuse and Neglect: When inflicted skin injuries constitute child abuse. Pediatrics 110:644, 2002.

Cheung, K: Identifying and documenting findings of physical child abuse and neglect. J Pediatr Health Care 13:142, 1999.

DiScala, M, et al: Child abuse and unintentional injuries: A 10-year retrospective. Arch Pediatr Adolesc Med 154:16, 2000.

Krugman, S, et al: Facing facts: Child abuse and pediatric practice. Contemp Pediatr August, 1998.

Murry, S, et al: Screening families with young children for child maltreatment potential. Pediatr Nurs 26:47, 2000.

Pressel, D: Evaluation of physical abuse in children. Am Fam Physician 61:3057, 2000.

Rubin, D, et al: Pulmonary edema associated with child abuse: Case reports and review of the literature. Pediatr 108:769, 2001.

Schizophrenia

Buck, M: Using the atypical antipsychotic agents in children and adolescents. Pediatr Pharm 7, 2001.

Gracious, B, and Findling, R: Antipsychotic medications for children and adolescents. Pediatr Ann 30:138, 2001.

Lott, D: Childhood-onset schizophrenia: Latest NIMH findings. Psychiatric Times 16, September, 1999.

Self-Injurious Behavior

American Academy of Child and Adolescent Psychiatry: Practice parameters for the assessment and treatment of children and adolescents with suicidal behavior. J Am Acad Child Adolesc Psychiatry 40:95, 2001.

American Academy of Pediatrics, Committee on Adolescence: Suicide and suicide attempts in adolescents (RE9928). Pediatrics 105:871, 2000.

Armstrong, M, et al: College tattoos: More than skin deep. Dermatol Nurs 14:317, 2002.

Borowsky, I, et al: Adolescent suicide attempts: Risks and protectors. Pediatrics 107:485, 2001.

Brook, I: Recovery of anaerobic bacteria from three patients with infection at a pierced body site. Clin Infect Dis 33:e12, 2001.

Carroll, S, et al: Tattoos and body piercings as indicators of adolescent risk-taking behaviors. Pediatrics 109:1021, 2002.

Favazza, A, and Rosenthal, R: Diagnostic issues in self-mutilation. Hosp Commun Psychiatry 44:134, 1993.

Khanna, R, et al: Body piercing in the accident and emergency department. J Accid Emerg Med 16:418, 1999.

Martel, S, and Anderson, J: Decorating the "human canvas": Body art and your patients. Contemp Pediatr 8:86, 2002.

Montgomery, D, and Parks, D: Tattoos: Counseling the adolescent. J Pediatr Health Care 15:14, 2001.

Pilowsky, D, et al: Panic attacks and suicide attempts in mid-adolescence. Am J Psychiatry 156:1545, 1999.

Roberts, T, and Ryan, S: Tattooing and high-risk behavior in adolescents. Pediatrics 110:1058, 2002.

Slap, G, et al: Adoption as a risk factor for attempted suicide during adolescence. Pediatrics 108:e30, 2001.

Stork, B: Medical complications of modern art: What you need to know about body piercing. ADVANCE NP 10:59, 2002.

US Food and Drug Administration, Center for Food Safety and Applied Nutrition, Office of Cosmetics and Colors Fact Sheet: Tattoos and Permanent Makeup. November 29, 2000.

Sexual Abuse

American Academy of Pediatrics, Committee on Adolescence: Care of the adolescent sexual assault victim. Pediatrics 107:1476, 200l.

American Academy of Pediatrics, Committee on Child Abuse and Neglect: Gonorrhea in prepubertal children (RE9803). Pediatrics 101:134, 1998.

American Academy of Pediatrics: Guidelines for the evaluation of sexual abuse of children. Pediatrics 87:87, 1988.

American Academy of Pediatrics: Guidelines for the evaluation of sexual abuse of children: A subject review. Pediatrics 103:186, 1999.

Anda, R, et al: Abused boys, battered mothers, and male involvement in teen pregnancy. Pediatrics 107:e19, 2001.

Christian, C, et al: Forensic evidence findings in prepubertal victims of sexual assault. Pediatrics 106:100, 2000.

Herendeen, P: Evaluating for child sexual abuse: Clinical skill and compassion guide the exam. ADVANCE NP 54, February, 1999.

Horner, G, and Ryan-Wenger, N: Aberrant genital practices: An unrecognized form of child sexual abuse. J Pediatr Health Care 13:12, 1999.

Knight, J, et al: Sexual abuse: Management strategies and legal issues. Contemp Pediatr 5:77, 2001.

McClain, N, et al: Evaluation of sexual abuse in the pediatric patient. J Pediatr Health Care 14:93, 2000.

Moody, C: Male child sexual abuse. J Pediatr Health Care 13:112, 1999.

Overstolz, G: Preventing child sexual abuse: It can start in primary care settings. ADVANCE NP 29:52, 2001.

Sleep Disorders

Brooks, L, et al: Adenoid size is related to severity but not the number of episodes of obstructive apnea in children. J Pediatr 132:682, 1998.

Brouillette, R, et al: Nocturnal pulse oximetry as an abbreviated testing modality for pediatric obstructive sleep apnea. Pediatrics 105:405, 2000.

Brouillette, R, et al: Efficacy of fluticasone nasal spray for pediatric obstructive sleep apnea. J Pediatr 138:838, 2001.

Corbo, G, et al: Snoring in 9- to 15-year-old children: Risk factors and clinical relevance. Pediatrics 108:1149, 2001.

Garcia, J, and Wills, L: Sleep disorders in children and teens: Helping patients and their families get some rest. Postgrad Med 107:161, 2000.

Gaylor, E, et al: Classification of young children's sleep problems. Am Acad Child Adolesc Psychiatry 40:69, 2001.

Gozal, D, and Pope, D: Snoring during early childhood and academic performance at ages thirteen to fourteen years. Pediatrics 107:1394, 2001.

Gozal, D, et al: Objective sleepiness measures in pediatric obstructive sleep apnea. Pediatrics 108:693, 2001.

Gozal, D: Sleep-disordered breathing and school performance in children. Pediatrics 102:616, 1998.

Guilleminault, C, et al: Sleepwalking and sleep terrors in prepubertal children: What triggers them? Pediatrics 111:e17, 2003.

McNamara, F, and Sullivan, C: Obstructive sleep apnea in infants: Relation to family history of sudden infant death syndrome, apparent life-threatening events, and obstructive sleep apnea. J Pediatr 136:318, 2000.

Ohayon, M, et al: Prevalence and patterns of problematic sleep among older adolescents. Am Acad Child Psychiatry 39:1549, 2000.

Owens, J, et al: Sleep and daytime behavior in children with obstructive sleep apnea and behavioral sleep disorders. Pediatrics 102:1178, 1998.

Pagel, J: Nightmares and disorders of dreaming. Am Fam Physician 61:2037, 2000.

Stein, M, et al: Sleep and behavior problems in school-aged children. Pediatrics 107:e60, 2001.

Thiedke, C: Sleep disorders and sleep problems in childhood. Am Fam Physician 63:277, 2001.

Yantis, MA: Assessing children for obstructive sleep apnea. J Pediatr Health Care 13:99, 1999.

Wake up! Treatments for childhood narcolepsy can prevent the development of serious social or academic problems. Drug Ther Perspect 17:5, 2001.

Substance Abuse

American Academy of Child and Adolescent Psychiatry: Substance abuse treatment for children and adolescents: Questions to ask. Facts for Families, #41, 2000.

American Academy of Pediatrics. Committee on Child Health Financing and

Committee on Substance Abuse: Improving substance abuse prevention, assessment, and treatment financing for children and adolescents. Pediatrics 10:1025, 2001.

American Academy of Pediatrics, Committee on Substance Abuse and Committee on Native American Child Health: Inhalant abuse (RE9609). Pediatrics 97, 1996.

American Academy of Pediatrics, Committee on Substance Abuse: Alcohol use and abuse: A pediatric concern (RE0060). Pediatrics 108:185, 2001.

American Academy of Pediatrics, Committee on Substance Abuse: Indications for management and referral of patients involved in substance abuse. Pediatrics 106:143, 2000.

Halpern, J, and Pope, H: Hallucinogens on the Internet: A vast new source of underground drug information. Am J Psychiatry 158:481, 2001.

Work Group on Quality Issues: Practice parameters for the assessment and treatment of children and adolescents with substance abuse disorders. J Am Acad Child Adolesc Psychiatry 37:122, 1998.

Temper Tantrums

American Academy of Pediatrics Committee on Psychosocial Aspects of Child and Family Health: Guidance for effective discipline. Pediatrics 101:723, 1998.

Green, M, et al: What to do with the angry toddler. Contemp Pediatr 8:65, 2001.

Stein, M: Temper tantrums, impulsivity, and aggression in a preschool-aged boy: Diagnosis and treatment of precocious puberty and congenital adrenal hyperplasia. J Dev Behav Pediatr 21:224, 2000.

Zurbrugg, E: When time-out fails, try Plan B. Contemp Pediatr January 1998.

Chapter 15

ENVIRONMENTAL DISORDERS

ANIMAL/HUMAN BITES

SIGNAL SYMPTOMS ▶ injury to skin (puncture, laceration, abrasions) by a bite of an animal or a human

Accidental animal/human bites	ICD-9 CM: E928.3 (add wound site)
Assault animal/human bites	ICD-9 CM: E968.7 (add wound site)

Description: Animal and human bites are injuries that cause disruption of skin integrity. A true bite may be occlusional or the result of a clenched fist injury, which results from the impact of a fist on teeth.

Etiology: Animal bites are most frequently caused by dogs (90%) and cats (10%), but other mammals, including rodents (1%), bite humans. Children usually cause human bites, but some forms of child abuse include bites by adults.

Occurrence: Each year, 1 to 2 million Americans are bitten, of which 70% are children younger than age 10 years. Bites constitute 1% of emergency department visits, and 90% of pets involved are owned by the victim's family or neighbors. Bites among children are common but rarely serious.

Age: Occurs in all pediatric age groups.

Ethnicity: Not significant.

Gender: Dogs bite males more often than females; cats bite females more often.

Contributing factors: Being ignorant of potential dangers is a primary factor, as well as provoking animals and engaging in fist fights.

Signs and symptoms: Presence of the wound. The history is important before initiating treatment. The following questions should be asked when evaluating a bite (Fig. 15–1).

What was the source of the bite—animal or human?

If animal, what kind, and is the animal known to the family?

What is the health status of the animal?

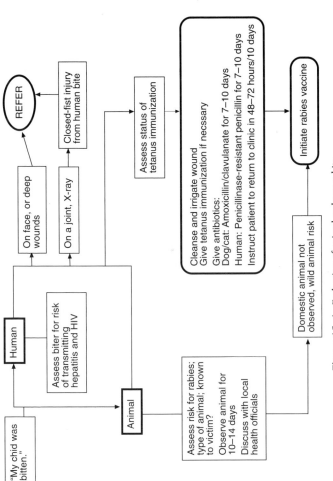

Figure 15–1. Evaluation of animal or human bite.

Was the attack provoked?

Can the animal be observed over the next 10 to 14 days?

How old is the wound?

What home treatment, if any, was initiated?

When was the last tetanus immunization?

Was the human bite from a child or an adult?

If from an adult, was the bite part of an abusive cycle, or the result of a physical altercation?

Assessment of the wound includes the following:

- Assessing for bleeding and signs of infection
- Determining the type of wound: puncture or laceration
- Determining the presence of infection

Infection is usually clinically evident within 24 hours. Clenched fist injuries usually result in lacerations over the fourth and fifth metacarpal joints.

Diagnostic tests:

Test	Results Indicating Disorder	CPT Codes
Radiographic studies	Possible fracture or foreign body, such as tooth, embedded in wound	Depends on body part
Culture wound	Presence of pathogenic bacteria	87070

Differential diagnosis: None.

Treatment:

Dog and Cat Bites

Cleanse wound with 1% povidone-iodine solution (Betadine) and rinse with normal saline. Débride wound as necessary. Assess for need for surgical closure. Delayed closure should be considered in wounds that are less than 1.5 cm in length, deep puncture wounds, infected wounds, and wounds seen less than 24 hours after bite. Take photographs of the wound if disfigurement or legal issues are a possibility.

 Clinical Pearl: Do not immediately suture deep puncture wounds, clinically infected wounds, bites on the hand, or wounds that are being seen 24 hours after injury.

Human Bites

Initial treatment includes irrigation of the open wound with normal saline, débridement of the area, assessment for possible presence of foreign body, and assessment of the need for surgical closure.

Tetanus Prophylaxis

The following are the recommendations for tetanus prophylaxis by the Advisory Committee on Immunization Practices.

If the wound is minor and clean, the history of tetanus immunizations is unknown, or the client has had fewer than three doses, administer tetanus and diphtheria toxoids (Td).

If last tetanus immunization was given more than 10 years earlier, administer Td.

Immunization is not required if the patient received three or more doses; tetanus immune globulin (TIG) is not required.

For all other wounds, if history of tetanus immunizations is unknown or the patient has had fewer than three doses, administer Td and TIG.

Administer Td if immunization occurred less than 5 years earlier. TIG is not required.

Antibiotics

ORAL

Amoxicillin/clavulanate (Augmentin): Amoxicillin, 45 mg/kg per day divided doses every 12 hours. Indicated for skin infections caused by β-lactamase-producing strains of *Staphylococcus aureus*.

Doxycycline (Vibramycin), 2 to 4 mg/lb per day in divided doses twice daily, then 1 to 2 mg/lb twice daily. Not for children younger than 8 years old or pregnant women.

INTRAVENOUS

Cefoxitin (Mefoxin), over 3 months, 80 to 160 mg/kg per day divided every 4 to 6 hours. This is an alternative drug indicated for infections caused by susceptible gram-positive cocci and gram-negative rods.

Postexposure rabies prophylaxis if indicated. For wild animals or domestic animals not observed or tested, administer human rabies immune globulin, 20 IU/kg intramuscular dose.

Human diploid cell vaccine, 1 mL on days 1, 3, 7, 14, and 28.

Perpetrator

Dogs, cats, wild carnivores, and bats are potentially rabid. Rodents and rabbits are usually not considered potentially dangerous. The following guidelines should be followed in dealing with the animal.

Assess, if possible, the immunization status of the animal.

Do not destroy the animal.

Pen the animal and observe for 10 to 14 days.

Report strays and other unknown animals; discuss with local health officials

Human perpetrators should be tested for hepatitis (A and B) and human immunodeficiency virus.

Follow-up: Examine the wound in 48 hours, and reassess at the end of antibiotic therapy for signs of infection. If rabies immunization is initiated, obtain a follow-up rabies antibody titer on day 42.

Sequelae: If not treated appropriately, infection or sepsis or both may result.

Prevention/prophylaxis: Educate children in the proper care and treatment of animals. Having an unneutered male dog or a German Shepherd or a Chow Chow poses an increased risk of having a non-household member being bitten.

Referral: Refer child for surgery if the lacerations are massive, involve the face, or require hospitalization. It is mandatory to report cases of suspected child abuse.

Fresh Start Surgical Gifts, Inc. (1-888-551-1003), an international, non-profit organization, provides free reconstructive surgery to children without financial means who have been disfigured by dog bites.

Education: Teach the child to be wary of unknown animals and not to provoke family pets or neighborhood animals. Instruct the child that any wild animal is to be considered dangerous, and direct contact is to be avoided.

HEAT CRAMPS

SIGNAL SYMPTOMS ▶ impaired heat loss

Heat cramps	ICD-9 CM: 922.2

Description: Heat cramps are brief muscle contractions, without rigidity of skeletal and abdominal muscles, resulting from sodium loss and inadequate fluid and sodium intake.

Etiology: Excessive sodium chloride loss from sweating.

Occurrence: Common in areas where climate factors indicate risk.

Age: Occurs primarily in adolescents and young adults.

Ethnicity: Not significant.

Gender: Occurs equally in males and females.

Contributing factors: Athletic activity and drinking excessive water in response to sweating are factors to be considered.

Signs and symptoms: The patient presents with complaints of painful muscle contractions and cramping of skeletal or abdominal muscles after exertion. Physical examination reveals painful muscles (Fig. 15–2).

Diagnostic tests: None.

Differential diagnosis: None.

Treatment: Supportive treatment, including rest, muscle massage, and oral replacement of sodium chloride. Severe cases may require administration of intravenous normal saline solution.

Follow-up: As warranted.

Sequelae: None.

Prevention/prophylaxis: Children should be preconditioned to the environmental stressor. Pre-exercise hydration is recommended and is usually 16 oz of fluid before exercise. During the activity, even though the athlete may not complain of thirst, provide 8 oz of cool water or sports

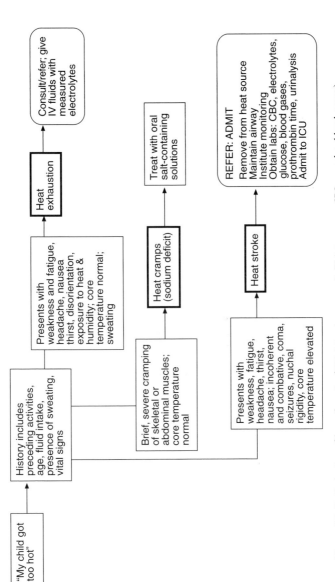

Figure 15–2. Evaluation of hyperthermia. (ICU, intensive care unit; IV, intravenous; CBC, complete blood count.)

drink, such as Gatorade Frost Thirst Quencher or Allsport Body Quencher, every 20 minutes.

Referral: None.

Education: Teach parents and children ways to keep electrolytes balanced during times of excessive sweating.

HEAT EXHAUSTION

SIGNAL SYMPTOMS▶ impaired heat loss

Heat exhaustion	ICD-9 CM: 922.5

Description: "Definite weakness produced by the excess loss of normal fluids and sodium chloride in the form of sweat" (*Tabor's Cyclopedic Medical Dictionary,* ed. 18, p 857).

Etiology: Depletion of plasma volume.

Occurrence: Common in adolescents and young adults in conducive environments.

Age: Primarily in adolescents and young adults.

Ethnicity: Not significant.

Gender: Occurs equally in males and females.

Contributing factors: Overexertion in a hot and humid environment, often during athletic activities or in the workplace.

Signs and symptoms: History of exposure to heat. The patient presents with complaints of general malaise, weakness, headache, anorexia, nausea, and vomiting. The body core temperature rises to greater than 100°F but less than 104°F. There is hypotension and tachycardia, and the patient continues to sweat (see Fig. 15–2).

Diagnostic tests: None.

Differential diagnosis: In heatstroke, the central nervous system dysfunction is increased (e.g., the heatstroke patient is incoherent and combative).

Treatment: Supportive treatment, such as rest in cool environment and restoration of fluids and salt. In severe cases, the patient may need hospitalization for cooling and intravenous rehydration.

Follow-up: None; patient usually recovers in 2 to 3 hours.

Sequelae: Usually none.

Prevention/prophylaxis: Can be avoided by acclimatization and increased fluid and salt intake.

Referral: In severe cases, refer patient for hospitalization.

Education: Teach parents and the general public of the dangers of fluid depletion in hot weather.

HEATSTROKE

SIGNAL SYMPTOMS ▶ impaired heat loss

Heatstroke	ICD-9 CM: 922.0

Description: Heatstroke is the failure of thermoregulation. Exertional heatstroke affects young, healthy persons who are not acclimated to heat or humidity. Classic heatstroke affects the elderly and debilitated persons.

Etiology: Exertional heatstroke is a result of engaging in strenuous muscular activity; classic heatstroke is a failure of thermoregulation that occurs during limited activity.

Occurrence: Common; responsible for approximately 4000 deaths in the United States each summer (adults and children) and is the third leading cause of death among high school athletes.

Age: Occurs in all pediatric age groups; more common in adolescent athletes.

Ethnicity: Not significant.

Gender: Occurs equally in males and females.

Contributing factors: Debilitating chronic illness, alcohol, medications (diuretics, β-blockers, antipsychotic drugs [e.g., haloperidol, chlorpromazine], major tranquilizers, anticholinergics), sports activities, and failure to acclimatize to hot and humid environments.

Signs and symptoms: The patient presents with a history of strenuous activity in a climate of high heat and humidity, complains of lack of sweating, and has a rectal temperature greater than 40°C (104°F). There is marked central nervous system dysfunction, and the patient is often incoherent and combative. The patient may lapse into a coma or have seizures and nuchal rigidity (see Fig. 15–2).

Diagnostic tests:

Test	Results Indicating Disorder	CPT Codes
Hematocrit	Elevated in dehydration	85104
BUN	Elevated in dehydration	84520
Urinalysis	Increase in urine specific gravity in dehydration Proteinuria, presence of red blood cells and casts	81000
Electrocardiogram	Conduction abnormalities Nonspecific ST-segment and T-wave changes	93042

BUN, blood urea nitrogen.

Differential diagnosis:

The differential includes hyperthyroid storm, neuroleptic malignant syndrome, pheochromocytoma, and central nervous system injury. Patients who have ingested a variety of drugs can present with hyperthermia and mental status changes.

Treatment:

Nonpharmacologic

Remove patient from the heat source and cool the body using cool water, cool mist, or fans. Maintain airway. Monitor cardiac function, urinary output, and temperature.

Pharmacologic

Administer intravenous fluids.

Follow-up: As warranted.

Sequelae: Transient personality changes occur when initiation of treatment is slow. If treatment is not prompt and appropriate, death may occur.

Prevention/prophylaxis:

 Clinical Pearl: Do not administer salt tablets.

Fans are helpful in low-humidity and ambient temperatures less than 90°F. Fans can increase heat stress, however, when ambient temperature is greater than 100°F. Offer patient the following guidelines.

Visit air-conditioned areas, such as malls or libraries.

Avoid excessive activity in extreme temperatures.

Take scheduled rest periods.

Wear lightweight and light-colored clothing, wear a hat, and use an umbrella.

Increase fluid intake.

Allow children to play in tub of cool water (59–61°F) during the summer.

Hydrate well before and during outdoor activities.

Referral: Immediate transfer to hospital.

Education: Teach above-listed preventive measures.

INSECT AND ARTHROPOD BITES AND STINGS

SIGNAL SYMPTOMS▶ injury to skin (puncture, laceration, abrasions) by insect/arthropod

Insect and arthropod bites and stings	ICD-9 CM (see under specific agent)
Insect bites and stings nonvenomous	ICD-9-CM: 906.4.
Black widow (*Latrodectus mactans*)	ICD-9-CM: 989.5
Brown recluse (*Loxosceles reclusa*)	ICD-9-CM: 989.5
Hobo spider (*Tegenaria agrestis*)	ICD-9-CM: 989.5
Scorpion (members of the *Vaejovis, Hadrurus, Anuroctonus,* and *Centruroides* groups)	ICD-9-CM 989.5

Description: Insect and arthropod bites and stings cause a toxic reaction resulting from the saliva, venom, or injury. Reactions may be classified as immediate or delayed. Bite site usually is associated with localized swelling and pruritus.

Immediate reactions are classified as follows:

Normal: Localized swelling, erythema, and transient pain are present. Children up to age 16 years have a 5% to 10% risk of a similar reaction if stung in the future.

Toxic: A toxic reaction is produced by exogenous vasoactive amines in the venom; usually occurs with multiple stings. Toxic dose of venom of a honeybee for a child is approximately 500 stings (19 stings/kg body weight).

Large local: Contiguous swelling lasts more than 24 hours.

Systemic: Generalized symptoms are remote from sting site. Delayed reactions are systemic, with varied manifestations, such as serum sickness–like reactions, myocarditis, transverse myelitis, and nephrosis.

Etiology: Bees, wasps, and ants cause most insect bites and stings. Common arthropods that bite or sting include spiders, scorpions, ticks, centipedes, and millipedes.

Occurrence: Common worldwide.

Age: All age groups.

Ethnicity: Not significant.

Gender: Occurs equally in males and females.

Contributing factors: Lightweight clothing; conducive environmental factors (e.g., wooded areas) and hiding places (e.g., dark closets).

Signs and symptoms: The patient presents with a skin lesion with or without specific knowledge of the time of bite or the specific agent. If the agent was an insect, the patient reports that there was immediate local pain with variable redness and later itching.

Nonvenomous Insect Bites and Stings

Patients with insect bites and stings present with skin lesions of varying sizes; the stinger may still be embedded, and redness and erythema are noted around the lesion site.

Spider Bites

Black widow (Latrodectus mactans*), ICD-9 989.5:* Envenomation has been categorized as grade 1, characterized by being asymptomatic with normal vital signs and pain at site. Grade 2 has normal vital signs but includes localized muscle pain and diaphoresis. Characteristics of a grade 3 envenomization include generalized muscle pain in back, abdomen, and chest; hypertension and tachycardia; nausea/vomiting; headache; and increased diaphoresis.

Brown recluse (Loxosceles reclusa*), ICD-9 989.5:* Local symptoms of itching, redness, and tenderness, with a target lesion, enlarging to form a necrotic central region that heals slowly. Systemic symptoms, often occurring 72 hours after the initial bite, may include fever, chills, headache, and malaise. Severe cases may involve a self-limited hemolysis.

*Hobo spider (*Tegenaria agrestis*), ICD-9 989.5:* Bite initially painless. Within 30 minutes, an indurated area appears with erythema measuring 5 to 15 cm. A blister appears 35 hours later that when ruptured reveals an encrusted cratered wound. Systemic reactions may include headache, nausea, and visual disturbances.

Scorpion (members of the Vaejovis, Hadrurus, Anuroctonus, *and* Centruroides *groups), (989.5):* The first three produce local edema and pain; the *Centruroides* produce burning paresthesia at the sting site. Other symptoms include hyperventilation, abdominal cramps, urinary incontinence, and respiratory failure.

Diagnostic tests: None for insect stings.

For a brown recluse spider bite, the following tests are useful.

Test	Results Indicating Disorder	CPT Code
Urinalysis	Red blood cells	81000
Complete blood count	Monitoring for hemodialysis	85007

Differential diagnosis: Primarily none.

Acute abdomen, renal colic, opioid withdrawal, organophosphate poisoning, and tetanus are part of the differential in black widow spider bites (grade 3). In black widow spider bites, the child is restless and moving about, whereas the child with other bites characteristically avoids movement.

Treatment:

Insect Stings and Bites

Initial treatment involves removing the stinger, cleansing the site with skin disinfectant, and giving supportive measures (e.g., cool compresses, elevation of the body part, if possible).

For mild allergic symptoms, systemic therapy includes diphenhydramine, 1 to 2 mg/kg intramuscularly or orally, one dose. Large local reactions may require a short course of prednisone.

For generalized urticaria, wheezing, chest or throat tightness, syncope, or dizziness, give epinephrine (1:1000, 0.01 mL/kg, to maximum of 0.3 mL) subcutaneously.

Spider Bites

Black widow spider: The severity of the envenomization may serve as a guide to treatment (Table 15–1).

Brown recluse spider: Supportive care is given. Wound care; check status of tetanus immunization; provide analgesics; and rest, immobilization, cold compresses, and elevation (RICE). Antibiotics are not given unless there is evidence of infection.

Table 15–1   Treatment of Black Widow Spider Bites

Treatment	Category 1	Category 2	Category 3
Monitor vital signs	X	X	X
Stabilize airway, breathing, and circulation	X	X	X
Cleanse wound with soap and water or chlorhexidine gluconate (Hibiclens)	X	X	X
Check status of tetanus; give booster if patient has not had immunizations or is unsure of status	X	X	X
Rest, immobilization, cold compresses or ice, and elevation (RICE)	X	X	X
Oral analgesics (acetaminophen, ibuprofen, or codeine)	X		
Relief for muscle pain and cramping; intravenous medications are recommended with admission to the hospital		X	X
Use of antivenom is considered controversial because of being derived from horse serum			X

Hobo spider: Supportive care is given. Wound care. Antibiotics generally are not given unless there is evidence of infection.

Scorpion: Sedation is the usual therapy. Maintain a patent airway. Most clinical signs subside within 48 hours.

Follow-up: Follow-up in 1 week if patient is prescribed antibiotics or prednisone or if patient requires hospitalization.

Sequelae: Anaphylaxis is always a possible. If this occurs, give subcutaneous epinephrine (1:1000), 0.01 mL/kg up to 0.5 mL and nebulized β-adrenergic agents for bronchospasm.

Prevention/prophylaxis: Provision of anaphylaxis kits for children at high risk. Automatic injectors, such as EpiPen, deliver 0.3 mg of epinephrine; EpiPen Jr. delivers 0.15 mg of epinephrine. Avoid wearing lightweight clothing, and exterminate contaminated areas.

Referral: In cases of upper airway obstruction, refer patient immediately for intubation.

Insect Stings

Refer high-risk patients to an allergist for diagnostic skin testing and possible immunotherapy. Patients with moderate or severe systemic symptoms should be admitted to the hospital.

Spider Bites

Refer patients for antivenom therapy. Black widow antivenom is available; it has significant side effects, such as anaphylaxis, but it can be used in children. Always test for hypersensitivity to horse serum before administering the drug. There is no antivenom for brown recluse spider bites or hobo spider. Refer to surgeon if a brown recluse or hobo spider bite needs débridement or wound is large enough to require plastic surgery.

Scorpion

Scorpion antivenom may be necessary for severe cases. Contact local poison control center for availability of specific antivenom.

Education: Ensure that parents know the dangers of insect and arthropod bites and stings, and teach them to call 911 when necessary. Teach parents and children to recognize stinging insects and venomous spiders and to avoid potential danger areas. If possible, capture the perpetrator and bring to the office for proper identification.

LEAD POISONING (PLUMBISM)

SIGNAL SYMPTOMS ▶ poisoning from lead

Lead poisoning	ICD-9 CM: 984.9

Description: Lead poisoning is toxicity caused by ingestion of lead; likely to occur when more than 0.05 mg of lead is absorbed.

Etiology: Ingestion of lead. Potential sources include lead-based paints, leaded gasoline, leaded objects, lead-based pottery glazes, leaded crystal, battery casings, and the occupations or hobbies of family members (e.g., painting, stained glass making, ceramics).

Occurrence: One in six children is at risk; one in two inner-city children is at risk. Children most at risk are primarily disadvantaged children from decaying neighborhoods.

Age: Usually affects children younger than age 5 years; children most at risk are 1 to 3 years old.

Ethnicity: Not significant.

Gender: Occurs equally in males and females.

Contributing factors: Older homes painted before 1960 with lead-based paint, lead water pipes, pica, and parental hobbies.

Signs and symptoms: The child has been found chewing on windowsills or crib, or family is remodeling an older house. Assessment of the child at risk involves a simple questionnaire that asks the following questions.

> Does your child live in or regularly visit a house with peeling or chipping paint that was built before 1957? (This might be a day care center, a preschool, or the home of a babysitter or relative.)

Does your child live in or regularly visit a house built before 1960 with recent, ongoing, or planned renovation or remodeling?

Does your child have a brother or sister, housemate, or playmate being followed or treated for lead poisoning (i.e., blood lead level >15 μg/dL)?

Does your child live with an adult whose job or hobby involves exposure to lead?

Does your child live near an active lead smelter, battery recycling plant, or other industry likely to release lead? (sample, CDC, 1991).

Does your child eat paint chips (pica)?

Does your child live next to a major highway?

The assessment should be completed at each early preventive screening diagnostic testing visit of children covered by Medicaid. Check with your local health department for the questionnaire developed by your state.

Physical examination reveals the following.

- *Early stages*—weakness, irritability, weight loss, vomiting, constipation, headache, colicky abdominal pain, Burton's blue lines, and bluish discoloration at the gingival margin
- *Late stages*—bradycardia, ataxia, lethargy, retarded mental and physical development, convulsions, and coma

Diagnostic tests:

Children at low risk should be screened for lead poisoning yearly until age 4 years.

Children at high risk should be screened at age 6 months and every 6 months thereafter.

When lead levels are greater than 20 μg/dL, complete additional testing:

Test	Results Indicating Disorder	CPT Codes
Complete blood count	Anemia	85007
Serum lead levels	Plumbism if >20 mg/dL	83655
Serum ferritin	Low in iron-deficiency anemia	82728
Whole blood lead level test	Blood lead burden	84655
Free erythrocyte protoporphyrin	High in iron-deficiency anemia	82135
Radiographs of the abdomen	Lead-containing foreign body	7400
Levels of essential metals such as calcium, magnesium, and zinc	Determines the effects of chelating agents	82310/ 83735/ 84630

Differential diagnosis:

Gastroenteritis has early symptoms of vomiting and diarrhea.

Attention-deficit/hyperactivity disorder needs to be differentiated.

Treatment:

Nonpharmacologic

Chelation is not recommended for levels of 25 to 45 µg; treatment consists of elimination of source, and removal of the child from contaminated area.

Pharmacologic

Children with blood lead levels greater than 45 µg/dL (class IV) should be hospitalized for chelation. Chelating agents include the following.

Succimer (Chemet), initial dose 10 mg/kg (350 mg/m^2) every 8 hours for 5 days, then every 12 hours for 14 days; wait at least 2 weeks before reinitiating therapy.

Dimercaprol (British antilewisite [BAL]), 4 mg/kg per dose (not preferred therapy).

Edetate calcium disodium (edathamil), usually given with dimercaprol; give 1 g/m^2 intravenously once daily or intramuscularly every 8 to 12 hours, treating for 5 days.

Treatment of associated iron-deficiency anemia includes supplemental iron, 4 to 6 mg/kg per day.

Follow-up:

Low-Risk Children

Children at low risk are screened at age 12 months. If lead levels are less than 10 µg/dL, screen yearly. If levels are 10 to 14 µg/dL, recheck every 3 to 4 months. Obtain a detailed environmental history when levels are 15 to 19 µg/dL. Begin educational and nutritional counseling. Recheck in 3 to 4 months; if level is still high, investigate the environment.

High-Risk Children

Children at high risk (positive answers to the risk questionnaire) are screened at age 6 months. If blood levels are less than 10 µg/dL, recheck every 6 months; if greater than 10 µg/dL, recheck every 3 to 4 months, begin educational and nutritional counseling, and obtain an environmental history. If blood lead level is equal to or greater than 20 µg/dL, recheck every 3 to 4 months and obtain a detailed history, including clinical symptoms, environmental sources, hand-to-mouth activities, pica, and family history of lead poisoning.

Sequelae: Effects of lead at levels of 35 to 40 µg/dL or less include learning disabilities, developmental delays, decreased hearing, and impaired growth. There also is impairment in vitamin D metabolism and hemoglobin synthesis. At blood lead levels greater than 70 µg/dL, encephalopathy, cerebral edema, seizures, coma, and death may occur. Lead is teratogenic to the fetus via placental transfer; it causes reduced birth weight and reduced gestational age.

Prevention/Prophylaxis: Use paint containing less than 1% lead for interior use. Remove other sources of lead. Remove the child from areas of environmental pollution. Wash the child's hands and face before eating. Wipe floors and windowsills with high-phosphate detergent solution.

Referral: Refer patient to a physician for chelation therapy when blood lead levels are greater than 45 μg/dL. Contact social services and health department for environmental assessments and family assistance.

Education: Teach parents the following protective measures for dealing with household lead dust.

Place furniture in front of peeling paint to make it less accessible to children.

Use sticky-backed tape to cover small peeling areas.

Damp dust and mop with a high-phosphate cleaner two times per week to decrease the amount of lead dust. Examples of cleaners are trisodium phosphate cleaners and some dishwasher detergents.

Remove paint chips with a disposable cloth dampened with the phosphate cleaner and dispose in an appropriate manner.

 Clinical Pearl: Do not dry sweep or vacuum: This only spreads the dust. Do not scrape, sand, or burn lead paint off the surfaces.

Provide a diet high in calcium and iron and a daily vitamin with iron.

Wash and dry toys and pacifiers frequently.

Wash hands frequently, especially before meals and bedtime.

NEAR-DROWNING

SIGNAL SYMPTOMS ▶ survival of a submersion episode in water

Near-Drowning	ICD-9 CM: 994.1

Description: Near-drowning is the survival for 24 hours or more after suffocation by submersion; there is aspiration and apnea resulting in hypoxemia. Illness and death are a result of hypoxic-ischemic injury to the brain. Of children who survive, 5% to 20% have permanent and severe neurologic sequelae. Children who are conscious after resuscitation have an excellent prognosis.

Etiology: Activities such as bathing and swimming place children at risk for drowning. The major sites for children younger than age 2 years are bathtubs and large buckets of water; for children older than age 2, private swimming pools are the major site. Industrial-type, 5-gallon buckets are half the height (14 inches) of an average toddler.

Occurrence: Near-drowning is a frequent emergency; children aged 1 to 3 years have the highest rate of drowning.

Age: Occurs in any age group; toddlers and teenagers are at greatest risk.

Ethnicity: African-American children are six times more likely to drown in a bucket than white children.

Gender: Occurs equally in younger boys and girls, but more often in adolescent boys than in adolescent girls.

Contributing factors: Poor supervision of young children, failure to teach children how to swim, swimming in unsupervised waters, and swimming alone. Children with epilepsy or developmental delays are at higher risk.

Signs and symptoms: The child presents with a history of submersion in water. The child may be or may not be awake or oxygenated. The child may present in a coma. Evaluate state of consciousness, pupils, size, and reaction to light. Whether the child is hypothermic or not depends on the temperature of the water and the length of time submerged. The longer the child is in a coma, the poorer the prognosis. The following are some predictors of a poor prognosis:

- Submersion greater than 10 minutes
- Delay in providing cardiopulmonary resuscitation (CPR)
- Severe metabolic acidosis: pH less than 7.1 after correction for partial pressure of carbon dioxide (PCO_2)
- Fixed, dilated pupils
- Glasgow Coma Scale score less than 5 (see Table 5–2)
- Asystole

Diagnostic tests:

Test	Results Indicating Disorder	CPT Codes
Arterial blood gases	Determine extent of hypoxemia	82803
Neck and skull radiographs	Determine associated injuries	70360/ 70250-72060

Differential diagnosis: None.

Treatment: The goal is to correct acidosis and hypoxia as soon as possible. Closed chest massage is initiated if no pulse is present. Intubation and positive end-expiratory pressure are often helpful to improve oxygenation. Treat hypothermia with warm blankets. Hyperventilate to maintain PCO_2 in the range of 25 to 28 mm Hg; use fluid restriction and osmotic diuresis. Drainage of ventricular fluid may be required to prevent cerebral ischemia resulting from intracranial hypertension.

Follow-up: The patient should return to the clinic after release from the hospital for evaluation of progress.

Sequelae: Cerebral edema may result from hypoxia. Pneumonia may result if the water was grossly contaminated. Treat with antibiotics.

Prevention/prophylaxis:

Constant adult supervision of young children: child younger than age 3 years and children with epilepsy should never be left unattended in a bathtub, wading pool, or near a swimming pool.

Proper fencing on all four sides of swimming pools and hot tubs.

The wearing of flotation devices for children when in boats or when playing near water.

Parents and older siblings should learn CPR.

Children age 3 to 8 years should take swimming lessons, but knowing how to swim does not mean they cannot drown.

Referral: Refer patient to a primary care physician for immediate admission to the hospital; near-drowning is always an emergency.

Education: Instruct parents in the basics of water safety. Instruct parents in safety measures to take in the home with toddlers, such as closing the toilet seat and not using 5-gallon buckets. Remind parents of the dangers of alcohol, drugs, and water sports for teenagers.

POISONING

SIGNAL SYMPTOMS ▶ state as a result of ingestion of toxic or hazardous substance

Poisoning	ICD-9 CM (see specific substance)

Description: Poisoning is the accidental or purposeful ingestion of toxic or hazardous substances.

Etiology: Any hazardous substance: chemical, medicinal, or botanical.

Occurrence: Common.

Age: Peak age range is 2 years to less than 5 years.

 Clinical Pearl: 25% of children with an initial case of poisoning have a second episode within 1 year.

In adolescents, these incidents are purposeful and usually represent either "acting out" behavior or a genuine suicide attempt.

Ethnicity: Not significant.

Gender: More common in males than females.

Contributing factors: Complex issues related to familial and environmental factors, such as (1) inadequate storage of drugs and chemicals in the home (prime factor in childhood poisonings) and (2) lack of knowledge that some houseplants, as well as common garden and wild plants, are poisonous when ingested. Occurs most frequently in kitchen, bathrooms, and garages.

Signs and symptoms: The child presents with a history of either known or suspected ingestion of a poisonous substance (Figs. 15–3 through 15–6).

The caregiver has often found the child engaged in the harmful activity. Adolescents may purposely ingest toxic substances as a means of attempting suicide (aspirin and acetaminophen). Gather information related to time of ingestion (noting time elapsed before parents began to seek health care), how the event happened, possible substance, where the event occurred, any previous episodes of drug abuse, possibility of suicide attempt, and what has already been done (e.g., home remedies)

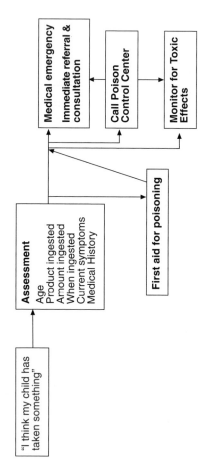

Figure 15–3. Evaluation of poisoning.

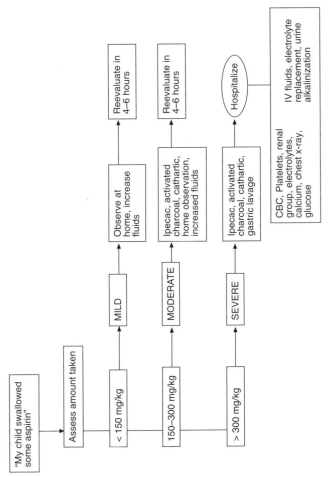

Figure 15–4. Evaluation of aspirin overdose. (CBC, complete blood count; IV = intravenous.)

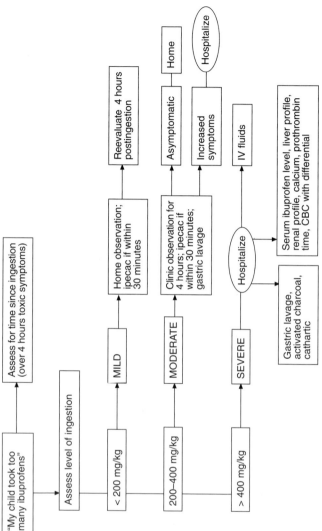

Figure 15–5. Evaluation of ibuprofen overdose. (CBC, complete blood count; IV, intravenous.)

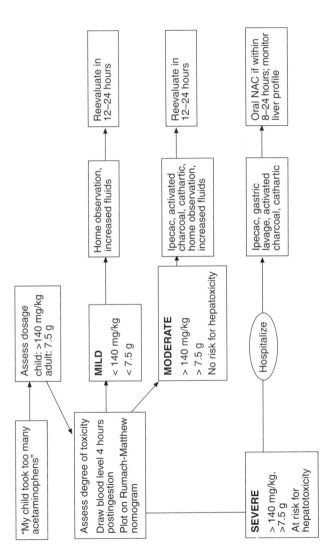

Figure 15–6. Evaluation of acetaminophen overdose. (NAC, *N*-acetylcysteine.)

to help the patient. Obtain a past medical history and a list of the substances that were present and accessible to the patient. *Note:* This history may not be reliable; patient may be asymptomatic or may present in an unconscious or agitated state.

A thorough physical examination can provide clues as to the substance and confirm the history. Conduct a review of systems, taking into consideration the following.

Vital signs: Blood pressure may be increased (amphetamine, lysergic acid diethylamide [LSD], cocaine, rhododendron) or decreased (barbiturates, imipramine, tricyclic antidepressants, monk's hood); pulse may be increased (atropine, aspirin) or decreased (digitalis, narcotics, organophosphates); respirations may be increased (aspirin, amphetamines) or decreased (alcohol, narcotics, yellow jasmine). Check for pattern of respirations (Kussmaul's, apneustic) and body temperature (hyperthermia or hypothermia).

Breath odors: Alcohol (ethanol); bitter almonds (cyanide); acetone (salicylate, methanol); garlic (arsenic, organophosphates); wintergreen (methyl salicylate); violets (turpentine).

Skin: Diaphoretic (aspirin, cocaine, organophosphates); dry (anticholinergic agents); mottled or track marks (heroin, phencyclidine [PCP], amphetamine); discoloration (lobster red, boric acid; red, belladonna alkaloids; yellow, delayed jaundice in acetaminophen toxicity).

Mouth: Dry (amphetamines, antihistamines); increased secretions (organophosphates, corrosives).

Eyes: Pupils characterized by miosis, mydriasis (irritant gases, organophosphates); conjunctivae injected, pale, and yellow (delayed jaundice, acetaminophen toxicity).

Central nervous system: Ataxia (alcohol, narcotics, phenytoin); coma (sedatives, salicylate, carbon monoxide, cyanide, poison hemlock); altered behavior (LSD, PCP, alcohol, cocaine, camphor).

Gastrointestinal system: Increased or decreased bowel sounds, constipation, colic (arsenic, lead); diarrhea (arsenic, iron, boric acid, castor bean, foxglove, lily of the valley); vomiting (larkspur, castor bean).

Diagnostic tests:

Test	Results Indicating Disorder	CPT Codes
Hematocrit	Determination of anemia	85104
Arterial blood gases	Determination of acid-base imbalances	82803
Oximetry	Extent of hypoxemia	82805
Serum electrolytes	Determination of acid-base imbalances	80051
Carboxyhemoglobin	Suggests carbon monoxide poisoning	82375–82376
Urine ferric acid	Evidence of ingestion of salicylate or phenothiazine, or isoniazid	82728
Blood calcium	Oxalates, fluoride, ethylene glycol	82310
Radiographs of kidney, ureter, bladder and abdomen	Radiopaque substances, chloral hydrate, heavy metals, iron, Playdoh	74400/ 74022
Electrocardiogram	Prolonged QT intervals suggest phenothiazine Widened QRS suggests ingestion of quinidine or tricyclic antidepressants Sinus bradycardia suggests digoxin, cyanide, or β-blocker ingestion	93042
Liver function tests	Acetaminophen poisoning	84450–84460

Differential diagnosis: If altered mental status consider:

- Metabolic disorders, with ketoacidosis
- Infectious problems, such as meningitis
- Structural diseases, such as an intracranial mass

An in-depth history rules out these problems.

Treatment (detoxification):

Cutaneous Exposure

Remove the clothing and wash the exposed areas to decontaminate. In cases of ocular exposure, rinse the eye with copious amounts of normal saline, paying particular attention to the conjunctival fornices.

Ingestion

Gastric emptying: Syrup of ipecac, 15 mL for children older than 1 year and 30 mL for adolescents (ipecac induces vomiting in about 20 minutes). Home ipecac administration, under the supervision of a physician or poison control center, is indicated for ingestion of acetaminophen, aspirin, toxic plants, and iron-containing substances, such as multivitamins. Induced vomiting within 30 minutes of ingestion can eliminate about 30% of the substance.

 Clinical Pearl: Ipecac is contraindicated in children who are comatose or who have ingested caustic agents or volatile petroleum distillates.

Lavage: Use a tube that approximates the size of the child's thumb and use 50 to 100 aliquots of fluid. Always protect the airway because vomiting does occur during the procedure. The effectiveness of lavage is inversely proportional to the length of time since toxic ingestion.

 Clinical Pearl: Do not initiate lavage when the substances contain caustics and solvents because of the risk of damage to the esophagus. Having the patient drink water or milk is a reasonable measure in these cases.

Absorbents: Activated charcoal, 1 g/kg. Mix the powder with enough liquid to make a drinkable slurry. Have the patient drink the solution, or administer it through a nasogastric tube. If ipecac was administered, wait 20 minutes before giving the charcoal. Not recommended for pure caustics, solvents, or iron. Serum concentrations of theophylline, salicylates, and barbiturates are reduced with multiple doses of activated charcoal.

Alkalinization of the urine to a pH of 7.8, combining fluid loading and diuresis (the principle of ion trapping), enhances the excretion of phenobarbital and salicylates.

Follow-up: Return in 24 hours for evaluation.

Sequelae: Permanent tissue injury or even death.

Prevention/prophylaxis: Proper storage of chemicals and medicines.

Referral: Call the regional poison control center for definitive antidotes. If necessary, refer patient immediately to a primary care physician for definitive treatment and hospitalization. Refer patients who have attempted suicide to a mental health center for counseling.

Education: Increase awareness to the dangers of childhood poisoning through parent education. Remind parents that children are curious and investigative. Instruct parents of young children to keep hazardous products out of sight and out of reach—under lock and key, if possible. Teach parents never to store medicine and chemicals in a cabinet used to store food and not to store these substances in a container normally used for food. Instruct parents to learn to use safety closures on packages, to read the labels on products, to avoid taking medicine in the presence of children, and never to tell a child that medicine is "candy." Advise parents to keep emergency phone numbers—physician, hospital, police department, fire department, and emergency rescue squad—by the telephone.

SNAKE BITES

SIGNAL SYMPTOMS ▶ injury to the skin (puncture) by the fangs of a snake

| Venomous snake bites | ICD-9 CM: E905.0 |
| Nonvenomous snake bites | ICD-9 CM: E906.2 |

Description: A snake bite is any puncture of the skin by the fangs of a snake, possibly with envenomization.

Etiology: Of bites by venomous snakes in the United States, 98% are caused by rattlesnakes, water moccasins, copperheads (pit vipers), coral snakes (elapids), and occasionally exotic, imported snakes. No envenomation occurs in 25% of all bites.

Occurrence: Rare to common, depending on the area.

Age: All pediatric age groups.

Ethnicity: Not significant.

Gender: Occurs equally in males and females.

Contributing factors: Living or participating in activities in rural, wooded areas.

Signs and symptoms: The patient reports having been bitten by a snake. Determine the time elapsed from the bite to the patient's arrival at the health care facility. Determine the type of snake; most bites are from nonvenomous varieties.

Pit vipers: There is a double-puncture wound surrounded by ecchymosis, immediate pain, discoloration, and edema.

Elapids: Initially there is little local pain, swelling, or necrosis around the double-puncture wound. In 5 to 10 hours, bulbar paralysis, dysphagia, and dysphoria may develop.

Diagnostic tests:

Test	Results Indicating Disorder	CPT Codes
Complete blood count	Depressed	85007
Platelets	Depressed	85585
Glucose	Normal	82947
BUN	Elevated	84520
Creatinine	Elevated	82565
Serum electrolytes	Normal	80051
Transaminases	Normal	84450/84460
Bilirubin	Normal	84520
Creatine kinase	Increase with cardiac involvement	82250
Prothrombin time	Prolonged: acquired deficiency in clot formation	85210
Partial thromboplastin time	Prolonged: acquired deficiency in clot formation	85730
Thrombin time	Degree of hemolysis	85670
Fibrinogen	Same as above	85384/85385
Cross-type in cases of hemolytic anemia	Treatment of hemolysis	86920

Differential diagnosis:

Differentiate by history, observation of fang marks (pit vipers have two long fangs, coral snakes have short fangs with teeth behind and leave multiple fang marks and small lacerations), and snake identification if possible.

Venomous snakes, in contrast to nonvenomous snakes, have a triangular head, elliptical pupils, and long fangs.

If there are no fang marks, envenomation did not occur.

Treatment: Transport to hospital immediately. Cleanse wound, and assess for tetanus immunization status. Measure the affected limb and remeasure every 30 minutes to assess progression of the injury or treatment.

 Clinical Pearl: Do not use a tight tourniquet or pack with ice.

Inpatient Treatment

Observe for development of severe symptoms of envenomation. Antivenom therapy should be started within 2 hours of the bite. Perform a skin test for sensitivity before initiating antivenom. Local envenomation includes bites involving digits and other tight fascial compartments; bites that are swelling rapidly; swelling involving more than half of the bitten limb; and bites from pit vipers, whose venom is known to be necrotic. Systemic envenomation is manifested by hypotension, shock, cardiac arrhythmias, impaired consciousness, neurotoxic signs, dark urine, tender and stiff muscles, and bleeding (spontaneous or excessive).

The dose of the antivenom is individualized based on the degree of envenomation. In moderate cases, give 3 to 5 vials intravenously; in severe cases, give 10 to 20 vials intravenously. Monitor for allergic reactions: Serum sickness is common 4 to 7 days after treatment.

Follow-up: Depends on the severity of illness.

Sequelae:

Pit vipers: In severe cases, respiratory difficulty, shock, and death (within 6–8 hours).

Elapids: In severe cases, total peripheral paralysis and death (within 24 hours).

Prevention/prophylaxis: Teach patients to wear boots and long pants, not to go barefoot, and not to explore under logs or crevices when walking in wooded areas.

Referral: Refer patient for immediate hospitalization. Consult with surgeon if bite is on a distal extremity. Consult the Antivenom Index, Tucson, AZ (24-hour hot line: 1-520-626-6016).

Education: Teach children the difference between venomous and nonvenomous snakes in their areas. Instruct them to wear appropriate clothing when engaging in activities in wooded areas.

REFERENCES

Animal/Human Bites

Advisory Committee on Immunization Practices Human Rabies prevention-United States: Recommendations of the Immunization Practices Advisory Committee (ACIP). 1999.

Bower, MG: Managing dog, cat, and human bite wounds. Nurse Pract 26:36, 2001.

Business Wire: Free reconstructive surgery for children disfigured by dog bites. March 20, 2001.

Le, T, and Dire, D: Managing human and animal bites. Clin Advisor 5:27, 2002.

McNamara, R: Bites, human. eMed J 2, April 25, 2001.

Presutti, J: Prevention and treatment of dog bites. Am Fam Physician 63:1567, 2001.

Heat Cramps, Heat Exhaustion, Heatstroke

American Academy of Pediatrics, Committee on Sports Medicine and Fitness: Climatic heat stress and the exercising child. Pediatrics July 2000.

Barrow, M, and Clark, K: Heat-related illness. Am Fam Physician 55, September 1, 1998.

Kunihiro, A, and Foster, J: Heat exhaustion and heat stroke. EMed J June 16, 2001.

Insect and Arthropod Bites and Stings

Arnold, T: Spider envenomations, brown recluse. eMed J 2, 2001.

Bahna, S: Insect sting allergy: A matter of life and death. Pediatr Ann 29:753, 2000.

Fernandez, M, and Arredondo, N: Bites, insects. eMed J 2, June 11, 2001.

Forks, T: Brown recluse spider bites. J Am Board Fam Pract 13:415, 2000.

Maher, J (Graft, D, et al [consultants]): Managing stinging insect allergies. Patient Care Nurse Pract June, 18,1998.

Metry, D, and Hebert, A: Insect and arachnid stings, bites, infestations, and repellants. Pediatr Ann 29:39, 2000.

Schexnayder, S, and Schexnayder, R: Bites, stings, and other painful things. Pediatr Ann 29:354, 2000.

Watson, J: Spider bites: Assessment and management. J Am Acad N P 11:215, 1999.

Vetter, R, and Visschner, PK: Bites and stings of medically important venomous arthropods. Int J Dermatol 37:481, 1998.

Lead Poisoning (Plumbism)

American Academy of Pediatrics, Committee on Environmental Health: Screening for elevated blood lead levels. Pediatrics 101:1072, 1998.

Centers for Disease Control: Preventing lead poisoning in children: A statement. Centers for Disease Control, Atlanta, GA, 1991.

Centers for Disease Control and Prevention: Recommendations for blood lead screening of young children enrolled in Medicaid: Targeting a group at high risk. MMWR Morb Mortal Wkly Rep 49:1, 2000.

Ellis, M: Lightening the lead load in children. Am Fam Physician 62:545, 2000.

Mendelsohn, A, et al: Low-level lead exposure and cognitive development in early childhood. J Dev Behav Pediatr 20:4225, 1999.

Near-Drowning

American Academy of Pediatrics: Policy statement: Drowning in Infants, children and adolescents. Pediatrics 92:292, 1993.

National Center for Injury Prevention and Control: Drowning prevention. August 28, 2001.

Reed, W: Near-drowning: Life-saving steps. Physician Sportsmed 26, July 1998.

Sheperd, S, and Martin, J: Submersion injury, near drowning. eMed J 2, 2001.

Thanel, F: Near drowning: Rescuing patients through education as well as treatment. Postgrad Med 103, June 1998.

Zuckerman, G, and Conway, E: Drowning and near drowning: A pediatric epidemic. Pediatr Ann 29:360, 2000.

Poisoning

American Academy of Pediatrics, Committee on Drugs: Policy statement: Acetaminophen toxicity in children. Pediatrics 108:1020, 2001.

Powers, K: Diagnosis and management of common toxic ingestions and inhalations. Pediatr Ann 29:330, 2000.

Shannon, M: Ingestion of toxic substances by children. N Engl J Med 342:186, 2002.

Snake Bites

Herman, B, et al: Bites that poison: A tale of spiders, snakes, and scorpions. Contemp Pediatr 8:41, 1999.

Shaw, B, and Hosalkar, H: Rattlesnake bites in children: Antivenin treatment and surgical indications. J Bone Joint Surg Am 84:1624, 2002.

Appendix 1
RESOURCES

	Name	Address & Phone	E-mail or Website
Chapter 4: Skin Disorders	Food Allergy Network	4744 Holly Avenue, Fairfax, VA 22030-5647 1-800-929-4040	www.food allergy.org
	Block the Sun, Not the Fun, American Academy of Dermatology	930 N Neacham Road, PO Box 4014, Shaumber, IL 60168 1-800-462-DERM; 312-856-8888	www.aad.org / www.copper-tone.com
	Solumbra by Sun Precautions	2815 Wetmore Avenue, Everett, WA 98201 1-800-882-7860	
	Stingray Bay Sun Protection	1-800-969-4SUN	www.stingrayby. com
Chapter 5: Head, Neck and Face	American Speech-Language-Hearing Association (ASHA)	10801 Rockville Pike, Department MO, Rockville, MD 20852 1-800-638-8255	www.asha.org
Chapter 6: Chest Disorders	American Lung Association	1740 Broadway, New York, NY 10019-4371 1-800-LUNG-USA	www.lung.usa.org
	National Sudden Infant Death Syndrome Resource Center	2070 Chain Bridge Road, Suite 450, Vienna, VA 22182 1-866-866-7437	www.sidscenter. org
Chapter 7: Abdominal Disorders	CDC Division of Bacterial and Mycotic Diseases Disease Information		http://www.ced. gov/ncidod/ dbmd/ diseaseinfo
	The Bad Bug Book		http://vm.cfsan. fda.gov/~mow/ intro.html
	FDA Center for Food Safety and Applied Nutrition		http://vm.cfsan. fda.gov

Name	Address & Phone	E-mail or Website
FoodNet		http://www.cdc.gov/ncidod/dbmd/foodnet
Gateway to Government Food Safety Information		http://www.food-safety.gov
Partnership for Food Safety Education		http://www.fight-bac.org
United States Department of Agriculture (USDA) Foodborne Illness Education Information Center		http://www.nal.usda.gov/fnic/foodborne/foodborn.htm
USDA Food Safety and Inspection Service		http://www.fsis.usda.gov
American Pseudo-Obstruction and Hirschsprung's Disease Society	PO Box 772, Medford, MA 02155 1-617-395-4255	
Capital Area Pediatric Heartburn Reflux Association	PO Box 1153, Germantown, MD 20875-1153 1-301-972-6128	
Pediatric Crohn's and Colitis Association	PO Box 188, Newton, MA 02168-0002 1-617-290-0902	
Chapter 9: Reproductive Disorders	National STD Hotline	1-800-227-8922	
	National Herpes Hotline	1-919-361-8488	
Chapter 10: Musculoskeletal Disorders	National Scoliosis Foundation	72 Mount Auburn Street, Watertown, MA 02172 1-617-926-0397	www.nichcy.org
Chapter 11: Central and Peripheral Nervous System Disorders	Epilepsy Foundation of America	4351 Garden City Drive, Landover, MD 20785 1-800-332-1000	www.efa.org
	United Cerebral Palsy Association, Inc.	1522 K Street, Suite 1112, Washington, DC 20006 1-202-842-1266, 1-800-USA-5UCP	www.ucpa.org
	National Reye's Syndrome Foundation	1-800-233-7393	nrsf@reyessyndrome.org

	Name	Address & Phone	E-mail or Website
Chapter 12: Endocrine, Metabolic, and Nutritional Disorders	Cystic Fibrosis Foundation	6931 Arlington Road, Bethesda, MD 20814 1-301-951-0902	www.cff.org
	Juvenile Diabetes Foundation	New York, NY 1-800-223-1138	www.jdf.org
	Overeaters Anonymous	World Service Office, PO Box 44020, Rio Rancho, NM 87174-4020 1-505-891-2664	
Chapter 13: Hematologic and Immunologic Disorders	National Hemophilia Foundation	The SOHO Building, 110 Greene Street, #303, New York, NY 10012 1-800-424-2634	www.hemo-philia.org
	Sickle Cell Disease Association of America	3345 Wilshire Boulevard, #1106, Los Angeles, CA 90010-1880 1-800-421-8453	www.sickle-celldisease.org
	AIDS Hotline	Atlanta, GA 1-800-551-2728	
Chapter 14: Psychosocial Problems	Academy for Eating Disorders	1-703-556-9222	www.acadeat-dis.org
	Eating Disorders Awareness and Prevention, Inc	1-800-931-2237	www. edap.org
	ADD Advocacy Group	15772 E Crestridge Circle, Aurora, CO 80015 1-303-690-7548	
	Children and Adults with Attention Deficit Disorder	499 NW 70th Avenue, #109, Plantation, FL 33317 1-305-587-3700	www.chadd.org
	National Attention Deficit Disorder Association	1-800-487-2282	www.add.org
	BASH—Bulimia Anorexia Self-Help	St Louis, MO 1-800-227-4785	
	American Sleep Disorder Association	1610 14th Street, NW, Suite 300, Rochester, MN 55901 1-507-287-6006	www.usda.org
	SNORE (Sleep Apnea Online Resource for Education)		www.newtech-pub.com/phantom/snore/snore/htm
	The Yale Center for Sleep Disorders		www.infomed.yale.edu/intmed/sleep

Name	Address & Phone	E-mail or Website
Autism Society of America	7910 Woodmont Avenue, #650, Bethesda, MD 20814-3015 1-800-328-8476; fax 1-301-657-0869	www.autism-society.org
800 Cocaine Information	Summit, NJ 1-900-262-2463	
The Munchausen by Proxy Survivors Network	PO Box 806177, Saint Clair Shores, MI 48080	www.mbps-network.com
The AsherMeadow MSP Resource Center	Producers of AsherMeadow MSP Magazine	www.asher-meadow.org
Marc Feldman, MD, Director of Adult Psychiatry and Medical Director, Center for Psychiatric Medicine	University of Alabama at Birmingham, Birmingham, AL	www.munchausen.com
Alcoholics Anonymous		http://www.alcoholics-anonymous.org/
National Inhalant Prevention Coalition		http://www.inhalants.org/
Office of National Drug Control Policy (ONDCP)		http://www.whitehouse-drugpolicy.gov/
Other Alpha Line	1-800-425-7421	
Alpha-1 National Association	1829 Portland Avenue, Minneapolis, MN 55404 1-612-871-1747	www.alpha1.org
Medic Alert Foundation	Turlock, CA 1-800-344-3226	www.medic-alert.org
Candlelighters Childhood Cancer Foundation	7910 Woodmont Avenue, #460, Bethesda, MD 20814-3015 1-800-366-2223	www.candle-lighters.org
Wish Upon a Star	Visalia, CA 1-800-821-6805	www.when-youwish-uponastar.org
National Center for Education in Maternal and Child Health	38th and R Streets, NW, Washington, DC, 20057 1-202-625-8400	
Association of Birth Defect Children	827 Ima Street, Orlando, FL 32803 1-407-245-7035	
Clearinghouse on Disability Information, The Council for Exceptional Children	1920 Association Drive, Reston, VA 22091-1589 1-703-620-3660	

Name	Address & Phone	E-mail or Website
National Asthma Educational Program, National Heart Lung/Blood Institute	1-301-251-1222	
National Center for Learning Disabilities	381 Park Avenue, #1420, New York, NY 10016 1-212-545-7510	
National Down Syndrome Congress	Park Ridge, IL 1-800-232-6372	
National Easter Seal Society for Crippled Children and Adults	70 East Lake Street, Chicago, IL 61601 1-312-726-6200	
National Information Center for Children and Youth with Handicaps	PO Box 1492, Washington, DC 20013 1-703-893-6061	
National Marfan's Foundation	382 Main Street, Port Washington, NY 11050 1-800-862-7326	www.marfan. org
National Multiple Sclerosis Information Hotline	New York, NY 1-800-227-3166	
ERIC Clearinghouse on Handicapped and Gifted Children	1920 Association Drive, Reston, VA 22091-1589 1-703-336-4797	
Learning Disabilities Association of America	4156 Library Road, Pittsburgh, PA 15234 1-412-341-1515	www.ldanall. org
National Organization on Fetal Alcohol Syndrome	1815 H Street NW, #1000, Washington, DC 20006 1-800-666-6327	www.nofas. org
National Stuttering Project	2151 Irving Street, Suite 208, San Francisco, CA 94122-1609 1-800-364-1677	www. nspstutter. org
ODPHP National Health Information Center	PO Box 1133, Washington, DC 20013-1133	
Office of Special Education and Rehabilitative Services, US Department of Education	Room 3132, Switzer Building, Washington, DC 20202-2524 1-202-732-1241	
Spina Bifida Association	Chicago, IL 1-800-621-3141	www....asso-famericas-boa.org
Stuttering Foundation of America	PO Box 11749, Memphis, TN 38111-0749 1-800-992-9392	www. stutersfa. org
TEF/Vater	15301 Grey Fox Drive, Upper Marlboro, MD 20772 1-301-952-6837	www.tef/vater .org
Tourette's Syndrome Association	Bayside, NY 1-800-237-0717	www.tsa_usa. org

INDEX

Entries followed by f reference figures. Entries followed by t reference table.

T